NGNA

CORE CURRICULUM for GERONTOLOGICAL NURSING

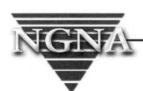

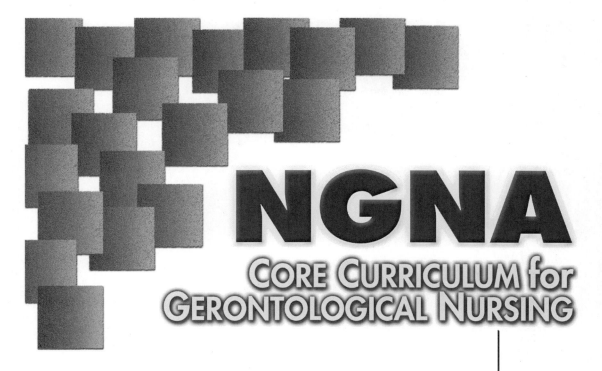

NGNA
CORE CURRICULUM for GERONTOLOGICAL NURSING

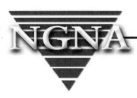

ANN SCHMIDT LUGGEN, PhD, RN, ARNP, CS, CNAA
Professor of Nursing
College of Professional Studies
Northern Kentucky University
Highland Heights, Kentucky

SUE E. MEINER, EdD, RN, CS, GNP
Former Research Patient Coordinator
Division of Geriatrics and Gerontology
Washington University School of Medicine
St. Louis, Missouri
Assistant Professor of Nursing
University of Nevada Las Vegas
College of Health Sciences
Las Vegas, Nevada

Second Edition

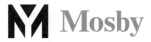 Mosby

A Harcourt Health Sciences Company

St. Louis   London   Philadelphia   Sydney   Toronto

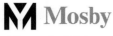

A Harcourt Health Sciences Company

Vice-President, Nursing Editorial Director: Sally Schrefer
Senior Editor: Michael S. Ledbetter
Developmental Editor: Lisa P. Newton
Project Manager: John Rogers
Senior Production Editor: Helen Hudlin
Designer: Kathi Gosche

Second EDITION

Mosby, Inc.
A Harcourt Health Sciences Company
11830 Westline Industrial Drive
St. Louis, Missouri 63146

Printed in the United States of America

ISBN 0-323-01098-9

00 01 02 03 04 CL/MV 9 8 7 6 5 4 3 2 1

Contributors

ANITA C. ALL, RN, PhD
Associate Professor
College of Nursing
University of Oklahoma Health Sciences Center
Oklahoma City, Oklahoma

MARGARET M. ANDERSON, EdD, RN, CNAA
Chair, Department of Nursing
Northern Kentucky University
Highland Heights, Kentucky

PHYLLIS ATKINSON, MS, RN, CS, GNP
St. Elizabeth Medical Center
Family Practice Center
Edgewood, Kentucky

NANCY HENNE BATCHELOR, MSN, RNC
Assistant Professor, Department of Nursing
Northern Kentucky University
Highland Heights, Kentucky

ROBERT BRAUTIGAN, MSN, ARNP, CS
Assistant Professor, Department of Nursing
Northern Kentucky University
Highland Heights, Kentucky

LaRae I. HUYCKE, RN, BSN
Graduate Student
University of Oklahoma Health Sciences Center
Oklahoma City, Oklahoma

PATRICIA M. KELLY, MSN, ARNP, CS
Associate Administrator
Wesley Manor Retirement Community
Louisville, Kentucky

MARY LOU LONG, RN, MSN
Director, Community Services
St. Luke's Regional Medical Center
Boise, Idaho

ANN SCHMIDT LUGGEN, PhD, RN, ARNP, CS, CNAA
Professor of Nursing
College of Professional Studies
Northern Kentucky University
Highland Heights, Kentucky

SUE E. MEINER, EdD, RN, CS, GNP
Former Research Patient Coordinator
Division of Geriatrics and Gerontology
Washington University School of Medicine
St. Louis, Missouri
Assistant Professor of Nursing
University of Nevada Las Vegas
College of Health Sciences
Las Vegas, Nevada

PATRICIA M. MEZINSKIS, MSN, RN, CS
Associate Professor
University of Cincinnati/Raymond Walters
College
Cincinnati, Ohio

MARY PAINTER-ROMANELLO, MSN, RN, GNP
Adult Nurse Practitioner
Geriatric Assessment
Good Samaritan Hospital
Cincinnati, Ohio

BEVERLY RENO, RNC, MSN
Associate Professor of Nursing
Northern Kentucky University
Highland Heights, Kentucky

ALICE G. RINI, JD, MS, RN
Associate Professor of Nursing
Adjunct Professor of Law
Department of Nursing
Northern Kentucky University
Highland Heights, Kentucky

JOANNE KRAENZLE SCHNEIDER, PhD, RN
Assistant Professor of Nursing
Saint Louis University School of Nursing
St. Louis, Missouri

DIANNE THAMES, DNS, RNC, APRN
Associate Professor
Division of Nursing
Dillard University
New Orleans, Louisiana

SHIRLEY S. TRAVIS, PhD, RN, CS
Dean W. Colvard Distinguished Professor
of Nursing
University of North Carolina
Charlotte, North Carolina

TAMARA J. WHITE, RN, MSN
Geriatric Nurse Practitioner
The Christ Hospital
Cincinnati, Ohio

Contributors to First Edition

MARY ANN ANDERSON, MS, RNC, CNA
Weber State University
Ogden, Utah

SISTER ROSE THERESE BAHR, ASC, PhD, RN, FAAN
Leadership Team
Adorers of the Blood of Christ
Wichita, Kansas

NANCY K. BEDFORD, MSN, RNCS, GNP
Department of Veterans Affairs
Medical Center
Nashville, Tennessee

NANCY R.S. BRAINARD, MSN, ARNP, CS
Department of Veterans Affairs
Medical Center
Gainesville, Florida

ANN BYERLY, RNC, MPH, CRRN, CNA
Louisiana State University Medical Center
New Orleans, Louisiana

JANE M. CAMPBELL, MSN, RN, CS
Gerontology Nursing Consultant
Hamilton, Ohio

RENEE M.A. CLERMONT, RN, CS-P
The Kennedy Krieger Institute
Baltimore, Maryland

KARLA DALLEY, MS, RN
Baccalaureate Nursing Program
Weber State University
Ogden, Utah

MARY ELLEN DELLEFIELD, MS, RN
University of Phoenix, San Diego Campus
San Diego, California

KEN DELLEFIELD, PhD, MN
Prospective on Aging
San Diego, California

JUDITH G. GOODWIN, MSN, RNC, GNP
Director of Nurses
Nashville Health Care Center
Nashville, Tennessee

SUSAN HERMANSEN
Old Town, Maine

ROSLYN A. JOHNNY, MEd, MSN, BSN
Geriatric Evaluation and Management
(GEM) Coordinator
Department of Veterans Affairs
Medical Center
New Orleans, Louisiana

MARY ANN JOHNSON, PhD, RN/CGNP
Salt Lake City VAMC/GRECC
Salt Lake City, Utah
Associate Professor
University of Utah College of Nursing
Salt Lake City, Utah

VIVIAN J. KOROKNAY, MS, RN, CRRN
Director of Rehabilitation and Restorative
Care
Asbury Methodist Village
Wilson Health Care Center
Rockville, Maryland

CLAIRE A. LINCOLN, MN, RN, CS
Psychiatric Mental Health Clinical Nursing
Specialist
New Orleans, Louisiana

MARY LOU LONG, MSN, RNC
St. Luke's Regional Medical Center
Boise, Idaho

ANN SCHMIDT LUGGEN, PhD, RN, CNAA
College of Professional Studies
Northern Kentucky University
Highland Heights, Kentucky

KAREN S. LUKACS, MSN, RNCS
Medical University of Southern California
Charleston, South Carolina

PATRICIA M. MEZINSKIS, MSN, RN, CS
University of Cincinnati/Raymond Walters
College
Cincinnati, Ohio

KAY MULFORD, MSW, BSW, LSW
Cincinnati, Ohio

LINDA NEGICH, BSN, RNC
Carmel Manor
Fort Thomas, Kentucky

MARIANNE QUIST O'BRIEN, MSN, RN
Northern Kentucky Nursing Services
Florence, Kentucky

CHRIS PEÑA, MSN, RN, CCRN
Nicholls State University
Department of Nursing and Allied Health
Technology
Thibodaux, Louisiana

DEMETRIUS PORCHE, DNS, RN, CCRN
Nicholls State University
Thibodaux, Louisiana

ALICE G. RINI, JD, MS, RN
Northern Kentucky University
Highland Heights, Kentucky

KAY T. ROBERTS, EdD, MSN, RNC, FAAN
Professor
University of Louisville School of Nursing
Louisville, Kentucky

JEANNE ROBERTSON SAMTER, MSN, CS
Geropsychiatric Nurse Specialist
Private Practice
Silver Springs, Maryland

MARCIA DALY SHAD, RNC
Meadowbrook Care Center
Cincinnati, Ohio

DIANNE THAMES, DNS, RN, CNS
Assistant Professor
Nicholls State University
Thibodaux, Louisiana

CAROL HRICZ TOWNSEND, MSN, ARNP, CS
Gainesville VA Medical Center
Gainesville, Florida

PREFACE

This is the second edition of the *National Gerontological Nursing Association Core Curriculum for Gerontological Nursing.* The first edition, which won the AJN Book of the Year Award, has been revised to include content found in the most recent American Nurses Credentialing Center (ANCC) Gerontological Nursing Certification Examination. In addition to this content, the new edition has two examinations the reader may use to test knowledge and comprehension.

The *NGNA Core Curriculum for Gerontological Nursing* is a resource for nurses working in varied settings where older adult patients receive care. With all the changes in America's health care system over the past few years, nurses are delivering, managing, and evaluating care to older adults. We recognize the need for nurses to be knowledgeable and skilled in gerontological nursing. This text provides basic knowledge for nurses to use in giving care.

The text provides an outline format that is useful for educators and administrators in planning educational programs for staff. Each chapter has useful references that can provide additional information in program preparation. The sample examination questions may be useful in testing learning after program completion.

The editors found that the outline format of the gerontological content was very much favored by readers of the first edition. This format allows the learner to review the book content at a much faster rate than would be possible with another format. Therefore, this format has been continued in the second edition. There are resources and references throughout the text for those who would pursue deeper study.

The editors wish to acknowledge the contributors of the first edition. These contributors are listed in the *front* of this text.

Ann Schmidt Luggen
Sue E. Meiner

CONTENTS

Unit Five Practice Examinations and Answers

PRIMARY CARE CONSIDERATIONS

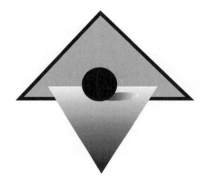

CHAPTER 1

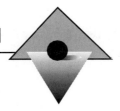

DEMOGRAPHICS

Ann Schmidt Luggen

LEARNING OBJECTIVES

Upon completion of this chapter, the reader will be able to:

- Describe major characteristics of older adults in the United States
- Identify the percentage of older adults who use home health services
- Discuss the percentage of older adults residing in nursing homes

I. GENERAL U.S. DEMOGRAPHICS

A. Populations age when the proportion of older adults vs. younger people increases
B. Percentage of U.S. adults 65+ years of age has doubled since 1950
C. By 2035, 20% to 25% of the U.S. population will be 65+
D. Frail older adults 85+ have increased four times the number since 1950
E. The fastest growing age group is the 85+ group
F. Because of a low birthrate from 1964-1970, older adults today do not have adequate family support
G. In advanced age, 22% of frail elders (85+) live in institutional settings

II. WOMEN VS. MEN

A. U.S. women can expect to live to age 78.3 years; males 71.4
B. Older women do not have spouses to assist in their care; only 40% live with a spouse compared to 77% of men
C. Most older women live alone
D. Most older women are in poorer health than men
E. Women use health care services more than men

III. DISABLED OLDER ADULTS

A. Adults 85+ have the highest rates of disability
B. Cognitive
- 4% of those 65-74 have moderate impairment
- 1% of those 65-74 have severe impairment
- 8% of those 75-84 have moderate impairment
- 3% of those 75-84 have severe impairment
- 11% of those 85+ have moderate impairment
- 8% of those 85+ have severe impairment

IV. HOME HEALTH RECIPIENTS

A. 66% are female
B. 72% are 65+ years of age

C. 65% are white

D. 29% are married; 35% are widowed

E. Home health agencies have increased from 8000 in 1992 to 13,500 in 1996

F. Services required for older adults, 65+

- Skilled nursing care   81%
- Personal care   57%
- Homemaker/companion   23%
- Physical therapy   17%
- Social services   9%

V. NURSING HOME RESIDENTS

A. 1.5 million people live in nursing homes today, increased 50% from 1973-1985

B. 89% are 65+

C. 72% are female

D. 44% of nursing home residents 65+ have bowel and bladder incontinence

E. 41% of nursing home residents 65+ are admitted from the hospital

F. 37% of nursing home residents 65+ are admitted from home

G. 12% are admitted from another nursing home

REFERENCES

Kinsella K: Aging and the family: present and future demographic issues. In Blieszner R, Bedford V, editors: *Handbook of aging and the family,* Westport, CT, 1995, Greenwood.

National Center for Health Statistics: *Health: United States 1998,* DHHS Publication No. PHS 98, Hyattsville, MD, 1998, Public Health Service.

US Bureau of the Census: *Current population reports, special studies, 65+ in the United States,* Washington, DC, 1998, US Government Printing Office.

CHAPTER 2

NORMAL AGING CHANGES

Nancy Henne Batchelor

LEARNING OBJECTIVES

Upon completion of this chapter, the reader will be able to:

- Describe the normal physiological phenomena that occur with aging
- Describe the normal psychological phenomena that occur with aging
- Explain the normal sociological processes that occur in older adulthood
- Identify disease processes that older adults are susceptible to as they age

I. PHYSICAL PHENOMENA

A. Integument changes
    1. Hair: thins, grays; sparse distribution; decreased amount: legs, axilla, pubis
    2. Skin: thin dermis; absence of subcutaneous fat; pigment spots; decreased collagen with increased skin tears; decreased turgor because of fewer elastic fibers; slowed healing time
    3. Nails: thickened, yellow nail plates; thinned cuticles; slowed growth
    4. Tissue elasticity: thinned epithelial layer; wrinkled, dry; collagen fibers shrunken and rigid; double chin; elongated ears
    5. Keratoses: scaly, raised areas darkening over time on exposed skin surfaces
    6. Skin cancer: from sun exposure over time; most prevalent: squamous cell, more prevalent in fair-skinned individuals

B. Neurological changes
    1. Brain size decreased; decreased neurons; ventricles dilated
    2. Nerve transmission slowed because of loss of dendrites affecting neurotransmitter release; accumulation of lipofuscin in cytoplasm
    3. Decreased amounts of dopamine and other enzymes with reduced response to environmental stimuli
    4. Cognition: acquired knowledge/intellect constant; abstract reasoning declines gradually; changes seen with complex tasks
    5. Memory: short-term memory decreases, long-term memory is maintained
    6. Sleep patterns: increased total daily sleep; decrease in sleep stages 3 and 4; more time spent alternating between rapid eye movement and light sleep
    7. Motor function: posture stooped, flexed; slow gait because of slowed motor reaction time; decreased fine motor skills because of decreased strength and muscle wasting
    8. Proprioception: decreased balance because of changes in nervous and musculoskeletal systems

C. Sensory changes
    1. Vision
        a. Anatomic: drooping eyelids; yellowed conjunctiva; arcus senilis; rigid and dense lens; decreased pupil size requiring brighter lighting; decreased corneal sensitivity; decreased

tear production from lacrimal ducts; yellowed lens skewing color discrimination; decreased ability to adapt to dark, affecting night vision; increased sensitivity to glare
   b. Susceptibility to glaucoma: may result in decreased peripheral vision and/or blindness
   c. Susceptibility to cataracts: diminished vision
   d. All visual changes may place patient at safety risk and decrease ability to carry out activities of daily living
2. Hearing
   a. Diminished acuity and sound discrimination
   b. Loss of eighth cranial nerve cells
   c. Loss of high frequency tones
   d. Deficits may lead to withdrawal, social isolation, suspicion, paranoia
   e. Changes within the ear involve hearing and balance, which have negative affect on ability to carry out activities of daily living
3. Taste and smell
   a. Tongue atrophy; olfactory receptors in roof of mouth develop decreased sensitivity; decreased renewal rate of taste buds
   b. Decreased sensory cells in nasal lining: losses affect reaction to the environment (decreased sensitivity to odors) and physical wellness (decreased appetite leading to nutritional problems)
4. Touch
   a. Decreased tactile sensitivity because of skin changes, decreased nerve endings
   b. Decreased ability to sense temperature and pressure, placing patient at risk for injury and misinterpretation of environment
D. Cardiovascular changes
   1. Cardiac output: decreased at rest and with exercise; decreased heart rate at rest
   2. Valves: loss of elasticity, narrowed lumens with increased rigidity of vessel walls
   3. Vascular system: decreased elasticity, atherosclerotic plaques in carotid and coronary arteries and aorta; narrowed lumens, producing increased resistance with decreased blood flow
   4. Patients at risk for
      a. Hypertension >140/90 and above secondary to increased peripheral vascular resistance, resulting in decreased blood flow to brain, kidneys, and heart
      b. Arrhythmias secondary to decreased contractility, decreased number of pacemaker cells, and decreased sensitivity of SA node, resulting in decreased blood flow
      c. Ischemic heart disease with decreased blood flow, causing myocardial infarction, congestive heart failure, angina, or arrhythmias
      d. Myocardial infarction, resulting in tissue hypoxia and cell death; lacking normal symptoms; may exhibit change in mentation; GI symptoms
      e. Congestive heart failure from backflow of blood, poor pumping capacity; results in restlessness, agitation, lethargy, and change in mental status secondary to tissue hypoxia
      f. Atherosclerosis in lower extremities, increasing risk for clots, ulcerations secondary to stasis and poor blood flow
      g. Thrombophlebitis secondary to decreased mobility and stasis, especially following acute illness or surgery
E. Respiratory changes
   1. Functional reserve capacity decreased: slow, shallow respirations; little response to increased demand
   2. Decreased vital capacity: less air exhaled
   3. Ventilation/perfusion ratio: decreased with less gas exchanged
   4. Anatomic and structural changes: decreased effectiveness of cilia; rigid thoracic cage with less mobile ribs; slight increase in AP diameter of chest; decreased muscle strength; increased use of accessory muscles

F. Gastrointestinal changes
1. Weakened jaw muscles and shrunken bony structures in mouth cause increased work of chewing, producing fatigue
2. Salivary gland production decreased; alkaline saliva; atrophy of taste buds
3. Decreased peristalsis with delayed stomach emptying, causing feeling of fullness
4. Decreased gastric acid secretions
5. Decreased intrinsic factor, increasing risk for pernicious anemia
6. Decreased esophageal sphincter tone, increasing risk for hiatal hernia and reflux, regurgitation, and aspiration
7. Increased risk for bleeding secondary to use of drugs that are gastric irritants—NSAIDs, ASA
8. Increased risk for colon cancer: monitor for obstruction or bleeding, constipation, or cramping

G. Endocrine changes
1. Hormone reduction: estrogen and testosterone
   a. Estrogen loss causing decreased breast tissue, reduced elasticity, increased fat and connective tissue
   b. Uterus and vulva shrink in size
   c. Benign prostatic hypertrophy because of tissue hyperplasia and decreased hormone production; symptoms: difficulty voiding, reduced stream, dribbling
2. Glucose metabolism: decreased sensitivity to circulating insulin or diminished insulin response
3. Thyroid: overall function adequate; slowed metabolic rate and oxygen use
4. Pituitary: 20% reduction in volume and hormone production

H. Renal changes
1. Decreased kidney size and weight
2. Decreased number of nephrons and glomeruli
3. Decreased renal blood flow, glomerular filtration rate, filtration, concentration, and dilution
4. Decreased glucose reabsorption and creatinine clearance
5. Decreased reabsorption of tubules with loss of water and electrolytes

I. Genitourinary changes
1. Loss of muscle tone in bladder and ureters, causing incomplete bladder emptying, urinary frequency, and nocturia
2. Female
   a. Relaxed pelvic muscles may result in urinary incontinence
   b. Urethral mucosa thins because of decreased estrogen, leading to urgency and frequency
3. Male
   a. Enlarged prostate results in changes in emptying, involuntary bladder contractions, dribbling, retention, reduced stream, and nocturia
   b. Bladder capacity decreased because of hypertrophy

J. Musculoskeletal changes
1. Decreased muscle mass
2. Muscle cells replaced by fibrous tissue
3. Narrowed intervertebral spaces (loss of height), flexed posture
4. Decreased bone/mineral mass
5. Less strength and tone
6. Limited joint activity; deteriorated cartilage and loss of elasticity

K. Immune system changes
1. Changes result in the inability of the older adult to resist disease processes: decreased white blood cell production

2. Older adults have delayed response to infection: greater morbidity and mortality than in younger patients
3. Greater number of autoimmune disorders with aging: decreased numbers of T lymphocytes and decreased ability of T lymphocytes to function
4. Nutritional factors, vitamin deficiencies, fat intake, psychosocial and lifestyle factors all play role in immune system functioning

II. PSYCHOSOCIAL PHENOMENA

A. Psychological changes
   1. Personality
      a. Consistent with earlier years
      b. Changes can result from pathology or responses to events affecting self-image
   2. Memory
      a. Long term intact; short term diminished
      b. Stress affects processing
   3. Learning
      a. Use of simple association rather than analysis
      b. Verbal and abstract abilities approximately equal
      c. Basic intelligence unchanged
      d. Spatial awareness and intuitive, creative thought declines
      e. Factors affecting learning: motivation, attention span, delayed transmission, perceptual deficits, illness
B. Sociological changes
   1. Sexuality and intimacy
      a. Sexual patterns persist throughout lifespan
      b. Maintenance and promotion of sexual functioning necessary for wellness, a sense of normalcy, and higher quality of life
      c. Normal aging variations, disabilities, medications, treatments affect an individual's ability to remain sexually active
      d. Environmental barriers: lack of privacy (living with adult children, institutionalization, assistive devices)
      e. Fears: rejection, boredom, failure, hostility
   2. Relationships
      a. Close sustaining relationships have a positive effect: lower stress, better mental health, life satisfaction; married have better support system, have better income and better nutrition
      b. Complex care issues: working, mobile families, changes in family patterns (divorce, remarriage of aging parents and adult children); fastest growing segment of population is the age group 85+
      c. Friends: shrinking social network
      d. Organizations and neighborhoods: promotion of social contacts
      e. Factors affecting social network: family members, friends, health, independence
   3. Loss
      a. Each loss requires individual to go through period of grieving and mourning
      b. Loss can result in social changes: may need to learn new roles and manage tasks of daily living
      c. Spiritual: search for meaning; may have crisis of faith and meaning

REFERENCES

Ebersole P, Hess P: *Toward healthy aging: human needs and nursing response,* ed 5, St Louis, 1998, Mosby.

Eliopoulos C: *Gerontological nursing,* ed 4, Philadelphia, 1997, JB Lippincott.

Lueckenotte A: *Gerontologic nursing,* St Louis, 1996, Mosby.

Luggen AS, Travis SS, Meiner S: *NGNA core curriculum for gerontological advanced practice nurses,* Thousand Oaks, CA, 1998, Sage.

Rosow I: The social context of the aging self, *Gerontologist* 12:82, 1972.

Stanley M, Beare P: *Gerontological nursing,* Philadelphia, 1995, FA Davis.

CHAPTER 3

ATTITUDINAL ISSUES, MYTHS, AND STEREOTYPES OF AGING

Mary Lou Long

LEARNING OBJECTIVES

Upon completion of this chapter, the reader will be able to:

- Define terms such as *attitude, stereotype, prejudice, ageism, discrimination,* and *myth*
- Recognize the major stereotypes that reflect negative prejudice and result in discrimination toward older persons
- Understand the consequences of ageism: gains to others, personal costs, economic costs, social costs
- Describe obstacles to health for older persons as a result of negative attitudes of nurses and other health professionals
- Describe strategies to reduce ageism

I. DEFINITIONS

- A. *Ageism:* process of systematic stereotyping, prejudice, or discrimination against or in favor of an age group
- B. *Myth:* ill-founded belief (positive or negative) about older persons
- C. *Stereotype:* standardized mental picture held in common by members of a group or population, representing mistaken or over-simplified beliefs and attitudes about older persons and the process of aging; negative stereotypes usually produce negative attitudes
- D. *Attitude:* feeling or emotion (positive or negative) toward older persons and the process of aging; negative attitudes support negative stereotypes
- E. *Prejudice:* beliefs or attitudes based on a stereotype about older people
- F. *Discrimination:* inappropriate negative treatment of older persons as a result of prejudice

II. CONSEQUENCES OF MAJOR STEREOTYPES

- A. Reflect negative prejudice and result in discrimination toward older persons
- B. Stereotypes and attitudes often go together; stereotypes are more cognitive, while attitudes are more affective
- C. Negative stereotypes produce negative attitudes, resulting in negative behavior or discrimination

III. Major Stereotypes Reflecting Negative Prejudice Toward Older Persons

A. Physical illness: the most common prejudice against older persons is that most are sick, disabled, and generally in poor health; many believe that older adults have more acute illnesses than younger persons
   1. FACT: most older adults (about 78% of 65+) are healthy and engage in normal activities
   2. Only about 5% are institutionalized; 81% of the non-institutionalized have no limitations in activities of daily living
   3. Older adults may have more chronic diseases than younger persons but older adults have fewer acute illnesses (102 acute illnesses per 100 persons 65+ compared to 230 for persons under 65)

B. Mental illness: a common stereotype is that most older persons are senile and/or that senility is an inevitable and untreatable mental illness among most elders; this belief is extremely dangerous when held by health professionals; it leads to lack of prevention and treatment, thus becoming a self-fulfilling prophecy
   1. FACT: mental illness is neither inevitable nor untreatable in older adults
   2. Only about 2% of 65+ are institutionalized with a primary diagnosis of psychiatric illness
   3. Most community studies show older persons have fewer mental impairments than do younger persons

C. Isolation: a majority of people believe that most older persons are socially isolated, lonely, and live alone
   1. FACT: Only about 4% of older adults are extremely isolated, and this is often a life-long pattern
   2. There may be a decline in total social activity but the total number of persons in the social network tends to remain steady

D. Depression: there is a belief that the typical old person is sick, useless, senile, lonely, and poor, which stereotypes older persons as miserable and thus depressed
   1. FACT: major depression is less prevalent among older persons than among younger persons
   2. Studies support the view that the majority of elderly are happy most of the time

E. Poverty: there is a common belief that the majority of older persons are poor
   1. FACT: most elderly have incomes above the poverty level
   2. The average 65+ person is more affluent than the average person under 65

F. Contribution to society: older adults are frequently viewed as frail or feeble, capable of making only a limited contribution to society
   1. FACT: 38 million aged 55+ contribute through volunteerism equal to 20 million full-time employees
   2. One out of five contributes a sizable portion to their children's or grandchildren's income

IV. Discrimination

A. Negative stereotypes lead to negative prejudice that can result in harmful discrimination
B. Discrimination can occur in the following institutions
   1. Health care: the belief that most illnesses and complaints by older adults are part of the normal aging process and are irreversible prevents treatment of illnesses that are reversible
      a. Studies show that most health professionals are prejudiced against older persons and prefer to treat younger persons
      b. Older adults are the only group in the U.S. population who have a national insurance option (Medicare)
      c. Significant access issues exist (e.g., unwillingness of health professionals to take Medicare patients, transportation problems, and financial barriers related to health expenses and services)

2. Family: there is less discrimination in the family than in other areas; however, about 4% of older adults are abused
   a. Less extreme discrimination is by practiced by families; nevertheless, they often ignore older adult members, insist on unnecessary restrictions, misuse older adults' property or finances, or commit older persons to a nursing home
   b. Of importance is the reality of limited resources or abilities to offer assistance appropriate to needs of older adults
3. Employment: this area involves possibly the most obvious and serious form of discrimination, ranging from hiring and promotions to firing and compulsory retirement
   a. Older persons' options for part-time employment are often limited to menial-type jobs with lower pay
   b. Older adults are frequently overlooked for jobs based on stereotypes and negative attitudes (e.g., sick more often, unable to learn new things, too set in their ways, not able to keep up)
4. Housing: an increasing number of older adults live in high concentrations in certain states and in communities with special age-restricted residences
   a. Self-imposed relocation to age-restricted residences may be by choice
   b. Discrimination against living in some areas is not by choice

V. CONSEQUENCES

A. Gains: other persons may gain from negative ageism and discrimination
   1. Employment discrimination gains include more jobs and promotions for younger workers, reduced wages, avoiding evaluating older workers, forcing the less able to retire
   2. Negative ageism gains include repressing the fear of aging and death, avoiding society's responsibilities toward older adults, satisfying pathological impulses for revenge
B. Personal costs: victims of prejudice and discrimination tend to adopt the negative image and behave in ways that conform to it
   1. Older persons tend to accept negative stereotypes, resulting in a self-fulfilling prophecy (e.g., avoiding sexual relations, new ideas, productivity, effective activity, and social engagement)
   2. Three specific personal costs can result
      a. Loss of freedom: loss of the freedom to be sexually active, creative, productive, effective, and engaged may lead to inactivity that may result in more rapid deterioration than normal, thus fulfilling the negative stereotype
      b. Loss of self-esteem and happiness: accepting the negative stereotype may lead to unhappiness, resulting in depression and suicide
         (1) One out of every four suicides in the United States is a person over 65
      c. Loss of access to health services: older persons may fail to seek proper medical and psychological services because they think deterioration in these areas is part of aging and there is nothing that can be done; when conditions get so bad that they are finally forced to seek treatment, it is often too late or there has been considerable loss of ability to function
C. Economic costs: a conservative estimate of the costs of ageism (negative and positive) is $178 billion a year; this estimate is based on the premise that services are offered based on age rather than need
   1. Tax breaks to middle class or affluent older adults are based on age not need
   2. Pensions are based on age not need
   3. Medicare goes to many older adults who could afford to pay for private insurance
   4. Loss of productivity (retired workers) occurs, which could have resulted in a significant contribution to the gross national product
   5. Cost of special programs incurred, needed, as the result of ageism

    D. Social costs: major types of social costs include the following
       1. Cost of social isolation caused by segregation, disengagement from organizations or social groups, unnecessary institutionalization, and other forms of discrimination
       2. Costs to the younger population because of loss of wisdom and guidance from older persons, development of unrealistic fears of aging, and loss of history as well as the emotional support and enjoyment of positive relationships with older persons

VI. Responses of Older Adults

    A. Society's negative attitudes about aging lead to negative expectations about how older persons should live and behave; unfortunately negative expectations emphasize what older persons should not do rather than what they can do; for example, some negative expectations indicate old people should not be interested in sex, should not marry younger persons, should not be creative or continue to work; older adults may become imprisoned in a "roleless role"
    B. Older adults respond in four basic ways
       1. Acceptance: it becomes easier to conform to the expectation of not working and of living in segregated areas
       2. Denial: many elderly refuse to identify themselves as old or may lie about their true age; attempts to pass for young or middle-aged are supported by the cosmetic market, plastic surgery, and false hair industries
       3. Avoidance: many older persons react to ageism by avoiding it through age segregation, isolation, drug or alcohol addiction, mental illness, or suicide
       4. Reform: some older persons choose to recognize prejudice and discrimination and try to do something about it
         a. Examples are the many organizations who focus their efforts to combat negative ageism, such as AARP, Gray Panthers, Older Women's League
    C. On an individual level, increasing self-responsibility is evidenced by people who engage in activities that do not conform to stereotypes (e.g., being active, employed, creative, romantic, healthy, and involved)

VII. Attitudes of Nurses and Other Health Professionals

    A. Nurses and other health professionals are no exception to general societal values and attitudes
       1. Nurses may have negative attitudes toward older adults based on experiences with specific patients such as the frail elderly and those in nursing homes
       2. Concern may exist over the number of nurses entering the field of gerontological nursing, with little progress being made to increase the number of nurses in long-term care
       3. Increased efforts are needed by nursing schools and educators to prepare professional nurses to meet the needs of caregiving for the future
    B. Lack of interest and/or negative attitudes toward the aged result in obstacles to health care for older persons
       1. The aged stimulate practitioners' fear about their own aging
       2. Older patients arouse practitioners' conflicts about their relationships with aging parents
       3. Nurses may think they have nothing to offer older adults because they cannot change the older person's behavior or health problems
       4. Nurses may not value skills required to provide care to older adults
         a. High touch vs. high tech
       5. Older adults might die during treatment, which may affect nurses emotionally
       6. Nurses' myths, stereotypes, and misinformation regarding older adults interfere with recognition of their problems
       7. Economic concerns, real and exaggerated, often provide an explanation or excuse for not offering full services to the elderly, including teaching

8. Nurses may be uneasy about the possibility of being overwhelmed by the diversity and complexity of problems older patients present

VIII. STRATEGIES TO REDUCE AGEISM
A. Individual actions
   1. Be informed about the facts on aging
   2. Examine and understand your own attitudes and the impact they may have on your behavior toward older patients
   3. Be proactive with family, friends, and peers about teaching the facts, especially when individuals express or imply prejudice toward older persons
   4. Do not use ageist terms or language
   5. Refuse to go along with any discrimination aimed at older persons
   6. Join or support groups that oppose ageism
B. Organized actions
   1. Gather and disseminate factual information on aging
   2. Write articles in newsletters or journals about the facts of aging
   3. Participate in programs to educate the public on the facts of aging and the harm of ageism
   4. Organize efforts to boycott products from companies with ageism practices
   5. Conduct voter registration drives for homebound persons or those in alternative residences or nursing homes
   6. Enlist cooperation or support of organizations to participate in campaigns against ageism (e.g., churches or schools)
C. Organizations opposed to ageism
   - Administration on Aging (AOA)
   - American Association of Retired Persons (AARP)
   - American Society on Aging (ASA)
   - Association for Gerontology in Higher Education (AGHE)
   - Gerontological Society of America (GSA)
   - Gray Panthers
   - National Institute on Aging (NIA)
   - Older Women's League (OWL)
   - Villers Foundation, Inc.
   - National Council on the Aging, Inc. (NCOA)
   - National Council of Senior Citizens (NCSC)
   - National Senior Citizens' Law Center (NSCLC)

REFERENCES
Anderson E, Rothenberg B, Zimmer J: *Assessing the health status of older adults,* New York, 1997, Springer Publishing.

Black J, Matassanin-Jacobs E: *Medical surgical nursing: clinical management for continuity of care,* ed 5, Philadelphia, 1997, WB Saunders.

Burke MM, Walsh MB: *Gerontological nursing: wholistic care of the older adult,* St Louis, 1997, Mosby.

Matteson MA, McConnell ES, Linton AD: *Gerontological nursing concepts and practice,* ed 2, Philadelphia, 1997, WB Saunders.

Nash D, Todd W: *Disease management: a systems approach to improving patient outcomes,* Chicago, 1997, AHA Publishing.

CHAPTER 4

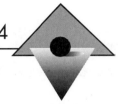

HEALTH PROMOTION AND DISEASE/DISABILITY PREVENTION

Patricia M. Mezinskis

LEARNING OBJECTIVES

Upon completion of this chapter, the reader will be able to:

- Describe the dimensions of wellness
- Identify risk factors for malnutrition in the older adult
- Discuss nursing interventions for the older adult with malnutrition
- Identify benefits of regular exercise for the older adult
- Identify screening tests and immunizations needed by older adults
- Discuss interventions that assist the older adult in returning to/maintaining self-care
- Differentiate types of alternative/complementary health care methods that may benefit the older adult

I. INTRODUCTION TO HEALTH PROMOTION AND DISEASE/DISABILITY PREVENTION

A. *Wellness:* an encompassing term that involves multiple dimensions: physical, emotional, mental, and spiritual

B. The wellness approach suggests that every person has an optimum level of functioning, even in chronic illness or the dying process

C. Wellness activities include several areas: nutrition, fitness, screening programs, immunizations, self-care skills, and complementary health care methods

D. The new millennium marks the target year for the initiative, *Healthy People 2000*
   1. Goals are set for health care, disease prevention, and health care standards (Box 4-1)
   2. Directions are laid out for ways to improve the quality of life, focused on prevention of illness and disease

II. NUTRITION

A. Malnutrition
   1. Older adults are at high risk for protein–calorie malnutrition (PCM); some studies show the rates to be as high as 59% to 65% for older adults who are institutionalized
   2. It is important to assess for and treat malnutrition in the older adult living at home as well as the older adult in long-term care

---

BOX 4-1 **Summary Objectives for Adults Age 65 and Older (*Healthy People 2000*)**

HEALTH STATUS

Reduce:

Suicide among white males

Death by motor vehicle accidents (age 70+)

Death from falls and fall-related injury, particularly age 85+

Death from residential fires

Hip fractures

Number of persons who have difficulty performing two or more personal care activities so as to enhance independence

Significant visual impairment

Epidemic-related pneumonia and influenza deaths

Pneumonia-related days of restricted activity

Increase:

Years of healthy life to at least 65 among African-Americans and Hispanics

RISK REDUCTION

Increase:

The percentage of individuals who regularly participate in light-to-moderate activity for at least 30 minutes a day

Immunization levels for pneumococcal influenza among the chronically ill older population

The percentage of older persons who receive, within appropriate intervals, screening and immunization services and at least one counseling service

SERVICES AND PROTECTION

Increase:

Percentage of recipients of home food service

Percentage of older adults who have the opportunity to participate yearly in at least one organized health promotion program through senior centers, life care facility, or community-based setting serving the older adult

Percentage of states in the United States that have design standards for signs, signals, marking and lighting, and other roadway environmental improvements to enhance visual stimuli and protect the safety of older drivers and pedestrians

The proportion of primary care providers who routinely review with their patients prescribed and over-the-counter medications each time a new medication is prescribed

The percentage of women who receive clinical breast examinations and mammograms

The number of women age 70+ with uterine cervix who receive Pap tests

Extend:

Long-term institutional facilities, the requirement for oral examinations, and service provided to new admissions no later than 90 days after entering a facility

From US Department of Human Services: *Healthy People 2000*, Washington, DC, 1991, Pub No (PHS) 91-50212, US Government Printing Office.

---

3. Malnutrition can delay the healing process, shorten the life span, diminish functional capacity, and lower the quality of life

4. Risk factors

   a. Loss of dentition

   b. Dysphagia

   c. Cognitive impairments (dementia, delirium)

   d. Neurological or musculoskeletal problems that make food preparation and eating difficult

   e. Inability to obtain food, insufficient income

   f. Gastrointestinal disturbances (constipation, anorexia, malabsorption diseases)

   g. Taste alterations (resulting from chemotherapy, age–related change in taste buds)

   h. Cultural dietary changes

   i. Living alone, emotional difficulties

   j. Inadequate knowledge

   k. Effects of medication

   l. Alcoholism

5. *Nutrition Screening Initiative:* a five–year project to promote early screening for malnutrition and better nutritional intake in the United States

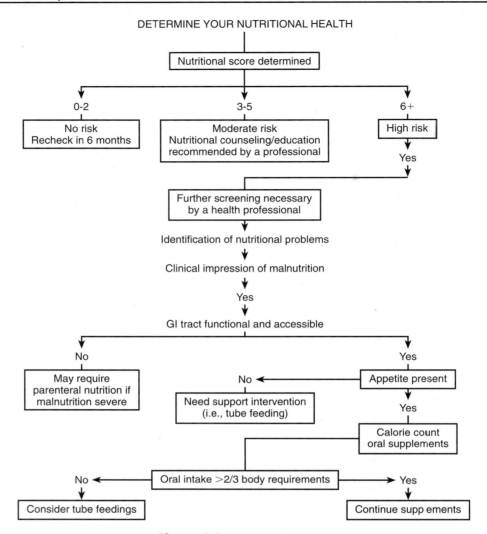

DETERMINE YOUR NUTRITIONAL HEALTH

Figure 4-1 Completed checklist.
(From National Research Council: *Diet and health implications for reducing chronic disease risk:
report of the committee on diet and health,* Food and Nutrition Board, Commission on Life Sciences,
Washington, DC, 1989, National Academy Press.)

B. Nursing management
   1. Assessment
      a. Evaluation of diet (usual intake), medical, drug, and social history data; anthropometric
         measurements (height, weight, mid-arm circumference, triceps skinfold measurements);
         physical exam; and laboratory data (hemoglobin, hematocrit, total protein, serum albumin,
         cholesterol)
      b. Tools to assess risk (*Nutrition Screening Initiative,* Figure 4-1); more detailed assessment by
         health professional should be done
      c. Nomogram for estimating body mass index (Figure 4-2)
      d. Important to assess for obesity as well as malnutrition

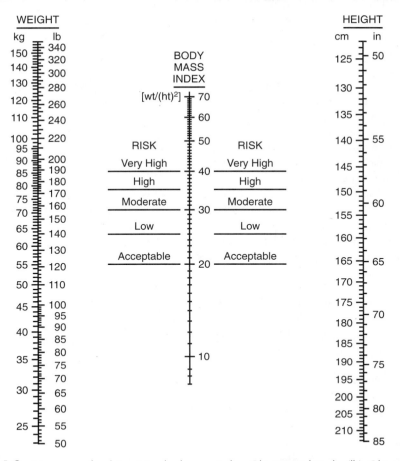

Figure 4-2   Nomogram for determining body mass index. Obtain weight in kg (lb). Obtain height
in cm (in). Hold ruler across weight and height. Read risk.
(From National Research Council: *Diet and health implications for reducing chronic disease risk:
report of the committee on diet and health,* Food and Nutrition Board, Commission on Life Sciences,
Washington, DC, 1989, National Academy Press.)

2. Planning/nursing diagnoses
   a. Nutrition, altered: less than body requirements, related to lack of adequate intake as
      manifested by 5% or more of body weight loss within a month (or 10% or more within
      6 months)
   b. Nutrition, altered: more than body requirements, related to increased intake as manifested
      by weight increase of 20% or more above ideal body weight
3. Goals (for avoiding PCM)
   a. Patient will eat at least 75% of each meal
   b. Patient will gain 2 lbs by _____ (target date)
   c. Patient will state recommended dietary intake from the food pyramid
4. Interventions
   a. Monitor weight and albumin levels (albumin less than 3.5 g/dl significant for PCM)
   b. Monitor patients with PCM for pressure ulcers; if a patient has a pressure ulcer,
      nutritional intake must be increased to aid in healing
   c. Teach patient and family members about the food pyramid and recommended
      servings/day for each of the five food groups

      d. Teach that intake of carbohydrates should be about 55%, fats 30%, protein 15%

      e. As a rule of thumb, most sedentary people can maintain their weight by consuming their weight in pounds times 10 calories (15 for moderate activity; i.e., 1600 calories for a 160 pound person); most older adults do not consume more than 1800 calories/day; therefore, the diet of an older adult should be nutritionally dense

      f. Teach that sodium should be limited to 2400 mg/day (one teaspoon equals about 2000 mg); sodium content information on label is important when shopping

      g. Have patient include high fiber foods in diet but when adding fiber to do so gradually to avoid gastrointestinal problems

      h. Teach that dietary iron is necessary to prevent iron deficiency anemia; sources of vitamin C will enhance iron absorption

      i. Dietary intake of calcium and vitamin D is needed to slow bone loss from osteoporosis; supplements may be needed (1500 mg of daily calcium is recommended); limit caffeine intake, which promotes calcium excretion

      j. Drink alcohol in moderation; alcoholism often ignored among the older population

      k. Vitamin supplements may be needed; thiamine is also necessary for the older adult with alcoholism

      l. Make referrals as needed (dentist for denture problems, psychological consult for depression and alcoholism, support services if unable to prepare meals)

      m. Treating obesity in the older adult is somewhat controversial; if no risk factors (hypertension, elevated blood lipids) are present and obesity is lifelong, no interventions may be recommended

   5. Evaluation

      a. Were goals met?

      b. What outcome criteria are present?

III. FITNESS

A. Physical activity

   1. Often used to judge a person's health and wellness

   2. Lack of exercise a risk factor for many chronic conditions, including obesity, diabetes, hypertension, coronary artery disease

   3. Benefits of regular exercise include improved appetite, improved muscle strength, increased bone density, improved balance, lowered cholesterol level, stabilized glucose tolerance, improved emotional health, decreased stress, decreased risk of medical problems

   4. One research study showed that only 30% of older adults exercise regularly and fewer than 10% exercise vigorously; another study showed that 31% of people 65 to 74 years engaged in regular walking, 24.3% of people over 75 years

   5. *Healthy People 2000: Midcourse Review* shows minimal changes in the area of exercise for older adults

   6. It is important to assess the older adult before an exercise program is recommended

B. Types of exercise

   1. Aerobic: swimming, brisk walking, cycling

   2. Water exercise is therapeutic for the person with limited mobility as a result of arthritis

   3. Regular exercise (3 times per week for 30 minutes) is recommended

   4. It is important to encourage wheelchair-bound people to use their arms and feet, whenever possible

   5. Passive and active range of motion should be encouraged for bed-bound patients when bathing, grooming

   6. Studies have documented the promotion of functional independence, balance, range of motion, flexibility, and spatial awareness from strengthening exercises

TABLE **4-1**

SUGGESTED EXAMINATIONS FOR PREVENTIVE HEALTH MAINTENANCE
FOR PERSONS 50 YEARS OLD AND OLDER

Examinations and Tests	Population Group	Frequency
Complete physical, including cholesterol check	All persons	Every 1-3 years until age 75; then every year thereafter
Pelvic examination and breast examination	Women	Annually
Breast self-examination	Women	Monthly
Clinical breast examination	Women	Yearly
Mammogram	Women	Annually after age 50
Digital rectal examination	All persons	Annually for women with pelvic examination; every 2 years for men
Sigmoidoscopy	All persons	Every 3-5 years after age 50
Stool for occult blood	All persons	Annually
Prostate examination	Men	Every 2 years
Blood pressure	All persons	Every office visit
Eye examination	All persons	Annually after age 50
Glaucoma test	All persons	Every 3 years after age 55; every year if family history
Dental examination and cleaning	All persons	Yearly for those with teeth; cleaning every 6 months, every 2 years for denture wearers
Hearing test	All persons	Every 2-5 years

Compiled from AARP strategies for good health; *Healthy People 2000,* US Government Printing Office, Washington, DC, 1991; Schmidt, RM: Preventive health care for older adults, societal and individual services, *Generations XVIII* (1), 1994; *Healthwise,* Kaiser Permanente, 1994; St. Mary's Medical Center, San Francisco, 1995; *Mayo Clinic Health Letter* 14(1), 1996.

IV. SCREENING PROGRAMS

 A. Nursing role
  1. Teaching the importance of self-responsibility in maintaining health
  2. Advocating for patients who are unable to avail themselves of screening
 B. Recommended screening (Table 4-1)
 C. Important for all residents of long-term care facilities: to have a two-step PPD test on admission because of the resurgence of tuberculosis; health care workers in these settings are also at risk

V. IMMUNIZATIONS

 A. Immunizations considered routine for children and young adults but not often for older adults
 B. Pneumonia and influenza fifth leading cause of death for older adults; 80% to 90% of influenza deaths in the United States are among the older population; only 30% of older adults get the influenza vaccine; especially important for long-term care residents
 C. Tetanus vaccinations are also important for older adults, especially those who have a pressure ulcer; less than 40% of older adults are protected against tetanus

TABLE **4-2**

GUIDELINES FOR IMMUNIZATIONS FOR OLDER ADULTS

Immunization	Indications	Frequency
Influenza	Aged 65 years and older, long-term care residents, anyone with chronic respiratory or cardiovascular disorders, health care workers	Annually, preferably between September and November (but they can be administered as late as January)
Pneumonia	Same groups as influenza, except for health care workers	Once in a lifetime, but people at very high risk may be revaccinated after 6 years
Tetanus toxoid	All adults, particularly debilitated adults with pressure ulcers	Initial series of three, then booster shot every 10 years (or after 5 years if at high risk)
Hepatitis B	Homosexual men, recipients of various blood products, patients receiving hemodialysis, people in health care–related jobs where exposure to hepatitis B is probable	A series of three doses should last for several years

    D. Hepatitis B vaccine is recommended for older homosexual men, people undergoing dialysis, those receiving blood products

    E. See guidelines for immunizations for the older population (Table 4–2)

VI. SELF-CARE SKILLS

    A. Definition: the practice of activities that individuals personally initiate and perform on their own behalf in maintaining life, health, and well-being

    B. Orem's Self-Care Deficit Theory

       1. Self-care is learned and requires knowledge, motivation, and skill

       2. Ability to perform self-care is by self-care agents; others who provide care are dependent agents

       3. Self-care deficit theory identifies when nursing is needed

    C. Nursing role: to assist the individual who is unable to meet self-care needs

       1. Assessment

          a. Important to obtain data about ability of older adult to perform self-care skills

          b. May also be necessary to assess the ability of the caregiver, particularly in the home; spouse or caregiver may be frail as well

          c. Even institutionalized older adults may have capacity to do self-care (i.e., bathe, administer their own medications, etc.)

          d. Several tools are available to measure ability to perform self-care as well as tools to describe functional health patterns

       2. Nursing diagnoses

          a. Should be patient-specific and based on data collected

          b. Identified as actual or high risk

          c. Examples

            • Case 1: Patient recently diagnosed with congestive heart failure: health maintenance, altered, high risk for: related to knowledge deficit of medication regimen

            • Case 2: New stroke patient: self-care deficit, bathing: related to neuromuscular impairment as manifested by inability to bathe self

3. Planning
   a. Goals are specific, measurable, and realistic for the patient
   b. Goals include outcome criteria, that is, what is expected
   c. Examples
      - Case 1: Patient will be able to verbalize action of digoxin and lasix, identify correct dosage, state what side effects may occur, and three implications of the drug therapy by _____ (target date)
      - Case 2: Patient will participate in self-care as evidenced by being able to wash upper part of body by _____ (target date)
4. Interventions (for Case 1)
   a. Assess learning needs and educational level of patient
   b. Develop a teaching plan that addresses medications patient will be on when discharged
   c. Include family or support system in teaching
   d. Use audiovisuals that are easy to read, patient can keep, and fit patient's educational ability
   e. When describing actions, side effects of drugs, use terminology that patient can understand
   f. Recognize that patient teaching is most effective when patient feels the need to learn and is encouraged to participate

D. Three variations in types of nursing systems
   1. Wholly compensatory: patients are entirely dependent on the nurse for the delivery of their care
   2. Partly compensatory: patients can and should perform some of their own care
   3. Supportive-educative: patients are able to perform and/or learn self-care but require assistance from the nurse
   4. Patients can move from one system to another as their needs change
      a. Example
         - Case 1: patient diagnosed with congestive heart failure may have acute pulmonary edema on admission and need total care
         - As the patient progresses, he becomes more able to perform self-care and eventually receives the teaching necessary to be able to be independent again
         - In this case, self-care would involve not only being able to care for himself independently but being able to maintain health by being accountable and responsible for the health care regimen

VII. ALTERNATIVE/COMPLEMENTARY HEALTH CARE

A. More people are using alternative methods to reduce stress in their lives and cope with chronic or disabling conditions
B. More than 40% of people in the United States are currently using alternative or complementary types of therapies
C. The National Institutes of Health (NIH) created the National Center of Complementary and Alternative Medicine (CAM), which funds $4 million in complementary and alternative medicine clinical centers
   1. Instruction in unconventional therapies is being added to health curricula, and we are now seeing reimbursement for such therapies
   2. In the future, many of these therapies will be conventional rather than alternative
D. Types of alternative/complementary health care
   1. Progressive relaxation: technique that teaches the person to alternately contract and then relax muscle groups in the body, starting with the feet and moving up to the face (used for pain control, sleep promotion, etc.)
   2. Visualization: also known as guided imagery, centering, focusing, distraction, and meditation; involves the creation of mental images as a way to deal with pain and anxiety and to promote relaxation and sleep

3. Hypnotherapy: uses therapist's power of suggestion to assist the patient to experience the imaginary as real, experience relaxation, and work through emotional conflicts
4. Biofeedback: used to gain control over involuntary functions, including pulse and blood pressure; by observing monitoring devices, the person can learn to control specific autonomic functions
5. Yoga: a system of mental and physical exercises, focusing on specific body postures, controlled breathing, and meditation; has shown to promote circulation and improve a sense of well-being
6. Therapeutic touch, healing touch: based on idea that disruption of one's energy field can lead to illness and disease; manipulation of this field can restore balance, reduce pain
7. Tai chi: an ancient Chinese form of simple, repetitive movements that emphasize a soft, flowing motion; helpful in maintaining balance and providing a safe form of exercise for older adults
8. Qigong (she-gong): a combination of movement, meditation, and breath regulation that enhances the flow of vital energy in the body
9. Acupuncture/acupressure: Chinese method used to relieve angina, treat respiratory problems, relieve pain through the use of hair-thin needles inserted at various sites or use of pressure at various body points
10. Aromatherapy: the use of essential oils of various plants to induce physical and emotional effects, including relieving headaches, boosting appetite, treating depression
11. Herbal therapy: the use of herbs for various effects, including relaxation, boosting the immune system, appetite stimulation, treatment of depression, treatment of skin conditions; unregulated and if taken with other drugs (prescription or over-the-counter) can cause harm; current research on many herbal treatments underway in the United States

REFERENCES

Allison M, Keller C: Physical activity in the elderly: benefits and intervention strategies, *Nurse Pract* 22(8):53-69, 1997.
Barry HC, Eathorne SW: Exercise and aging: issues for the practitioner, *Med Clin North Am* 78(2):357, 1994.
Brill PA: Effective approach toward prevention and rehabilitation in geriatrics, *Activ Adapt Aging* 23(4):21-32, 1999.
Carpenito LJ: *Nursing diagnosis: application to clinical practice,* ed 7, Philadelphia, 1997, JB Lippincott.
Dossey B: Using imagery to help your patient heal, *AJN* 95(6):41-47, 1995.
Ebersole P, Hess P: *Toward healthy aging: human needs and nursing responses,* ed 5, St Louis, 1998, Mosby.
Eliopoulos C: *Gerontological nursing,* ed 4, Philadelphia, 1997, JB Lippincott.
Evans BM: Complementary therapies in HIV infections, *AJN* 99(2):42-45, 1999.
Good M: Relaxation techniques for surgical patients, *AJN* 95(5):39-43, 1995.
Healthy People 2000, Washington, DC, 1991, US Department of Health and Human Services, No. 91-50212, Public Health Service, US Government Printing Office.
Healthy People 2000: Midcourse Review and 1995 Revisions, Washington, DC, 1995, US Department of Health and Human Services, Public Health Service, US Government Printing Office.
Hoffart MB, Keene EP: The benefits of visualization, *AJN* 98(12):44-47, 1998.
Hutchison CP: Healing touch: an energetic approach, *AJN* 99(4):43-48, 1999.
Kaufmann MA: Wellness for people 65 years and better, *J Gerontol Nurs* 23(6):7-9, 1997.
Lueckenotte AG: *Gerontologic nursing,* St Louis, 1996, Mosby.
Mackey RB: Discover the healing power of therapeutic touch, *AJN* 95(4):27-32, 1995.
Miller CA: Preventive care should address immunizations for older adults, *Geriatr Nurs* 18(1):42-43, 1997.
O'Neill CK, et al: Herbal medicines, *Nursing '99* 29(4):58-61, 1999.
Orem DE: *Nursing: concepts of practice,* ed 5, St Louis, 1995, Mosby.
Phaneuf C: Screening elders for nutritional deficits, *Am J Nurs* 96(3):58-60, 1996.
Schaller KJ: Tai chi chih: an exercise option for older adults, *J Gerontol Nurs* 22(10):12-17, 1996.
Shinkarovsky L: Hypnotherapy, not just hocus-pocus *RN* 59(5):55-57, 1996.

Siegel PZ, Brackbill RM, Heath GW: The epidemiology of walking for exercise: implications for promoting activity among sedentary groups, *Am J Pub Health* 85(5):706, 1995.

Tyson SR: *Gerontological nursing care,* Philadelphia, 1999, WB Saunders.

Wold GH: *Basic geriatric nursing,* ed 2, St Louis, 1999, Mosby.

Yen PK: Complementary therapies: fad or fact? *Geriatr Nurs* 20(1):52-53, 1999.

Yen PK: Herbal foods, *Geriatr Nurs* 20(2):111-112, 1999.

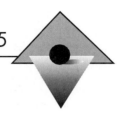

CHAPTER 5

ENVIRONMENT

Mary Painter-Romanello ● *Ann Schmidt Luggen*

LEARNING OBJECTIVES

Upon completion of this chapter, the reader will be able to:

- Analyze and discuss how various environments affect the living arrangement and lifestyle of the older adult
- Describe the impact of relocation on the life of the older adult
- Use strategies to reduce the stress of relocation
- Discuss the need of the older adult for personal space
- Describe the effects of loss of personal space

I. LIVING ARRANGEMENTS

A. General conditions
1. Older adults want to stay in their own homes independently as long as possible
2. Mobility, transportation, and safety factors often affect the living patterns of older adults
3. Factors that may cause older adults to change living arrangements
- Death of a spouse
- Divorce
- Change in economic circumstances
- Loss of health; reduced cognitive or functional status
- Availability of family
- Personal preference
4. 6.5 million older adults need assistance with daily activities
5. Most common chronic conditions affecting older adults
- Arthritis
- Hypertension
- Heart disease
- Hearing impairments
- Cataracts
- Orthopedic impairments
- Sinusitis
- Diabetes
6. To maintain independence, identification of needs and appropriate interventions are essential; the assessment is ideally performed in the home setting
B. Living environments
1. Home
a. Approximately 70% of older adults live in a family setting; 4% to 6% live in a nursing home
b. 78% of older householders own their own home; 22% are renting

      c. 36% of older homeowners are single

      d. 79% of older homeowners are female

      e. Majority of older males are married and live in a family setting

      f. 44% of older women are widowed and live outside a family setting

      g. Home ownership rates of minority households are lower than the rates for all other older households

- 66% for older African Americans
- 59% for older Hispanics

      h. Even though home ownership is viewed as an asset, it also represents a burden because of the cost of ownership and maintenance

  2. Assisted living

      a. Assisted living is the fastest growing type of senior housing in the United States

      b. The goal is to maintain or enhance the frail elder's capabilities to remain as independent as possible

  3. Homelessness

      a. Housing needs of homeless older adults are often ignored

      b. Older people who are homeless as a result of uncontrollable circumstances often do not receive a range of services and support

      c. Factors that promote older adult homelessness include

- Frailty and poor health
- Mental health problems that produce isolation among the homeless
- Reluctance of medical practitioners to accept homeless older adults as patients
- Inadequate discharge planning from emergency rooms and hospitals
- Lack of social service interventions to provide adequate long-term support and housing accommodations

C. Housing

  1. Housing needs of older adults often differ and must accommodate specific means of mobility and environmental conditions

      a. 40% of community-based elderly Americans age 70+ have modified their homes because of physical limitations caused by chronic illnesses or conditions

      b. The most common home modifications are bathroom grab bars or shower seats, those that allow indoor wheelchair use, railings, and wheelchair ramps

  2. Use of assistive devices, such as walkers, canes, wheelchairs, must be considered when assessing safety, adequacy of housing units, and environmental barriers

II. SAFETY AND SECURITY ISSUES

A. Crime

  1. Approximately 25% of older adults live in fear of crime

  2. Fear of crime is associated with

- Being female
- Being a frail male
- Low socioeconomic status
- Living alone in an urban, high-crime area

  3. Consequences of fear of crime

- Social isolation
- Impaired function
- Decreased quality of life

B. Safety

  1. Driving

      a. Older adults are involved in more motor vehicle accidents than younger people

      b. Sensory and cognitive changes have adverse effects on driving ability

      c. Safety assessment should include asking if the older adult uses safety belts

2. Physical environment
   a. Home visits are the most effective way to assess safety in the physical environment
   b. Look for barriers to effective functioning
   c. Assess the patient's ability to perform IADLs necessary for independent functioning (Box 5-1)
3. Fall risk
   a. Approximately 30% of community-based older adults fall each year
   b. Most falls occur in the home
   c. Key areas to assess
      • Adequate lighting and access to switches
      • Safe flooring; look for cords
      • Safe stairways; secure handrails; adequate toilet height, grab bars
      • Kitchen: access to items
      • Smoke alarms
      • Clutter
      • Medications labeled
      • Safety of the neighborhood
      • Barriers to optimum functioning: distance to bathroom, ease getting in and out of chair
   d. Interventions
      • Highlight thresholds, stairs, and level changes with contrasting tape or paint
      • Reds and oranges are seen best
      • Use non-skid, non-glare flooring
      • Apply sheers to all windows to eliminate glare
      • Provide adequate lighting
      • Eliminate throw rugs, electrical cords

III. RELOCATION

A. Major psychosocial adjustment
B. Older adults may perceive relocation as relief from responsibility of home ownership
C. Only 5% of adults 65+ in the United States move to a nursing facility; however, the chance of being admitted at some time is about 50%
D. Degree of willingness to relocate and level of involvement in decision-making are important variables in successful relocation

IV. TRANSPORTATION

A. Transportation is assessed as part of IADL
   • 0 = independent, drives a car
   • 1 = arranges own transport, depends on others for transport except for walking
   • 3 = assists in own transport but needs special accommodation, e.g., wheelchair
   • 5 = completely homebound even for medical care

BOX 5-1   Instrumental Activities of Daily Living (IADLs)

Ability to use telephone
Shopping independently
Food preparation
Housekeeping
Laundry
Using modes of transportation
Responsibility for taking own medications
Handling finances

   B. Title II: Public Services and Transportation
      1. Prohibits discrimination in public transportation programs
      2. Services must be provided for disabled who cannot use public ground transport
      3. Bus and rail systems must be accessible
   C. Title III: Public Accommodations
      1. Privately owned enterprises must provide public accommodation for the disabled
      2. Exempt are private clubs and religious organizations
   D. Alternatives to driving
      1. Reduced-fare taxis
      2. Volunteer drivers
      3. Public transportation
      4. Chartered buses
      5. Dial-a-ride programs

V. TERRITORIALITY/PERSONAL SPACE

   A. Institutionalized older adults need to gain, maintain, and defend an area of space to preserve security
   B. Territoriality exists when individuals exhibit behaviors to claim or defend an area of space from others
   C. Individuals in densely populated institutions may exhibit behaviors of less involvement
   D. Loss of space or invasion of territory may be anxiety provoking
   E. Types of territory
      1. Body: anatomical space of human body
      2. Home: area where person has freedom of behavior and control over the area
      3. Interactional: area where social gathering may occur
      4. Public: area that individuals have freedom to access
   F. Institutional territoriality concepts
      1. Crowding: number of persons per living area
      2. Density: number of persons in a geographic area
      3. Increased number of persons per area reduces personal space
      4. Acute anxiety behaviors occur as a result of diminished personal space or overcrowding of territory
      5. Individuals requiring chronic institutionalization are often deprived of personal space and may exhibit behaviors to gain space
         a. Body manipulation to gain more than one area, e.g., sitting on 2 chairs
         b. Adorning body with atypical clothing or tattoos
         c. Gaining freedom through penetration of inner space, e.g., daydreaming
         d. When chronically deprived of space, converting public territory into home territory

VI. COMMUNITY RESOURCES: FEDERAL, STATE, LOCAL GOVERNMENTS

   A. Agency on Aging
      1. Congregated nutrition programs
      2. Home-delivered meals
      3. Adult day care
      4. Senior centers
      5. Services for dementia cases
      6. Home repairs
   B. County Welfare Office
      1. Food stamps to financially qualifying older adults
   C. Distribution Agencies
      1. Food distribution to maintain and improve nutrition in older adults and promote independent living

    D. Departments of Social Services, Human Resources
       1. Public housing
       2. Public assistance
       3. Medicaid
    E. Department of Health
       1. Immunization programs
       2. Health care programs
       3. Programs for Alzheimer's disease and related dementias
    F. Services for Visually and Hearing Impaired
       1. Education
       2. Guide dog training
       3. Home and medical appliances to ensure safety
       4. Talking books
       5. Magnification and amplification devices
    G. Department of Mental Health
       1. Evaluation services
       2. Day treatment programs
       3. Clinics for treatment
       4. Adult homes
    H. Adult Protection Agency
       1. Guardianship
       2. Financial management
       3. Residence placement

REFERENCES

Boettcher EG: Boundary marking: a social ecological study of human need satisfaction among institutionalized elderly persons, *J Psychosoc Nurs Ment Health Serv* 23(8):25-30, 1985.

Cooper KM: Territorial behavior among the institutionalized: a nursing perspective, *J Psychosoc Nurs Ment Health Serv* 22(12):6-11, 1984.

Haight BK, Michel Y, Hendrix S: Life review: preventing despair in newly relocated nursing home residents: short- and long-term effects, *Int J Aging Hum Dev* 47(2):119-142, 1998.

Iwasiw C, Goldenberg D, MacMaster E, et al: Residents' perspective of their first two weeks in a long-term care facility, *J Clin Nurs* 5(6):381-388, 1996.

King K, Dimond M, McCance K: Coping with relocating, *Geriatr Nurs* 8(5):258, 1987.

Kovach CR: Nursing home dementia care units: providing a continuum of care rather than aging in place, *J Gerontol Nurs* 24(4):30-35, 1998.

Lander SM, Brazill AL, Ladrigan RM: Intrainstitutional relocation: effects on residents' behavior and psychosocial functioning, *J Gerontol Nurs* 23(4):809-816, 1997.

Petrou M, Obenchain J: Reducing incidents of illness post transfer, *Geriatr Nurs* 8(5):264, 1987.

Rodgers BL: Family members' experiences with the nursing home placement of an older adult, *Appl Nurs Res* 10(2):57-63, 1997.

CHAPTER 6

PERSONAL AND CULTURAL INFLUENCES

Sue E. Meiner

LEARNING OBJECTIVES

Upon completion of this chapter, the reader will be able to:

- Describe variables that should be considered when caring for individuals of diverse cultural backgrounds
- Name an activity that can promote intergenerational involvement between older adults and children
- List four areas of focus in a spiritual assessment
- Differentiate relationship from companionship
- Discuss elements of autonomy that can lead to limitation of decision-making

I. CULTURE/ETHNICITY

A. Cultural sensitivity involves
1. Avoiding the belief that one's own culture is the best one (ethnocentrism)
2. Relying on patient-centered nursing to understand the unique cultural needs of a pluralistic society (multiculturalism)
3. Seeking cultural competence through understanding interpersonal and clinical competence
4. Identifying barriers to health care associated with cultural diversity
B. Ethnicity: basic concepts
1. Time
    a. *Past-oriented cultures* value tradition and do things as they always have been done; they have a reluctance to try new procedures and are not concerned about the future
    b. *Present-oriented cultures* focus on the here and now and are often unconcerned about preventive health measures; past or future events may be recognized but are not emphasized
    c. *Future-oriented cultures* value change and progress
2. Social structure
    a. *Egalitarian social structure* views everyone as an equal; status and power depend on personal qualities rather than other characteristics; equality is seen as an ideal even though things in reality may operate differently
    b. *Hierarchical social structure* allows that inequalities exist among individuals based on certain characteristics (age, gender, or occupation); people of higher status command respect
3. Communication issues
    a. There are verbal and nonverbal means by which people share information, signals, or messages

      b. Barriers to communication: language, communication style or pattern differences, knowledge, education, dialect, and silence elements
   4. Personal space
      a. Territoriality: cultural factors, which might include encroaching into private space, that may be uncomfortable for those in some cultures
      b. Social and public distance: rarely encountered as a problem in the health care setting
      c. Personal distance: 18 inches to 4 feet, norm for the health interview
      d. Intimate distance: most commonly encroached upon in a health care setting (e.g., using the ophthalmoscope)
  C. Cultural/ethnic variables affecting health care of the older adult
   1. A goal of health care is to analyze the knowledge/practices of cultural variations in an effort to develop insight and prevent misunderstanding or misjudgment of the individual
   2. An understanding of ethnocentrism and cultural relativism may help to determine why differences occur among cultures
      a. Ethnocentrism: views one's own ways of doing things as the right and natural way
      b. Cultural relativism: recognizes other ways of doing things as different but equally valid
  D. Intergenerational issues
   1. A breadth of cohort groups interacting through community involvement programs such as adopt-a-grandparent and day care (children and elderly) interactions
   2. Opportunities for young children and older adults to interact accompanied by an intermediary support person (to prevent exhaustion among the older persons and provide needed supervision of children)

II. SPIRITUALITY

  A. A quality that transcends a particular religious affiliation
  B. Encompasses religion and one's own interpretation of life and inner resources
   1. A sense of meaning and purpose
   2. Finding meaning in suffering
   3. Forgiveness
   4. Source of love and relatedness
   5. Sense of transcendence
   6. Awe and wonder about life
   7. Trustful relatedness to God or a Supreme Being
  C. Religion is a personal way of externally expressing spirituality through affiliations, rites, and rituals based upon creeds and communal practices
  D. Spirituality and religious meaning for the older adult
   1. Promotes acceptance of the past, allows enjoyment of the present, and provides hope for the future
   2. Provides a basic human need
   3. Over time the practice that was habit in earlier years may become stronger
   4. Spirituality and religion can help in stressful life events, in understanding the meaning of life, and in preparation for death
   5. A strong sense of hope in spirituality or religion can provide support during phases of multiple losses and the grieving process
  E. Nursing assessment
   1. Highly unique to each older adult
   2. Nurses traditionally have limited spiritual assessment to religious affiliation
   3. Spiritual assessment can include
      a. Concept of God or deity
      b. Sources of hope and strength

   c. Religious practices

   d. Relation between spiritual beliefs and health

  4. In assessing the cognitively impaired older adult's needs

   a. Personal manner sets the tone

   b. Use gentle touching, eye contact, patience, and listening

   c. Promote the need for identity through encouraging discussion of long-term memories, using hymns, prayers, icons, or other specific religious items

III. RELATIONSHIPS, COMPANIONSHIP, INTIMACY/SEXUALITY

 A. Relationship: short or long-term, personal or impersonal, intimate or superficial

 B. Companionship: spousal, life partners, family members, and/or friends

 C. Intimacy/sexuality: provides an opportunity to express passion, affection, admiration, and loyalty

 D. Sexual dysfunction: state in which an individual experiences a disruption of satisfactory sexual activity; there is a perceived problem in achieving desired satisfaction of preferred sexuality

  1. Changing sexual performance and/or expression that are self-identified as unfulfilling

  2. Women experience a decline in hormonal levels after menopause, leading to changes in the vaginal wall (thinness) and to inelasticity that can cause pain

  3. Men have a gradual decline in testosterone, leading to a longer refractory time between erections

  4. Decline in sexuality/marital intimacy can be related to disease processes

   a. Women: osteoporosis, cancer of the reproductive organs, Alzheimer's disease

   b. Men: benign prostatic hypertrophy, prostate cancer, and Alzheimer's disease

IV. AUTONOMY (CONTROL, POLITICAL ACTIVITY)

 A. Autonomy (self-determination) is an issue of personal freedom and the right to choose for oneself

  1. Autonomy is one of the highest valued rights of older adults

  2. Protection against abuse, social problems, and financial concerns may limit autonomy; judgment must be made about balancing protection against limiting the older adult's personal freedom

  3. Elevation of the individual's rights over the wishes or opinions of others

  4. Respect for autonomy means consideration of the right of another person for self-governance

  5. Lost autonomy often in one area of life is compensated for in another area (e.g., decline in correctable vision may result in listening to audio books)

  6. Competency as an issue of autonomy: The Patient Self-Determination Act of 1991

  7. Diminished autonomy because of incompetence

   a. Remedies through court-appointed guardian or conservator, usually a relative, friend, or attorney

   b. Proxy directive or power of attorney

   c. Informal delegation of a family member to assist in decision-making

 B. Control issues

  1. Remaining in independent housing that was established during mid-life or younger into the ninth decade of life (aging in place)

  2. Personal choice regarding end-of-life decisions and advanced directives

 C. Political action

  1. Older adults are an active political group

  2. 70% of all voters 65+ voted in the 1996 election

REFERENCES

Ebersole P, Hess P: *Toward healthy aging: human needs and nursing response,* ed 5, St Louis, 1998, Mosby.

Lester N: Cultural competence: a nursing dialogue, *AJN* 98(8):26–33, 1998.

Luggen AS, Travis SS, Meiner SE: *NGNA core curriculum for gerontological advanced practice nurses,* Thousand Oaks, CA, 1998, Sage.

Stone JT, Wyman JF, Salisbury SA: *Clinical gerontological nursing: a guide to advanced practice,* ed 2, Philadelphia, 1999, WB Saunders.

Sumner CH: Recognizing and responding to spiritual distress, *AJN* 98(1):26–30, 1998.

Tyson SR: *Gerontological nursing care,* Philadelphia, 1999, WB Saunders.

Wold GH: *Basic geriatric nursing,* St Louis, 1999, Mosby.

CHAPTER 7

NURSING PRACTICE THEORIES

Ann Schmidt Luggen

LEARNING OBJECTIVES

Upon completion of this chapter, the reader will be able to:

- Discuss two nursing theories that are useful in caring for older patients
- Name five biological aging theories and state the tenets of each
- List the prominent sociological theories of aging and discuss each one
- Delineate differences among the three important developmental theories of aging
- Describe the six stages of the family life cycle
- Discuss the major tenets of systems theory

I. NURSING THEORIES

    A. Orem: Self-Care Deficit Theory

        1. Definitions

            a. Self-care: actions to maintain one's health and well-being

            b. Self-care deficit: inability to meet one's self-care demands

            c. Self-care demands: actions needed to meet self-care requisites

        2. Nursing systems

            a. Wholly compensatory: patient depends on nurse for care

            b. Partly compensatory: patient can perform some self-care

            c. Supportive-educative: patient can perform and/or learn self-care but requires nursing assistance

        3. Assessment

            a. Focus on maintenance of self-care behaviors

            b. Identify illness-imposed demands, effects of illness on physical function

            c. Identify illness-imposed demands, social effects

            d. Identify caregiver ability and available support systems

        4. Diagnosis

            a. Include actual and potential problems

        5. Plan

            a. Nurse assists patient to restore self-care

            b. Patient participates in plan of care

            c. Measurable outcomes

        6. Interventions

            a. Universal life demands (e.g., circulation, nutrition, ventilation) determine interventions

            b. Change interventions as patient progresses from wholly compensatory to partly to supportive self-care

       c. Consider patient values and beliefs in interventions
       d. Knowledge provided so patient has control of outcome
    7. Evaluation
       a. Modify plan of care to meet goals
       b. Determine that goals are met

B. Roy's Adaptation Theory
    1. Definitions
       a. Adaptation systems: regulator—physiological, such as endocrine, nutrition, oxygenation
       b. Adaptation systems: cognator—symbolic meanings used to relate events; perceptual such as selective attention; insight, problem solving; attachments
       c. Contextual stimuli: situational elements such as noise, pain
       d. Focal stimuli: immediate confronting stimulus, internal or external
       e. Residual stimuli: other factors affecting current situation such as self-esteem, spiritual beliefs, attitudes, personal ethics
    2. Adaptation modes
       a. Physiological mode: physical response to environment
       b. Self-concept mode: perception of physical and personal self
       c. Role function: primary or secondary roles, position, performance
       d. Interdependence: nurturing, affection, support systems, significant others
    3. Patients assessed in different systems, modes, considering stimuli; plans and interventions: consider same and evaluation of effect of outcome in each

II. AGING THEORIES

A. Biological theories
    1. Biological clock: "programmed" theory that each of us has predetermined number of cell divisions that play out with graying hair, thymus atrophy, menopause, etc.; influenced by heredity
    2. Gene theory: existence of one or more harmful genes that can activate over time and cause cell mutations that are self-perpetuating, resulting in organism failure
    3. Free radical theory: free radicals, substances produced during normal metabolism, are not eliminated and interfere with normal body function, resulting in cell damage
    4. Error theory: errors in protein synthesis result in errors in cells, causing progressive decline in biological functioning
    5. Cross-link theory: cellular DNA and connective tissue interact with free radicals damaging the DNA; normal defense mechanisms are weakened over time and eventually irreparable damage occurs

B. Sociological theories
    1. Disengagement theory: Cumming and Henry wrote in 1961 that social equilibrium is achieved by a reciprocal withdrawal from society by older people and by society; older adults are said to be happy when this disengagement occurs
    2. Activity theory: Havighurst, 1963, believed that social role participation in old age indicated a positive adjustment to aging; if older adults remain active, they will remain psychologically and physically fit
    3. Continuity theory: Neugarten, 1968, proposed a personality continuity or development theory of aging; personality is dynamic and evolving; one can predict adjustment to aging by viewing adjustment through life
    4. Subculture theory: Rose, 1965, believed that older people have their own norms, habits, beliefs—their own subculture; they interact well among themselves rather than with other age groups; the subculture is a response to loss of status
    5. Age stratification theory: focuses on the relationship between age as an element of social structure and aging people as a cohort; it purports that
       a. There are age cohorts that age socially, biologically, and psychologically
       b. Each cohort experiences a unique history

c. Society continually changes and those in each age strata do also

d. There is a dynamic interplay between social change and individual aging

C. Developmental theories

1. Erikson: aging is a normal stage in life in which the older adult either accepts his/her past life and maintains integrity or cannot accept it and experiences despair

2. Havighurst: there are specific tasks connected with aging—adjusting to loss, adapting to change, accepting life's experiences, undergoing role changes, and preparing for death

3. Maslow: each of us has an innate hierarchy of needs that motivates us; basic needs must be met first to move on to the next levels

a. Basic needs: shelter, food, temperature, ventilation

b. Safety, security: adequate lighting, door locks, smoke detectors

c. Belonging: love, comfort, being surrounded by favorite things

d. Trust: control over lifestyle, pain, choices

e. Self-esteem: status, pride, confidence

f. Self-actualization: satisfying relationships, creativity, values, self-direction

III. FAMILY THEORIES

A. Family life cycle: six stages

1. Unattached young adult: parents and young adults successfully separate

2. New marriage: commitment to new family system

3. Family with young children: accept new members into family system

4. Family with adolescents: remold boundaries to allow independence

5. Launching the children: accept exits and entrances into the family

6. Later life: accepting shifting generational roles and death

B. Systems theory

1. von Bertalanffy, 1986, developed systems theory; basic to understanding family stress and impact of illness on family

2. Basic tenets

a. Family viewed as a complex social system

b. Family unit constantly exchanges information, energy, materials with the environment

c. Family unit socializes members by establishing roles, influencing basic values, beliefs, attitudes, aspirations of individuals

d. Family provides physical maintenance, such as food, clothing, shelter, care

e. Family shares intense emotional ties that influence emotional development of children and the whole family

3. Illness is a potential hazard that may be the product of family interactions

REFERENCES

Chinn P, Kramer M: *Theoretical nursing: development and progress,* ed 2, Philadelphia, 1995, JB Lippincott.

Ebersole P, Hess P: *Toward healthy aging: human needs and nursing response,* St Louis, 1998, Mosby.

Eliopoulos C: *Gerontological nursing,* ed 4, Philadelphia, 1997, JB Lippincott.

Fawcett J: *Analysis and evaluation of conceptual models of nursing,* ed 3, Philadelphia, 1995, FA Davis.

Nicoll L: *Perspectives on nursing theory,* ed 3, Philadelphia, 1997, JB Lippincott.

CHAPTER 8

COMMUNICATION PROCESS

Margaret M. Anderson

LEARNING OBJECTIVES

Upon completion of this chapter, the reader will be able to:

- Discuss four learning theories
- Discuss the relationship between learning style and learning theory
- Explain how core learning and teaching principles drive the teaching/learning environment
- Identify effects of the aging process on learning
- Identify four methods to combat memory decline
- Discuss the impact of aging on the educational process

I. THEORIES OF LEARNING

A. Common learning theories
  1. Behavioral theory (Skinner, Pavlov, and Thorndike)
     a. Based on the concept that behavior is learned and, therefore, can be shaped and molded for desired results; a system of rewards and punishments is used to shape the behavior in the desired direction; the discomfort of punishment encourages the learner to seek rewards and, therefore, to behave in a way to obtain rewards and avoid punishment
     b. The learner is in a passive, reactive role while the teacher is in an active role, directing the learning with rewards and punishment
  2. Cognitive theory (Bloom, Gagne, and Ausubel)
     a. Basic premise is problem-solving as a means to achieving goals; the conditions of the learning environment determine the acquisition and retention of knowledge by impacting existing cognitive knowledge; learning builds from and on concepts used in previous experiences
     b. Learning processes include such basics as assimilation, accommodation, and construction of knowledge
     c. Motivation to learn is based on the individual's need to solve problems
     d. The learner is active in determining the experience and how experiences occur; the teacher is active in structuring the experiences to impact cognition
  3. Humanistic theory (Rogers, Maslow, and Dewey)
     a. Conceptual notion of the individual's responsibility for self; the need to learn is the basis of self-actualization; there is a natural desire to learn; education is needed for the development of human potential
     b. Knowledge is transferable from one situation to another; the assumption is that individuals can determine their learning needs and the methods for meeting those needs

      c. The learner is active in efforts to impact self-growth and self-concept; the teacher is a facilitator in encouraging the learner and directing the learner to appropriate resources

   4. Adult education theory (Knowles, Schon, Cross, and Caffarella)

      a. Belief is that adults learn differently from children

      b. Andragogy is used to refer to adult theory rather than pedagogy, which is related to how children learn; adults are more self-directed and are not interested in knowledge that does not meet a specific problem they have or are going to have in the future; adults want useful, real, and immediately applicable information

      c. The learner is active in determining his/her needs as well as devising methods of meeting them; the teacher guides or coaches the learner to meet the goals; often uses thoughtful questioning as a means of guidance

   5. Depending on the material to be taught, the teacher may apply different learning theories

      a. Teaching methods and learning style affect the theory selected

      b. Behavioral theory is useful for psychomotor skills and habit cessation

      c. Cognitive theory is often used to change cognitive abilities as seen in skills or lifestyle changes

      d. Humanistic theory encourages self-reflection and study to make major life changes

      e. Adult education theory is applicable to most teaching situations with adults and can be used in combination with other theories

B. Learning styles

   1. Learning style is the unique way an individual learns

   2. Learning style has biological and sociological components and varies from one individual to another (styles may be similar; each learner is unique in processing information in various situations)

      a. Principles related to learning styles

         (1) Both the teacher's style and the learner's style can be identified

         (2) Teachers need to guard against using only their own style

         (3) Teachers are helpful when they teach in the learner's style; students should have the opportunity to learn with their own style

         (4) Diversification of learning styles should be encouraged in the learner

         (5) Learning activities can be developed by teachers to enhance each of the learner's learning styles

      b. Learning styles can be learned and developed through practice, confidence, and self-direction

C. Core learning principles (Braungart and Braungart)

   1. New learning must relate to what the learner already knows

   2. Environmental factors (e.g., type of stimuli, effectiveness of role models, feedback mechanism for correct and incorrect responses, and opportunities to practice new learning) impact the actual learning process

   3. It is important to consider motivational need or desire of the learner to learn

   4. The learner is in control of what and how much is learned and is affected by many factors, including developmental stage, cultural conditioning, socialization, prior experiences with education, and personality

   5. Knowledge of the material and the learner and the teaching competence and educational methodologies the teacher has or is perceived to have affects what or how much the learner learns

   6. Other barriers to learning might include a lack of clarity and meaningfulness of material to be learned, harsh punishment for incorrect responses, confusing reinforcement, and lack of readiness on the part of the learner

   7. Responsibilities of the learner include acceptance of responsibility for learning, determining goals of learning, active participation in the learning situation, and monitoring own progress and pace in the learning situation

D. Core teaching principles
1. Respect and value learners
2. Establish an environment conducive to learning (non-threatening, pleasant, related to material to be learned)
3. Make learning active by involving learners in what they need to know and what they already know; help them to establish reasonable and realistic learning goals
4. Include learners in planning content and teaching strategies
5. Help learners to relate new material to information already known
6. Encourage learners to make use of available resources and to engage others in the learning situation
7. Facilitate self-directed inquiry
8. Use positive reinforcement rather than negative

II. AGING PROCESS AND ITS IMPACT ON LEARNING

A. Barriers to learning in the aging population can include memory impairment, vision and hearing impairment, fatigue, and delayed cognitive processing
B. Methods to combat memory decline
1. Increase amount of time allowed for teaching, especially for psychomotor skills
2. Help the learner identify association between items
3. Promote physical comfort (toileting, fluid intake) and eliminate distracters (AV equipment, noise, traffic)
4. Make sure glasses are clean and on and hearing aids are working
5. Set realistic and achievable mutual goals
6. Encourage verbal responses and allow time for response
7. Reinforce correct responses immediately and correct incorrect responses immediately
8. Use examples that relate to the learner's everyday life
9. Use simple, black on white, large-lettered visual aids
10. Include a family member whenever possible and appropriate
11. Make sure information is in writing and at a level the learner can understand
12. Treat the learner with respect and dignity at all times

III. EDUCATIONAL PROCESS AND THE OLDER ADULT

A. Assessment
1. Mutually identify knowledge deficits
2. Assess physical changes that impact learning and the level of impact
3. Assess the learner's attitude and feelings about the material to be learned; look for threats to compliance and opportunities for adherence
4. Determine learner's orientation to time, place, and person and the ability to carry out simple instructions or directions
B. Set goals and expected objectives of the teaching process
1. Appropriate time frame to achieve learning goals
2. Amount and type of resources available to achieve goals
3. Congruency of goals with the learner's physical, mental, and emotional status
4. Timeliness, practicality, and realism of goals
5. Value and importance the learner places on goals
C. Instructional process
1. Make sure the setting is appropriate and instruction is not rushed
2. Learner should not be tired, hungry, in pain, or uncomfortable
3. Determine if a family member should be present
4. Teaching techniques should fit the material to be taught
5. Use real equipment or equipment the learner will be using if teaching a skill

6. Use lecture, demonstration, return demonstration, role-play, case studies, questioning, and reinforcement for accurate learning
7. Keep the session short, factual, and to the point
8. Use common vocabulary and simple sentences
9. Look at the learner when talking to get verbal cues to understanding, confusion, tiredness, boredom, or physical discomfort
10. Ask questions and ask for questions frequently
11. Observe for low-literacy issues and use techniques that aid in teaching the low-literacy learner
    a. Present the most important and relevant information necessary
    b. Limit the number of points made and increase the number of sessions to achieve goals
    c. Present the information in the same order the patient will use it
    d. Repeat and summarize main points often
    e. Be concrete and specific
    f. Use the very same vocabulary each time (e.g., mm, cc, or tsp)
    g. Use short, descriptive sentences
    h. Maintain respect and dignity
D. Methods for evaluation of effectiveness of the teaching plan
    1. Oral testing
    2. Questioning about content
    3. Written testing
    4. Return demonstration
    5. Interview

REFERENCES

Beare PG: Health teaching and compliance. In Stanley M, Beare PG, editors: *A health promotion/protection approach,* ed 2, Philadelphia, 1999, FA Davis.

Braungart MM, Braungart RG: Learning theory and nursing practice. In Bastable SB, editor: *Nurse as educator,* Sudbury, MA, 1997, Jones and Bartlett.

Kitchie S: Determinants of learning. In Bastable SB, editor: *Nurse as educator,* Sudbury, MA, 1997, Jones and Bartlett.

Norton B: From teaching to learning: theoretical foundations. In Billings DM, Halstead JA: *Teaching in nursing: a guide for faculty,* Philadelphia, 1998, WB Saunders.

Richardson V: The diverse learning needs of students. In Billings DM, Halstead JA: *Teaching in nursing: a guide for faculty,* Philadelphia, 1998, WB Saunders.

CHAPTER 9

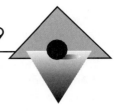

DEATH AND DYING

Tamara J. White ● *Sue E. Meiner*

LEARNING OBJECTIVES

Upon completion of this chapter, the reader will be able to:

- Identify care provided by the team of hospice professionals
- State the role of Medicare in hospice care
- Discuss the role of cultural/ethnic traditions in the grieving process
- Describe the physical and psychosocial losses of older adults that may produce grief
- Discuss assessment of the patient in grief

I. HOSPICE

A. Philosophy of hospice is to provide high-quality comfort (palliative) care for the terminally ill or dying patient and support for the patient's family

B. Main goal is to provide comfort, relieve pain, and promote quality of life rather than extending the length of life

C. Care is provided by a team, which includes nurses, physicians, social workers, a chaplain, nursing assistants, and volunteers (others are added as specific needs arise, such as speech therapists, physical therapists, respiratory therapists, etc.)

D. A highly qualified team of health care professionals and volunteers provide care
1. Meeting physiologic, psychologic, social, spiritual, and economic needs of patient/family
2. Collaborating with the primary care provider for an individualized plan of care
3. Coordinating a program of palliative and supportive care
4. Focusing on keeping the patient in the home setting for as long as possible
5. Providing services 24 hours, 7 days a week, in any setting of care delivery
6. Accounting for appropriate allocation and use of resources for optimal care
7. Maintaining a comprehensive record of services

E. Hospice care can be provided in the home, nursing care facility, or the inpatient unit in the hospital

F. Members of the hospice team are available to the patient and family every day and around the clock as well as providing follow-up after the death of the patient

G. Hospice care financing: since the 1980s, Medicare part A, Medicaid, and private insurance companies will reimburse for hospice services; no out-of-pocket expenses are requested of the hospice patient or family for services

H. Eligibility for hospice services are limited to patients with the following
- End-stage cardiovascular disease
- End-stage lung disease
- Cancer

- HIV-related conditions
- Debility, unspecified
- End-stage dementia
- Multiple-system organ failure

I. Symptom management includes pain, anorexia, dyspnea, nausea/vomiting, dysphagia, profound weakness, bowel obstruction, and multisystem deterioration

J. Enrollment in a hospice program is available through several systems
   1. The patient's primary care provider determines if the patient meets the criteria for hospice services and submits a referral
   2. The patient must have a terminal diagnosis with a 6-month or less prognosis
   3. The patient and family must agree to a palliative plan of care
   4. After 6 months, a reevaluation will be made to determine if the patient still qualifies for recertification of hospice to continue to manage the symptoms of the disease process

II. INDIVIDUAL CULTURAL BELIEFS/ETHNIC TRADITIONS

A. Variation across cultural/ethnic traditions

B. General emotional transitions and phases of grief (not all phases may be experienced)
   - Denial
   - Anger
   - Bargaining
   - Depression
   - Acceptance

III. GRIEVING PROCESS

A. Grief: subjective physical, emotional, and social response to a loss

B. General information
   1. Grief occurs in phases
   2. Individuals move in and out of phases during the grief process
   3. Grieving is an individual response to an event
   4. Grieving can be both functional and dysfunctional
   5. Normal grieving can occur up to 3 months or more after the loss of a significant other

C. Physical losses
   1. Loss of physical abilities
   2. Loss of physical attractiveness
   3. Loss of mobility
   4. Loss of cognitive abilities

D. Psychosocial losses
   1. Loss of spouse or significant other, which may result in increased morbidity and mortality
   2. Loss of social activities
   3. Loss of financial security
   4. Loss of a roommate in a nursing home

E. Types of grief
   1. Acute grief: can last up to 6 weeks
      a. Somatic symptoms of distress that cycle throughout this time
      b. Experiencing a sensation similar to daydreaming, accompanied by unreality
      c. Feelings of self-blame or guilt can be present but not always obvious
      d. Motivation and zest toward daily activities and friends disappear
   2. Chronic grief
      a. Abnormal or maladaptive grief
      b. Normal evolution of grieving may be interrupted
      c. Feelings of guilt, anger, hostility, or ambivalence need to be resolved before proceeding through the grief process

      3. Anticipatory grief
        a. Response to a real or perceived loss before the actual loss
        b. Preparation for a potential loss
        c. When the loss does not happen as anticipated, anger or hostility may replace this response (can deprive the family of completing unfinished business with the dying person)
      4. Disenfranchising grief
        a. Not recognized or validated by others
        b. Occurs with unresolved family discord
        c. Hidden relationships that are not revealed
      5. Dysfunctional grieving
        a. Prolonged interference with life functioning
        b. Repetitive use of ineffective behaviors associated with attempts to reinvest in relationships
        c. Developmental regression
        d. Unrealistic idealization of the deceased person

F. Multiple factors affect the grief process
      1. Physical process is affected by type of loss, preexisting conditions (rest, nutritional state, exercise, and medications)
      2. Psychological process is affected by the unique meaning of each loss, past experiences with loss, timeliness, number and type of secondary losses, presence of concurrent stresses, and health state

G. Support for the grieving process
      1. Important to grieve a significant loss
      2. Indicators of effective coping include realistic good and bad memories, ability to support other grieving persons, and ability to revive social relationships

H. Grief work: the process or experience of mourning
      1. Time must pass for the grief work to be accomplished
      2. Anniversary dates can exacerbate a grief response (birthdays, holidays, etc.)
      3. Older adults may take longer to complete grief work
      4. Older adults may exhibit confusion, depression, preoccupation with thoughts of the deceased
      5. Multiple losses may complicate the grieving process through layering of grief—one loss must be resolved before another loss can be handled

I. Nursing assessment
      1. Assess for physical signs of loss: anorexia, insomnia, immobilization, fatigue
      2. Assess for psychosocial signs of loss: sadness, depression with or without anxiety, guilt, loneliness, social withdrawal, unkempt appearance, decreased desire for sex, inability to experience or express feelings about the painful loss
      3. Assess for other recent losses
      4. Assess previous coping mechanisms when dealing with losses
      5. Assess support groups: family, friends, neighbors, religious, economic, community, and medical
      6. Assess for pathological grieving: greater than 6 months, failure to acknowledge and accept the loss(es)
      7. Assess for increased depression with suicidal ideation
      8. Assess for significant weight loss and/or alcohol abuse

J. Nursing management
      1. Caregiver must have spiritual strength or strength from within to support the needs of the grieving person/family
      2. Caregiver needs to have a personal philosophy of life and a positive belief in self

   3. Comfort with one's own mortality is essential to support the grieving person/family
   4. There must be active listening to the verbalizations of the grieving person/family
 K. Nursing management: interventions
   1. Support the grieving process
   2. Encourage the bereaved to grieve a significant loss
   3. Monitor for effective coping throughout the grieving process
 L. Nursing diagnoses
   1. Anxiety: related to increased decision-making responsibility
   2. Social isolation: related to the loss of a spouse
   3. Grieving, anticipatory
   4. Communication, impaired verbal: related to grieving
   5. Grieving, dysfunctional: related to repetitive use of ineffective behaviors

REFERENCES

Abrams W, Beers H: *The Merck manual of geriatrics,* ed 2, Whitehouse Station, NJ, 1995, Merck Research Laboratories.

Dunn H: *Hard choices for loving people: CPR, artificial feeding, comfort measures only, and the elderly client,* ed 4, Herdon, VA, 1994, A & A Publishers.

Durham E, Weiss L: How patients die, *AJN* 97(2):41-46, 1997.

Ebersole P, Hess P: *Toward healthy aging: human needs and nursing response,* ed 5, St Louis, 1998, Mosby.

Kim MJ, McFarland GK, McLane AM: *Pocket guide to nursing diagnoses,* ed 7, St Louis, 1997, Mosby.

Otto S: *Oncology nursing,* ed 3, St Louis, 1997, Mosby

Stuart B, Herbst L, Kinzbrunner BM: *Medical guidelines for determining prognosis in selected non-cancer diseases,* Alexandria, VA, 1995, National Hospice Organization.

MAJOR HEALTH PROBLEMS

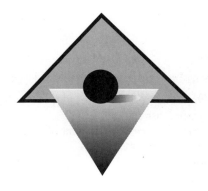

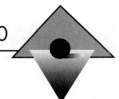

CHAPTER 10

ASSESSMENT OF OLDER ADULTS

Sue E. Meiner

LEARNING OBJECTIVES

Upon completion of this chapter, the reader will be able to:

- Describe special considerations needed for assessing the older adult
- Identify purposes of psychosocial assessment
- Name elements of lifestyle, nutrition, and environmental assessment
- Identify components of the functional assessment
- Discuss elements of a cultural assessment

I. PHYSICAL ASSESSMENT

   A. Special considerations

      1. Environmental modifications may be needed to respond to sensory or musculoskeletal changes of aging (see Chapter 16)

      2. Check to see that assistive devices (sensory or mobility aids) are available and in working condition

      3. Measure all parameters under the most favorable conditions (eliminate distractions and reduce excess noise levels)

      4. Provide privacy throughout the assessment

      5. Provide a toilet nearby

   B. Provide for an unhurried experience for the health care provider and the patient

      1. Allow time for the older adult to answer questions; respect silence

      2. Provide personal comfort to avoid fatigue; use the older adult's peak energy time (usually early in the day)

II. PSYCHOSOCIAL ASSESSMENT

   A. Home situation: daily life experiences and rituals

   B. Psychological assessment

      1. General appearance

      2. Level of consciousness, flow of speech and thought

      3. Emotional state (e.g., depression, anxiety, insomnia, fearfulness, nervousness)

      4. Cognitive domains (memory, language, attention span)

      5. Concentration difficulties leading to decision-making inabilities

      6. General outlook in the present and in the future

C. Social support
   1. Formal social support: private organizations, institutions, government agencies (senior centers, AARP, Gray Panthers, church affiliation)
   2. Informal social support: family members, neighbors, and friends
   3. Socialization patterns (e.g., how often and level of satisfaction)

III. FAMILY/NETWORK ASSESSMENT

A. Close ties with family
B. Ritualized contact with family
C. Group or community activities (frequency and degree of satisfaction)

IV. LIFESTYLE ASSESSMENT

A. Widowed, divorced, or single
B. Living alone, with spouse, with life partner of either sex, with children
C. Sexual preference: heterosexual or homosexual

V. NUTRITION ASSESSMENT

A. Determine if food intake is adequate and appropriate
   1. Knowledge level of daily nutritional needs of the older adult
   2. Co-existing health problems that might compromise eating habits
   3. Diet evaluation (e.g., personal nutrition history of likes and dislikes, 24–hour dietary and fluid intake recall, 72–hour food diary including one weekend day)
   4. Fluid intake per day (separating water intake from other liquids)
      a. What, when, how much, and daily patterns of intake
      b. Determine intake of caffeine, tea, colas, and/or alcohol
      c. Clinical observations (percent of food eaten per meal)
      d. Biochemical tests (Table 10–1)
      e. Anthropometrics
         (1) Weight, height, body mass index (BMI = 22–27) (see Chapter 4), and body frame (using elbow breadth and wrist circumference)
         (2) Alternative anthropometric assessment for non–ambulatory patients (Box 10–1)

TABLE **10-1**

LABORATORY TESTS

Test	Value
Urine creatinine	0.5-1.0 mg/dl
BUN	10-30 mg/dl
Serum albumin	3.5-5.0 g/dl
Pre-albumin (PAB)	2%-7%
Hemoglobin	14-18 g/dl (men)
	12-16 g/dl (women)
Hematocrit	40%-50% (men)
	38%-44% (women)
Thyroid-binding protein	12-25 mg/L (men)
	14-30 mg/L (women)
Serum transferrin	250-450 mg/dl
Total iron-binding capacity (TIBC)	200-310 µg/dl
Ferritin	20-250 ng/dl (men)
	10-120 ng/dl (women)
Calcium	9-11 mg/dl
Folic acid	3-25 mg/dl
Glucose	70-120 mg/dl

BOX 10-1   **Alternative Anthropometric Assessment for Non-Ambulatory Older Adults**

HEIGHT MEASUREMENT

Total arm length: Measure the arm length from attachment at the shoulder to the end of the arm at the wrist

Arm span: Full arm-span measure is an alternative to height measurement in older adults using a metric measure from fingertps to fingertips, with the tape in front of the clavicles (may use fingertip to middle of sternal notch × 2)

Knee height (KH):   Knee-to-floor height with patient in a sitting position: measure from just under the kneecap to the floor surface

With patient lying in a supine position: measure with the left knee and ankle bent at a 90-degree angle, using a special caliper (Ross Laboratories)

Height calculation for men: $64.19 + (0.04 \times age) + (2.02 \times KH)$

Height calculation for women: $84.88 + (0.24 \times age) + (1.83 \times KH)$

WEIGHT MEASUREMENT USING FOUR PARAMETERS

Calf circumference: With patient in the supine position with the left knee bent at a 90-degree angle: measure the calf circumference (CC) at the largest point

Also measure knee height (KH), mid-arm circumference (MAC), and subscapular skinfold (SSF) to determine the body weight value

Weight calculation for men: $(0.98 \times CC) + (1.16 KH) + (1.73 \times MAC) + (0.37 \times SSF) - 81.69 = weight$

Weight calculation for women: $(1.27 \times CC) + (0.87 KH) + (0.98 \times MAC) + (0.4 \times SSF) - 62.35 = weight$

Modified from Williams SR: *Essentials of nutrition and diet therapy*, ed 7, St Louis, 1999, Mosby.

VI. ENVIRONMENTAL ASSESSMENT

  A. Falls

    1. Intrinsic causes (Box 10-2)

      a. Vision and/or balance problems

      b. Reduced or interrupted cerebral oxygenation

      c. Fatigue factors

      d. Drop attacks

    2. Extrinsic causes

      a. See home safety issues discussed following

      b. Institutional causes: room assignment, call light issues, high bed position, side rails (up or down), lack of attention to comfort measures, bedside obstacles, unlocked wheels on mobility aids, unmet oral fluid or toileting needs

    3. Assessment of institutional risk for falls

      a. History of previous falls

      b. Untreated visual impairment or new-onset impairment because of interventions (medication and/or surgery)

      c. Impaired judgment (cognitive deficit or iatrogenic)

      d. Unsteady gait or disorientation to surroundings

    4. Interventions for institutional risk for falls

      a. Complete a *Fall Risk Assessment* tool

      b. Implement actions: patient instructions on admission and as needed, call light within reach, bed in lowest position, locks on wheels when bed is not being moved, caregivers alerted to risks, risk notices posted in and outside of room, hourly checks that may or may not include offering assistance with fluids, transferring, or toileting needs

---

BOX 10-2   **Classification of Falls (Gray-Miceli, 1997)**

Multifactorial falls
Premonitory falls
Prodromal falls
Extrinsic falls
Isolated falls
Cluster falls

From Ebersole P, Hess P: *Toward health aging: human needs and nursing response,* St Louis, 1998, Mosby. Reprinted with permission of the author.

B. Neighborhood safety assessment and instruction guide for older adults
   1. Determine awareness of crimes against the elderly
   2. Assess frequency of nearby street crimes and protective practices
      a. Install peepholes in solid main entrance doors
      b. Keep doors locked, install deadbolt locks on all entrance doors
   3. Home safety issues
      a. Adequate home maintenance (e.g., heating; cooling; ventilation; entrances accessible, uncluttered, with secure handrail)
      b. Electrical safety
         • Replace frayed electrical wires
         • Do not overload electrical circuits
         • Conduct annual inspection
      c. Lighting (non-glare) in hallways, stairwells, and in entrance areas
      d. Special modifications to the home environment
         • Grip bars, elevated toilet seats, and slip-proof floors in bathrooms
         • Handrails in stairwells
      e. Hot water temperatures within a safe level (not to exceed 120° F)
C. Safety issues in other environments
   1. Risk factors for injuries
      a. Impaired physical mobility
      b. Sensory deficits
      c. Incontinence (bowel or bladder)
      d. Hazardous environment (room clutter, blocked doors, slick floors)
      e. History of accidents
      f. Unsupervised smoking associated with forgetfulness or carelessness
      g. Hurried behaviors (walking fast or running, rushing to an activity)

VII. DRIVING SAFETY ASSESSMENT

A. Assess for safe driving practices
   1. Always plan trips, daily or long distance
   2. Wear appropriate hearing aids and glasses
   3. Use extra caution when approaching intersections
   4. Drive at a safe distance behind other cars
   5. Avoid road rage by defensive driving practices
B. Assess for driving avoidance behavior
   1. If medications can impair driving skills
   2. During rush hours
   3. At night (low lighting) or in bad weather
   4. On busy streets and in congested traffic areas

VIII. THERMOREGULATION SAFETY ASSESSMENT

A. Excessive cold (hypothermia)
  1. Mental confusion
  2. Decreased pulse and respiratory rate
  3. Decreased body temperature with cool/cold skin
  4. Pallor or cyanosis
  5. Swollen or puffy face
  6. Changes in gait or balance and muscle stiffness
  7. Altered coordination and fine tremors
  8. Lethargy, apathy, irritability, hostility, or aggression
B. Excessive heat (hyperthermia, heat exhaustion, or heat stroke)
  1. Heat exhaustion: feeling hot, listless, or uncomfortable
  2. Heat stroke: life-threatening
      a. Hot, dry skin without perspiration
      b. Tachycardia with or without chest pain
      c. Throbbing headache with or without dizziness
      d. Profound weakness
      e. Changes in mentation
      f. Nausea, vomiting, abdominal cramps, and/or diarrhea

IX. MENTAL STATUS ASSESSMENT

A. Tests
  1. Folstein MiniMental State Examination (MMSE) (Box 10-3)
  2. Short Portable Mental Status Questionnaire (SPMSQ)
  3. Information–Memory–Concentration Test (IMCT)
  4. Short Blessed Test

X. FUNCTIONAL ASSESSMENT

A. Physical functioning assessed for issues of mobility (balance, flexibility, endurance, and strength)
B. Activities of daily living (ADLs)
  1. Bathing
  2. Dressing (clothing and appropriateness)
  3. Transferring (bed to chair, chair to standing, and reverse)
  4. Toileting (use and hygiene)
  5. Bowel continence (frequency and control)
  6. Feeding (serving self, readying food for consumption, use of utensils)
C. Instrumental activities of daily living (IADLs)
  1. Use of a telephone
  2. Preparation and self-administering medication as directed
  3. Traveling appropriately outside of the home
  4. Driving a motor vehicle appropriately for health status
  5. Housework (unless it is provided by someone else)
  6. Food planning, shopping, and preparation (unless it is provided)
  7. Managing finances through banking, paying bills, and record-keeping

XI. CULTURAL ASSESSMENT

A. Sensitivity to the knowledge of similarities/differences between people of different cultural backgrounds is needed to establish positive relationships and communication
B. Structured assessment tool is beneficial when cultures that differ from that of the assessor are being done

BOX 10-3 MMSE (MiniMental State Examination)

NAME OF SUBJECT _____ Age _____

NAME OF EXAMINER _____ Years of School Completed _____

Approach the patient with respect and encouragement   Date of Examination _____
Ask: Do you have any trouble with your memory?   ☐Yes ☐No
May I ask you some questions about your memory?   ☐Yes ☐No

SCORE	ITEM

5 ( ) TIME ORIENTATION

Ask:

What is the year _____ (1), season _____ (1),
month of the year _____ (1), date _____ (1),
day of the week _____ (1)?

5 ( ) PLACE ORIENTATION

Ask:

Where are we now? What is the state _____ (1), city _____ (1).
part of the city _____ (1), building _____ (1).
floor of the building _____ (1)?

3 ( ) REGISTRATION OF THREE WORDS

Say: Listen carefully. I am going to say three words. You say them back after I stop.

Ready? Here they are: PONY (wait 1 second). QUARTER (wait 1 second). ORANGE (wait 1 second). What were those words?
_____ (1)
_____ (1)
_____ (1)
Give 1 point for each correct answer, then repeat them until the patient learns all three.

5 ( ) SERIAL 7s AS A TEST OF ATTENTION AND CALCULATION

Ask: Subtract 7 from 100 and continue to subtract 7 from each subsequent remainder until I tell you to stop. What is 100 take away 7? _____ (1)

Say:

Keep going._____ (1), _____ (1).
_____ (1), _____ (1).

3 ( ) RECALL OF THREE WORDS

Ask:

What were those three words I asked you to remember?
Give 1 point for each correct answer _____ (1).
_____ (1), _____ (1).

2 ( ) NAMING

Ask:

What is this? (show pencil) _____ (1). What is this? (show watch)_____ (1).

From Folstein MF, Folstein SE, McHugh RP: MiniMental State: a practical method for grading the cognitive state of patients for the clinician, *J Psychiatr Res* 12:189-198, Elsevier, Oxford, England, 1975, Pergamon Imprint.   *Continued*

1 ( ) REPETITION

Say:

Now I am going to ask you to repeat what I say. Ready? No ifs, ands, or buts.

Now you say that _____(1)

3 ( ) COMPREHENSION

Say:

Listen carefully because I am going to ask you to do something:

Take this paper in your left hand (1), fold it in half (1), and put it on the floor. (1)

1 ( ) READING

Say:

Please read the following and do what it says but do not say it aloud. (1)

Close your eyes

1 ( ) WRITING

Say:

Please write a sentence. If patient does not respond, say: Write about the weather. (1)

_____

_____

1 ( ) DRAWING

Say: Please copy this design.

TOTAL SCORE _____ Assess level of consciousness along a continuum

	Alert	Drowsy	Stupor	Coma

	YES	NO		YES	NO	FUNCTION BY PROXY
Cooperative:	☐	☐	Deterioration from Previous			Please record date when patient was last able to perform the following tasks.
Depressed:	☐	☐	Level of Functioning:	☐	☐	Ask caregiver if patient independently
Anxious:	☐	☐	Family History of Dementia:	☐	☐	handles:
Poor Vision:	☐	☐	Head Trauma:	☐	☐	
Poor Hearing:	☐	☐	Stroke:	☐	☐	
Native Language:			Alcohol Abuse:	☐	☐	
			Thyroid Disease:	☐	☐	

	YES	NO	DATE
Money/Bills:	☐	☐	_____
Medication:	☐	☐	_____
Transportation:	☐	☐	_____
Telephone:	☐	☐	_____

From Folstein MF, Folstein SE, McHugh RP: MiniMental State: a practical method for grading the cognitive state of patients for the clinician, *J Psychiatr Res* 12:189-198, Elsevier, Oxford, England, 1975, Pergamon Imprint.

C. Basic understanding of differing values, experiences, social networks, communication styles, and perceptions of health and illness is needed

D. Health beliefs of various subcultures include a wide range of concepts related to health and illness

1. African Americans with Carribean roots often see health as being in harmony with nature and illness as being in disharmony

2. Native American/Native Alaskans often subscribe to rules that govern the symbiotic relationship among the individual, the group, and the earth (a survival pact that has led many of the members of these groups to prosper in consort with the earth)

3. Asian Americans often subscribe to the Yin and Yang (flow of life forces) with illness being an imbalance

4. Hispanic Americans often see health as a balance between hot and cold, with illness being an imbalance

5. European (White) Americans often see achievement as a high priority, occurring within a certain time frame, leading to internal and external pressures that can be the basis for illness

REFERENCES

Ebersole P, Hess P: *Toward healthy aging: human needs and nursing response,* St Louis, 1998, Mosby.

Folstein MF, Folstein SE, McHugh RP: MiniMental State: a practical method for grading the cognitive state of patients for the clinician, *J Psychiatr Res* 12:189-198, 1975.

Gray-Miceli D: Falling among the aged: exploring psychological issues, *ADVANCE Nurs Pract* 5(7):41-44, 1997.

Jarvis C: *Physical examination and health assessment,* ed 2, Philadelphia, 1996, WB Saunders.

Seidel HM, Ball JW, Dains JE, et al: *Mosby's guide to physical examination,* ed 3, St Louis, 1995, Mosby.

Weber J, Kelley J: *Health assessment in nursing,* Philadelphia, 1998, JB Lippincott.

Williams SR: *Essentials of nutrition and diet therapy,* ed 7, St Louis, 1999, Mosby.

CHAPTER 11

CARDIOVASCULAR PROBLEMS

Phyllis Atkinson

LEARNING OBJECTIVES

Upon completion of this chapter, the reader will be able to:

- Identify age-related changes of the cardiovascular system
- Define hypertension, coronary heart disease, heart failure, arrhythmias, and peripheral vascular disease
- Identify the risk factors for hypertension, coronary heart disease, heart failure, arrhythmias, and peripheral vascular disease
- Identify signs and symptoms of hypertension, coronary heart disease, heart failure, arrhythmias, and peripheral vascular disease
- Identify appropriate nursing measures for hypertension, coronary heart disease, heart failure, arrhythmias, and peripheral vascular disease

I. AGE-RELATED CHANGES: CARDIOVASCULAR SYSTEM

A. Heart
1. Size: essentially unchanged except for an increase in heart wall thickness
2. Connective tissue: increase in interstitial collagen and elastin
3. Ventricular wall thickness: increase in ventricular septal thickness
4. Valves: aortic and mitral valves thicken, become fibrotic and calcified
5. Coronary arteries: become tortuous, dilated, with calcifications
6. Heart rate: maximal heart rate decreases with age
7. Electrophysiologic changes
   a. Increased elastin and collagen in all parts of the heart
   b. Fat accumulation around SA node
   c. Decreased number of pacemaker cells

II. HYPERTENSION (HTN)

A. Definition
1. A persistent elevation of systolic blood pressure (SBP) and/or diastolic blood pressure (DBP) at/or above the normal parameters of 139 SBP and 89 DBP on at least three consecutive readings (National Heart, Lung, and Blood Institute, 1993)
B. Classification of blood pressure *(Sixth Report of the Joint National Committee on Prevention, Detection, Evaluation, and Treatment of High Blood Pressure [JNC VI])*
1. Optimal: SBP <120 and DBP <80
2. Normal: SBP <130 and DBP <85
3. High normal: SBP 130-139 or DBP 85-89

       4. HTN
         a. Stage 1: SBP 140-159 or DBP 90-99
         b. Stage 2: SBP 160-179 or DBP 100-109
         c. Stage 3: SBP $\geq$180 or DBP $\geq$110
C. Isolated systolic HTN
   1. SBP of 140 mm Hg or greater with DBP of <90 mm Hg
   2. Most prominent form of HTN in the elderly
D. Primary HTN (85%-90% of all HTNs)
   1. Etiology
      a. Increased weight
      b. Increased sodium intake: older adults have less ability to maximally retain and excrete sodium
      c. Increased peripheral vascular resistance secondary to decrease in connective tissue elasticity and atherosclerosis as well as possible increase of calcium within smooth muscle cells
      d. Decreased vessel wall compliance and atherosclerosis
      e. Left ventricular hypertrophy
      f. Decreased renal mass and function
      g. Decreased relaxation of small vessels
      h. Decreased plasma renin levels seen in older adults without HTN; with HTN, the older adult has higher renin levels; therefore, angiotenson-converting enzyme (ACE) inhibitors are effective
   2. Signs and symptoms
      a. Asymptomatic: most common
      b. Subcortical headache in the morning
      c. Epistaxis
      d. Tinnitus
      e. Fatigue
      f. Nervousness and irritability
      g. "Cardiac awareness": seen in severe disease, usually presenting as tachycardia/palpitations
      h. Target organ damage symptoms: resulting diseases affect kidneys, heart, and brain
E. Secondary hypertension
   1. Etiology
      a. Renovascular: renal artery stenosis, which is one of the most common causes of resistant hypertension
      b. Renal parenchymal: resulting from chronic pyelo- or glomerulonephritis
      c. Hormonal
         • Decreased ability of the kidney to maximally respond to antidiuretic hormone
         • Hypothyroidism or hyperthyroidism
      d. Coarctation of the aorta
      e. Drugs, chemicals, and foods, primarily alcohol, salt, over-the-counter products especially cold preparations
      f. Secondary to specific therapy such as steroids and antidepressants
   2. Nursing measures
      a. Relieve signs and symptoms
      b. Report significant changes to the primary care provider
      c. Keep blood pressure under control
         • Monitor at specific intervals
         • Teach patient and family to monitor
   3. Medications
      a. Monitor responses
      b. Observe for side effects, such as depression, confusion, and orthostasis, resulting in falls and fractures

    c. Teach about rationale, compliance, and side effects

    d. Most common causes of ineffective blood pressure control
- Inadequate drug regimens
- Patient factors, such as noncompliance, obesity, cigarette smoking, or alcoholism
- Office hypertension: rise in BP due to anxiety related to visit to physician

    e. All major classes of antihypertensive medications are effective in lowering blood pressure among Caucasians; calcium channel blockers are most effective among African Americans

4. Lifestyle changes/reduce risk factors, keeping patient's finances in consideration
    a. Diet
    b. Weight loss
    c. Sodium restriction
    d. Exercise
    e. Relaxation therapy

5. Follow-up

6. Preventing complications

7. Return to independence

III. CORONARY HEART DISEASE (CHD)

A. Definition

1. Occurs when the coronary arteries are not able to meet the demand of the myocardium for blood supply; simply stated, there is an imbalance between myocardial oxygen supply and demand

2. Caused by atherosclerosis, which is a lesion of the inner wall of blood vessels, resulting from increased amounts of connective proliferated smooth muscle tissue, increased amounts of connective tissue, and accumulation of intracellular and extracellular lipids

B. Prevalence

1. Varies substantially by geographic region and state (more prevalent in South)

2. Leading cause of death and disability in those >65

C. Risk factors for elderly

1. Family history: immediate family members with cardiovascular disease before age 65

2. Cigarette smoking
    a. Substantial risk factor
    b. Acts synergistically with other known risk factors

3. HTN
    a. Increased SBP single greatest risk factor
    b. Presence of HTN and hyperlipidemia increases risk for myocardial infarction (MI) 15 times
    c. Elevated blood pressure often associated with other risk factors

4. Hyperlipidemia
    a. LDL increase has been predictive of CHD in men >50
    b. In women >50, increased triglycerides are a better predictor
    c. HDL <50 mg/dl in men to age 79 and in women to age 69 indicates increased risk
    d. Hypertriglyceridemia

5. Diabetes
    a. Independent risk factor, especially in women, with two times the risk for MI; with hyperlipidemia, 15 times the risk; 30 times the risk if HTN as well
    b. Glucose intolerance is a direct effect of overweight, often associated with hypertriglyceridemia, HTN, elevated LDL cholesterol, and depressed HDL

6. Physical inactivity
    a. Affects other risks factors, such as HTN, diabetes, stress, and hyperlipidemia

7. Obesity
    a. More likely to lead to sudden death in men
    b. More likely to contribute to congestive heart failure in women

8. Psychological stress
   a. Related risk factor
   b. Signal of other problems such as asymptomatic disease
   c. Impacts other health maintenance issues such as medication compliance
9. The "deadly quartet"
   a. Hypertension
   b. Hypercholesterolemia
   c. Diabetes
   d. Obesity
10. Potential new risk factors for CHD
   a. Homocysteine, a naturally occurring amino acid found in dietary protein; elevated levels are thought to induce adverse pathological changes both in the arterial walls and in clotting factors; this leads not only to atherosclerosis but peripheral vascular disease as well as venous thromboembolism; use of folic acid and the B vitamins, especially B_6, is helpful
   b. Plasma fibrinogen was found to be higher among patients with acute thrombosis; it is uncertain if this is a cause or consequence of atherosclerosis
   c. Lipoprotein (a), a unique lipoprotein particle with both proatherogenic and prothrombotic properties, competes with plasminogen for plasma-binding sites; this inhibits fibrinolysis, reduces endothelium-dependent vasodilatation, and contributes to LDL oxidation
   d. Inflammation, particularly C-reactive protein; it is uncertain if this is a cause or a consequence
D. Signs and symptoms of CHD
   1. Angina pectoris: discomfort brought on by exertion and relieved by rest
      a. Atypical pain
      b. Dyspnea caused by age-associated myocardial and pericardial changes
      c. Associated symptoms
         • Diaphoresis
         • Fatigue
         • Shortness of breath (SOB)
         • Heart palpitations
         • Anxiety
   2. Myocardial infarction (MI): necrosis of myocardial tissue caused by an obstruction of blood flow in a coronary artery
      a. Atypical presentation (vague): signs and symptoms are masked by other diseases such as alcohol abuse and drug toxicity; silent MIs and asymptomatic CHD are common because of decreased sympathetic response
      b. Fatigue
      c. Dyspnea
      d. Low-grade fever
      e. Chest pain
      f. Nausea/vomiting
      g. Anxiety
      h. Diaphoresis, clammy skin, pallor
      i. Impending feeling of doom
E. Signs and symptoms in women
   1. Current research suggests there are significant differences in the manifestation and clinical features of coronary artery disease in women
      a. Most common initial symptom of coronary artery disease in women is angina
      b. Women tend to have fewer Q waves and ST changes with chest pain
      c. Initial signs and symptoms of coronary artery disease are more atypical, including epigastric pain and shortness of breath

---

BOX 11-1   Relieving Symptoms of Unstable Angina

DECREASE MYOCARDIAL OXYGEN CONSUMPTION	INCREASE CORONARY BLOOD FLOW AND OXYGEN SUPPLY
Rest; incline of head of bed should be increased 20-30 degrees	Oxygen
Small frequent meals	Nitroglycerin
Stool softeners	Calcium channel blockers
Stress management	Revascularization with PTCA, TPA
Exercise program	Coronary artery bypass graft
Risk factor modification	Heparin/coumadin
Nitroglycerin and long-acting nitrates	Exercise program
Narcotics and analgesics	Risk factor modification
Beta-blockers	Vasoactive drugs that improve systemic hemodynamics
Calcium channel blockers	
Sedatives/tranquilizers	
Antihypertensives	
Diuretics	

   F. Nursing measures for unstable angina
     1. Relieve symptoms by decreasing demand and increasing blood flow and oxygen supply (Box 11-1)
     2. Decrease potential complications such as congestive heart failure and arrhythmias
     3. After acute phase is over, focus should be on education
       a. Disease process and basic cardiac function
       b. Risk factors and modification
       c. Medications
       d. Coping behaviors and stress reduction (encourage treatment of depression)
       e. Lifestyle changes, such as diet, exercise, and smoking cessation
       f. Recurring signs and symptoms of unstable angina

IV. HEART FAILURE (HF)

   A. Definition
     1. Syndrome where the heart cannot pump an adequate supply of blood in relation to venous return to meet the metabolic needs of the tissues; simply stated, when cardiac output is insufficient to meet metabolic demand
     2. Characterized by
       a. Signs and symptoms of intravascular and interstitial volume overload, including shortness of breath, rales, and edema
       b. Manifestations of inadequate tissue perfusion, such as fatigue or poor exercise tolerance
   B. Pathophysiology
     1. Four determinants of myocardial performance
       a. Preload: changes in preload can lead to peripheral edema, pulmonary vascular congestion, pulmonary edema, and/or decreased alveolar oxygenation complications
       b. Afterload: decreased afterload is linked to decreased arterial oxygenation and decreased oxygen saturation while increased afterload can cause reduced peripheral tissue perfusion because of arterial vasoconstriction
       c. Contractility: reduced contractility is linked to increased cardiac workload, fluid volume excess, increased sodium retention, and activity intolerance
       d. Heart rate: increased heart rate leads to reduced myocardial oxygen demand complications
     2. Systolic dysfunction
       a. Inadequate ventricular pumping function
       b. Cardiac enlargement with decreased ejection fraction

3. Diastolic dysfunction
    a. Ventricular underfilling because of abnormal ventricular relaxation
    b. Should be suspected in those with pulmonary congestion without cardiac enlargement
    c. Systolic function preserved

C. Incidence
  1. One of the most common cardiac conditions in the older adult
  2. Men > women

D. Risk factors for HF
  1. CHD
  2. Hypertensive heart disease
  3. Less common factors
    a. Valvular heart disease
    b. Cardiomyopathy
  4. Factors that influence HF
    a. Impedance to left ventricular ejection
      • Systemic arterial hypertension
      • Aortic valve stenosis
      • Cardiomyopathy
      • Pulmonary hypertension
    b. Medications
      • Drugs that depress myocardial function, such as beta-blockers, calcium channel blockers
      • Drugs that promote sodium retention, such as nonsteroidal antiinflammatories (NSAIDs)
      • Inability to follow therapy
    c. Arrhythmias: especially atrial fibrillation where there is a loss of atrial/ventricular synchrony, resulting in the loss of atrial contribution to ventricular filling
    d. Anemia: hematocrit of 25% to 35% may aggravate underlying heart failure; hematocrit below 25% can produce signs and symptoms of heart failure without underlying cardiac abnormalities
    e. Fever
    f. Hyper- or hypothyroidism
    g. Fluid overload
    h. Renal insufficiency or failure may cause volume overload that mimics heart failure or exacerbates underlying left ventricular dysfunction
    i. Increased dietary sodium
    j. Alcohol, which depresses myocardial contractility in patients with known heart disease

E. Signs and symptoms of HF
  1. Left-sided failure: characterized by elevated pulmonary venous pressure and decreased cardiac output (congestion in lungs)
    a. Anxiety, restlessness, mental status changes secondary to hypoxemia
    b. SOB/dyspnea (can be absent)
    c. Orthopnea, paroxysmal nocturnal dyspnea
    d. Cough, hemoptysis, frothy white sputum
    e. Basilar rales, bronchial wheezes
    f. Fatigue, decreased exercise tolerance; often not reported because believed to be secondary to age and to be expected with aging process
    g. Weight gain
    h. Cyanosis or pallor
    i. Tachycardia, palpitations, especially atrial fibrillation with rapid ventricular response
    j. S_3, S_4, or summation gallop, which usually indicates excess volume and myocardial stretching
    k. Increased blood pressure, which is a catecholamine-induced compensatory mechanism, causing vasoconstriction

l. Compensatory mechanisms, involving sodium and water retention, may mimic gastrointestinal disease and produce anorexia, nausea, early satiety, and abdominal discomfort

2. Right-sided failure: increase of systemic venous pressure because of the inability of the right side of the heart to effectively pump blood from the body into the lungs
   a. Anorexia, nausea
   b. Weight gain
   c. Oliguria during the day with increased nocturia may be initial symptoms, related to low cardiac output with increased nocturnal venous return and renal perfusion at night caused by the recumbent position
   d. Dependent peripheral edema
   e. Weakness
   f. Jugular venous distention
   g. Enlarged liver and spleen
   h. Ascites

3. Atypical, nonspecific signs and symptoms of HF in the elderly
   a. Somnolence
   b. Confusion
   c. Disorientation, which may be presenting symptom
   d. Dizziness
   e. Syncope
   f. Some typical signs and symptoms may be attributed to other causes
      • Rales: pulmonary disease
      • Ankle edema: venous stasis, malnutrition

F. Nursing measures for acute HF
   1. Monitor for arrhythmias
   2. Bedrest initially with appropriate cardiac rehabilitation program
   3. Provide assistance with ADLs
   4. Daily weights and I & O
   5. Oxygen therapy as needed
   6. Calm environment
   7. Medications
      a. Observe for side effects: orthostatic blood pressure secondary to decreased baroreceptor responsiveness; decreased potassium can predispose to arrhythmias and digoxin toxicity
      b. Digoxin is unlikely to provide benefit for older adults with preserved systolic function and maintenance of sinus rhythm; digoxin is contraindicated in older adults with diastolic dysfunction as it can actually worsen the condition

G. Nursing measures for chronic HF
   1. Education
      a. Disease process
      b. Signs and symptoms of worsening failure, including orthopnea, paroxysmal dyspnea, leg edema, exercise intolerance, or a 3-5 pound weight gain
      c. Medications, including their function/purpose and side effects
      d. Individualized activities plan; consider quality of life
      e. Energy-saving techniques
      f. Self-monitoring with daily weights
      g. Dietary recommendations, including sodium restriction of 2 to 3 g of sodium per day (individualized), avoidance of excessive fluid intake, and alcohol restriction (no more than one drink per day)
      h. Follow-up
      i. Yearly influenza vaccination and pneumovax every 7 years
      j. Encouraging completion of Advanced Directives

V. ARRHYTHMIAS

A. Four most common arrhythmias
   1. Atrial fibrillation
      a. Can lead to heart failure because of loss of atrial systolic contribution to cardiac output and a rapid and irregular ventricular rhythm
      b. Strokes can occur from emboli caused by left atrial thrombi
      c. Atrial fibrillation may potentate ventricular arrhythmias by irregular and shortened RR intervals as well as by inducing ischemia and autonomic imbalances with increased circulating catecholamines
   2. Heart block
   3. Sick sinus syndrome
   4. Stokes–Adams syndrome (syncope secondary to arrhythmia)
B. Risk factors
   1. Coronary atherosclerosis
   2. Ventricular hypertrophy (especially with HTN)
   3. Atrial dilatation
   4. Myocardial fibrosis
C. Signs and symptoms of arrhythmias
   1. ECG changes
   2. Pre-syncope/syncope
   3. Dizziness
   4. Palpitations
   5. Fatigue
   6. Exacerbation of angina or CHF
   7. Nausea
   8. Restlessness
   9. Claudication
   10. Numbness, tingling in arms
   11. Diaphoresis; cool, clammy skin
D. Nursing considerations
   1. Patient teaching
   2. Follow–up contact

VI. PERIPHERAL VASCULAR DISEASE (PVD)

A. Definition
   1. Condition affecting the lower extremities in which there is an abnormal narrowing or dilatation of the veins and/or arteries
   2. Common conditions of PVD
      a. Arterial occlusive disease
      b. Claudication
      c. Venous insufficiency
      d. Thrombophlebitis
B. Arterial occlusive disease
   1. Etiology
      a. Atherosclerosis
   2. Risk factors
      a. Smoking
      b. Obesity
      c. Hyperlipidemia
      d. Hypertension
      e. Diabetes mellitus
      f. Positive family history

g. Plasma homocysteine
3. Incidence
   a. Very common in men ages 50 to 70
   b. Increased in women after menopause
4. Signs and symptoms
   a. Six Ps
      - **P**ain: acute, sudden, and severe; intermittent claudication
      - **P**allor: when limb is elevated and red when dependent
      - **P**aresthesia: possible
      - **P**ulselessness: or diminished, weak pulse
      - **P**aralysis: results when there is total occlusion
      - **P**olar: cold sensation
   b. Hair loss
   c. Shiny skin
   d. Ulcer formation, which is painful
C. Venous disease
   1. Etiology
      a. Results from obstruction, such as a thrombus, or from inflammation or incompetent valves
   2. Risk factors
      a. Complications of surgery, especially orthopedic
      b. Obesity
      c. Prolonged sitting or standing; immobility
      d. Trauma
      e. Tight-fitting garments
      f. Family history
   3. Incidence
      a. 50% of all surgical patients
      b. Seven million have chronic venous insufficiency
   4. Signs and symptoms
      a. Little or no pain
      b. Brawny (reddish-brown) skin color; cyanotic if dependent
      c. Warm skin
      d. Stasis ulcers, usually ankle area, mild pain
      e. Edema
      f. Veins visible
      g. Mottled skin
      h. Stasis dermatitis
   5. Nursing measures for PVD
      a. Relieve symptoms
         (1) Position
            - Dependent for arterial
            - Elevated for venous
            - Provide analgesics as needed
            - Progressive exercise
            - Decrease risk factors
      b. Protect from further damage
      c. Education
         - Skin care
         - Pulse checks
         - Disease process, risk reductions
         - Signs and symptoms

REFERENCES

Agency for Health Care Policy and Research: *Diagnosing and managing unstable angina,* Rockville, MD, 1994, Publication No 94-0602, Department of Health and Human Services.

Agency for Health Care Policy and Research: *Heart failure: evaluation and care of patients with left-ventricular systolic dysfunction,* Rockville, MD, 1994, Publication No 94-0612, Department of Health and Human Services.

Aronow WS, Ahn C: Association between plasma homocysteine and peripheral arterial disease in older persons, *Coron Artery Dis* 9(1):49-50, 1998.

Austin MA, Hokanson JE, Edwards KL: Hypertriglyceridemia as a cardiovascular risk factor, *Am J Cardiol* 81(4A):7B-12B, 1998.

Dahlen R, Roberts S: Acute congestive heart failure: preventing complications, *Dimen Crit Care Nurs* 15(5):226-241, 1996.

Fleg JL, Lakatta EG: Role of muscle loss in the age-associated reduction in $\dot{V}O_2$ max, *J Appl Physiol* 65:1477-1151, 1988.

Futterman L, Lemberg L: Atrial fibrillation: an increasingly common and provocative arrhythmia, *Am J Crit Care* 5(5):379-387, 1996.

Hahn R, Heath G, Chang MH: Cardiovascular disease risk factors and preventive practices among adults—United States, 1994: a behavioral risk factor atlas, *MMWR* 47(SS-5):35-48, 1998.

Hamel L, Oberle K: Cardiovascular risk screening for women, *Clin Nurs Special* 10(6):275-281, 1996.

Hennekens C: Increasing burden of cardiovascular disease: current knowledge and future directions for research on risk factors, *Circulation* 97:1095-1102, 1998.

Hughes S, Berra K: Emerging risk factors for coronary heart disease. In Murphy JL, editor: *Nurse practitioners' prescribing reference: clinical management of dyslipidemia,* New York, 1998, Philips Healthcare Communications.

Jacobsen B: Signs of a tiring heart: congestive heart failure, *JEMS,* November, 1996, pp 86-96.

Jensen L, King K: Women and heart disease: the issues, *Crit Care Nurs* 17(2):45-53, 1997.

Kannel WB, Wolf PA, Benjamin EJ, et al: Prevalence, incidence, prognosis, and predisposing conditions for atrial fibrillation: population-based estimates, *Am J Cardiol* 82(8A):2N-9N, 1998.

Kaplan N: Hypertension in the elderly, *Ann Rev Med* 46:27-35, 1995.

Kitzman D, Edwards W: Mini review: age-related changes in the anatomy of the normal human heart, *J Gerontol* 45(2):M33-39, 1990.

LaPalio L: Hypertension in the elderly, *Am Fam Phys* 52:1161-1165, 1995.

LaRosa J: Cholesterol and atherosclerosis: a controversy resolved, *ADVANCE Nurs Pract,* May, 1998, pp 37-41.

Lip G, Beevers M, Potter J, et al: Malignant hypertension in the elderly, *Q J Med* 88:641-647, 1995.

Maynard C, Every N, Martin J, et al: Association of gender and survival in patients with acute myocardial infarction, *Arch Inter Med* 157:1379-1384, 1997.

Miller S: Hypertension update, *ADVANCE Nurs Pract,* January, 1999, pp 53-56.

Moser DK: Pathophysiology of heart failure update: the role of neurohumoral activation in the progression of heart failure, *AACN Clin Issues* 9(2):157-171, 1998.

Musselman D, Evans D, Nemeroff C: The relationship of depression to cardiovascular disease, *Arch Gen Psychiatr* 55:580-588, 1998.

Papademetriou V, Narayan P, Rubins H, et al: Influence of risk factors on peripheral and cerebrovascular disease in men with coronary artery disease, low high-density lipoprotein cholesterol levels, and desirable low-density lipoprotein cholesterol levels, HIT investigators, Department of Veterans Affairs HDL, Intervention Trial, *Am Heart J* 136(4 Pt 1):734-740, 1998.

Rosamond WD, Chambless LE, Folsom AR, et al: Trends in the incidence of myocardial infarction and in mortality due to coronary heart disease, 1987-1994, *N Engl J Med* 339(13):861-867, 1998.

Ross B, Fischer R: Management of hypertension, *ADVANCE Nurs Pract,* April, 1998, pp 27-35.

Safar M: Ageing and its effects on the cardiovascular system, *Drugs* 39(Suppl 1):1-8, 1990.

Schwabauer N: Retarding progression of heart failure: nursing actions. *Dimen Crit Care Nurs* 15(6):307-317, 1996.

Singh BN: Controlling cardiac arrhythmias: an overview with an historical perspective, *Am J Cardiol* 80(8A):4G-15G, 1997.

Tresch D: The clinical diagnosis of heart failure in older patients, *J Am Geriatr Soc* 45:1128-1133, 1997.

Turner S, Bechtel G: Homocysteine and the heart, *ADVANCE Nurs Pract,* March, 1999, pp 71-73.

CHAPTER 12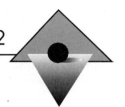

RESPIRATORY PROBLEMS

Sue E. Meiner

LEARNING OBJECTIVES

Upon completion of this chapter, the reader will be able to:

- Identify normal age changes in the respiratory system of older adults
- Identify components that comprise chronic obstructive pulmonary disease (COPD)
- Discuss nursing assessment and interventions associated with specific respiratory disorders
- Describe the differences between obstructive and restrictive airway diseases
- Identify signs and symptoms of tuberculosis

I. RESPIRATORY SYSTEM

A. Definition
   1. Organs and structures responsible for respirations
   2. All body cells require oxygen (O_2) for survival
   3. Respiratory system provides oxygen through inspiration and diffusion and then clears the respiratory waste product carbon dioxide (CO_2) through diffusion and expiration
B. System structure (Figure 12-1)
   1. Upper tract
   2. Lower tract

II. RESPIRATORY CHANGES IN THE NORMAL OLDER ADULT

A. Decreased exchange of O_2 and CO_2 caused by decreased pulmonary circulation
B. Increased anteroposterior diameter of chest
C. Degeneration and decreased strength in the respiratory accessory muscles, resulting in increased rigidity
D. Muscle atrophy of the larynx and pharynx
E. Decreased vital capacity, residual volume, and functional capacity
F. Increased airway resistance
G. Less ventilation at the base of the lungs and increased ventilation at the apex of the lungs
H. Impaired cough mechanism
I. Diminished mucociliary transport

III. CHRONIC OBSTRUCTIVE PULMONARY DISEASE (COPD)

A. COPD: blanket term for three separate yet overlapping conditions: asthma, chronic bronchitis, and emphysema
   1. Asthma: a reversible, intermittent response by the tracheobronchial tree to an irritant or stimulus; response is characterized by bronchial smooth muscle constriction, mucosal edema, and increased mucus production

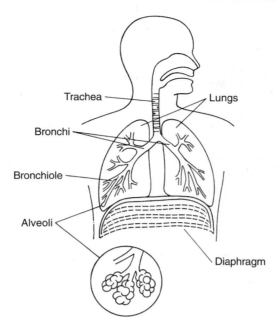

Figure 12-1 The respiratory system.

2. Chronic bronchitis: based on clinical criteria of a chronic productive cough for three consecutive months in two consecutive years; hypersecretion can lead to chronic obstructive bronchitis with a rapid deterioration of pulmonary function
3. Emphysema: based on morphologic features, there is irreversible dilation and destruction of alveolar ducts and air spaces distal to the terminal bronchiole; results in air trapping

B. Incidence
   1. 16 million persons are affected by COPD in the United States
   2. COPD is the fifth leading cause of death in the United States
   3. Mortality from COPD has risen substantially over the past 20 years
   4. Men are affected more than women
   5. Mortality rates are higher among Caucasians than among other ethnic groups

C. Typical clinical presentation
   1. Asthma: tightness in the chest, wheezing, chronic cough (non-productive progressing to productive), dyspnea, cyanosis in severe attacks, intercostal muscle retractions, fatigue
   2. Chronic bronchitis: intermittent dyspnea, severe productive cough of mucopurulent sputum, obesity, cyanosis (blue bloaters)
   3. Emphysema: progressive dyspnea/dyspnea on exertion, mild hypoxia, cough with clear sputum, muscle wasting, weight loss (pink puffers)

D. Nursing management of asthma
   1. Nursing assessment: subjective
      a. General: anxiety, restlessness, fatigue, weakness, insomnia, lethargy, weight gain or loss
      b. Pulmonary: breathlessness, dyspnea at rest or on exertion, orthopnea, dyspnea while recumbent, paroxysmal nocturnal dyspnea, episodic coughing, wheezing, chest tightness, sputum production, history of rhinitis, COPD, emphysema, sinusitis, childhood injury to airways, childhood allergies
      c. Cardiovascular: tachycardia, arrhythmias, palpitations
      d. Musculoskeletal: dependent edema, muscle weakness
      e. Neurological: confusion, acute behavior change, anxiety, dizziness, changes in dementia state

      f. Environmental: pollens, dust, pollutants, pets, occupational exposure

      g. Habits: smoking, alcohol

  2. Nursing assessment: objective

      a. Vital signs: tachypnea, tachycardia, hypotension or hypertension, weight gain or loss

      b. Pulmonary: crackles, wheezes, prolonged inspiratory phase, distant breath sounds, increased resonance on chest percussion, increased AP chest diameter, accessory muscle hypertrophy, tachypnea, abnormal function tests

      c. Cardiovascular: tachycardia, arrhythmias, pulsus paradoxus of 10 mm/Hg or greater

  3. Nursing interventions

      a. Position patient in a high Fowler's position

      b. Start oxygen if indicated

      c. Use relaxation techniques

      d. Encourage oral fluids to liquefy secretions unless contraindicated

      e. Teach deep-breathing exercises

      f. Perform chest physiotherapy if condition permits

      g. Plan periods of rest and exercise

      h. Assess nutritional status and make appropriate adjustments

      i. Advise yearly influenza immunization and pneumococcal vaccine

      j. Instruct in use of metered-dose inhaler (Box 12-1)

      k. Advise rinsing mouth with water after using inhaler of cortisone

E. Nursing management of chronic bronchitis

  1. Nursing assessment: subjective

      a. General: anxiety, restlessness, fatigue, weakness, insomnia, lethargy, fever, weight loss or gain (usually overweight)

      b. Pulmonary: breathlessness, dyspnea on exertion, orthopnea, dyspnea while recumbent, paroxysmal nocturnal dyspnea, coughing, wheezing at rest or on exertion, history of asthma, emphysema, recurrent pulmonary infections

      c. Cardiovascular: tachycardia, arrhythmias, palpitations

      d. Musculoskeletal: dependent edema, muscle weakness

      e. Neurological: confusion, acute behavior changes, anxiety, dizziness, changes in dementia state

      f. Environmental: exposure to asbestos, pollution, passive smoking

      g. Habits: smoking, alcohol

BOX 12-1   Correct Use of a Metered-Dose Inhaler

1. Remove the cap and hold the inhaler upright
2. Shake the inhaler well
3. Tilt the head slightly back
4. Position the inhaler in one of the following ways:
   a. Open mouth with the inhaler 1 to 2 inches away (best)
   b. Use spacer between inhaler and mouth
   c. Place lips tightly around inhaler mouthpiece
5. Take a big breath, then blow it all out
6. Breathe in slowly, this time pressing down on the inhaler to release medication at the same time
7. Hold breath for 10 seconds to allow medication to reach deeply into the lungs
8. Repeat puffs as directed; waiting 1 minute between puffs may permit second puff to penetrate the lungs better
9. When using both bronchodilator and corticosteroid, use the bronchodilator first
10. Rinse the mouth well with water following each use of corticosteroids to prevent oral candidiasis
11. To use a dry powder inhaler, it is important to close the mouth tightly around the inhaler mouthpiece and inhale rapidly

   2. Nursing assessment: objective
      a. Vital signs: may have hypertension or hypotension
      b. Pulmonary: crackles, wheezes, prolonged expiratory phase of respiration, distant breath
         sounds, increased resonance, AP diameter of chest is less than the transverse diameter,
         abnormal rib movement, minimal use of accessory muscles of respiration, tracheal
         descent on inspiration, central cyanosis, cough
      c. Cardiovascular: tachycardia, arrhythmias
      d. Gastrointestinal: hepatosplenomegaly
   3. Nursing interventions
      a. Encourage smoking cessation
      b. Instruct in the correct use of inhalation medications as ordered
F. Nursing management of emphysema
   1. Nursing assessment: subjective
      a. General: anxiety, restlessness, fatigue, weakness, insomnia, lethargy, weight loss, depression
      b. Pulmonary: breathlessness, dyspnea at rest or on exertion, orthopnea, dyspnea while
         recumbent, coughing, wheezing, history of: bronchitis, asthma, upper respiratory
         infections
      c. Cardiovascular: tachycardia, arrhythmias, palpitations
      d. Musculoskeletal: edema, muscle weakness
      e. Neurological: confusion, acute behavior change, anxiety, dizziness, change in dementia
         state
      f. Environmental: current or previous occupational exposure to pollutants, passive
         smoking
      g. Habits: smoking, alcohol
   2. Nursing assessment: objective
      a. Vital signs: tachycardia, tachypnea, hypotension or hypertension, usually weight loss
      b. Pulmonary: crackles, wheezes, prolonged inspiratory phase of respiration, distant breath
         sounds, hyperresonance to percussion, barrel-shaped chest, accessory muscle hypertrophy,
         tracheal descent on inspiration, pursed lip breathing (pink puffers)
      c. Cardiovascular: tachycardia, arrhythmias, palpitations
      d. Musculoskeletal: muscle wasting, decreased diaphragmatic excursion
   3. Nursing interventions
      a. Encourage smoking cessation
      b. Instruct in cough and deep-breathing exercises
      c. Assist as needed with positional changes at least every 2 hours if patient is confined to
         bed
      d. Perform chest percussion if condition permits
      e. Encourage po fluids
      f. Encourage good nutrition
      g. Provide frequent small meals if condition requires
      h. Perform low-flow oxygen therapy, if indicated
   4. Nursing diagnoses
      a. Breathing pattern, ineffective
      b. Airway clearance, ineffective
      c. Tissue perfusion, altered
      d. Anxiety
      e. Activity intolerance

IV. PNEUMONIA (SIXTH LEADING CAUSE OF DEATH IN THE UNITED STATES)

A. Causes
   1. Virulent organisms (bacterial, mycobacterial, fungal, protozoal, helminthic, or viral agents)
   2. Large inoculum

     3. Vulnerable health state of the individual or group
- Immunocompromised persons
- Chronic health conditions

     4. Aspiration pneumonia etiology
- Gastric achlorhydria leaving large colonies of bacteria in the stomach
- Frequent use of antacids or H_2-receptor antagonists leaving large colonies of bacteria in the stomach
- Regurgitation or vomiting leading to aspiration of bacteria into the lungs
- Eating disorders leading to aspiration of food or fluids
- Altered state of mind (advanced dementia, achalasia, seizures, anesthesia, alcohol consumption, iatrogenic causes)
- Altered anatomy (CVA, tracheostomy, tracheal fistula, esophageal stricture, nasogastric [NG] tube placement or management)

     5. Bacterial pneumonia etiology (see 1 and 2 previously)

B. Route of entry
1. Inhalation
2. Ambient air
3. Aspiration of bacteria from a previously colonized upper airway
4. Direct spread from other infected sites
5. Hematogenous spread
6. Aspiration of bacteria from food sources or stomach contents

C. Community-acquired pneumonia: refers to organisms found in the environment outside of the home or institutional setting
1. Pneumococcal pneumonia: most common form
2. Legionnaires' disease: form of bronchopneumonia resulting from water sources, including water cooling systems for buildings

D. Institutional-acquired pneumonia: refers to organisms found in health care facility environments
1. Immunocompromised persons are at high risk
   a. Patients receiving chemotherapy for cancer treatment
   b. *Pneumocystis carinii* pneumonia among HIV-positive persons

E. Presentation
1. Typical clinical presentation
   a. Gradual onset
   b. Cough, sputum production
   c. Wheezing, shortness of breath (SOB), with or without fever
   d. Tightness in the chest
   e. Fatigue and anorexia
2. Atypical clinical presentation
   a. 25% to 30% of older adults will not have a temperature elevation
   b. >20% will not have leukocytosis
   c. 25% will not have cough and sputum production

F. Nursing management of the patient with pneumonia
1. Nursing assessment: subjective
   a. General: malaise, lethargy, apathy, weakness, fatigue, fever, deterioration in mobility, deterioration in general performance
   b. Pulmonary: dyspnea, cough, pleuritic pain, history of upper respiratory infection (URI), dysphagia, chronic lung disease
   c. Cardiovascular: tachycardia, palpitations, cyanosis
   d. Neurological: acute confusion, acute behavior change, memory lapses, anxiety, dizziness, change in dementia state
2. Nursing assessment: objective
   a. Vital signs: low-grade fever or normal, tachypnea, tachycardia, blood pressure may be low or normotensive

      b. Pulmonary: (early) slight crackles, (later) crackles and wheezes, tachypnea, intercostal and substernal retractions, nasal flaring, use of accessory muscles to breathe, percussed dullness, positive tactile fremitus

    3. Nursing interventions

      a. Elevate head of bed 45 degrees

      b. Perform frequent position changes

      c. Instruct in cough and deep-breathing exercises

      d. Encourage fluids orally

      e. Ensure good nutrition

      f. Ensure proper placement of NG tubes

      g. Perform patient/family teaching

- Disease course and expected outcome
- Medication management (purpose and side effects)
- Deep-breathing exercises, cough when congested
- Need for good nutrition and fluid intake
- Proper handling of expectorated secretions
- Chest physiotherapy
- Smoking cessation

    4. Nursing diagnoses

      a. Airway clearance, ineffective

      b. Tissue perfusion, altered

      c. Breathing pattern, ineffective

      d. Thought processes, altered

      e. Anxiety: related to difficulty breathing

G. Medical management

    1. Diagnostic tests: complete blood count with differential, sputum smear, culture and sensitivity, chest radiograph (x-ray)

    2. Medications: antibiotics, expectorants, cough suppressants (if sleep is difficult), acetaminophen for fever or myalgia

    3. Nutritional support: increase fluid intake (assist in liquefying secretions), airway humidification, and oxygen as needed

V. CANCER OF THE LUNG

A. Prevalence

    1. Second most common cancer in the United States

    2. Leading cause of cancer death for both men and women as well as a major cause of morbidity and mortality in the aging population

    3. When current aging population were young adults, cigarette smoking was seen as glamorous, not hazardous

B. Pathophysiology

    1. Bronchogenic: 90% to 95% of lung cancers; others 5% to 10%

    2. Cell differentiation

      a. Small-cell lung carcinoma, 20% to 25%

      b. Non-small cell, squamous cell carcinoma, 25% to 40%

      c. Non-small cell, adenocarcinoma, including bronchioalveolar carcinoma, 25% to 40%

      d. Large-cell, 10% to 15%

      e. Combined patterns, 5% to 10%

    3. Metastatic spread

      a. Exists in 50% of patients presenting with signs and symptoms

      b. Eventually will occur in 90% of diagnosed lung cancers

      c. Most common sites are brain, bone, and liver

C. Risk factors

- Tobacco smoking

- Asbestos exposure
- Air pollution
- Passive smoke inhalation
- Alcohol intake
- Elevated cholesterol levels
- Lung scars
- Arsenic
- Diesel exhaust
- Radon
- Nickel

D. Nursing management of the patient with cancer of the lung
   1. Nursing assessment: subjective
      a. Dyspnea
      b. Bone pain
      c. Headache
      d. Malaise, fatigue
      e. Anorexia
   2. Nursing assessment: objective
      a. Persistent cough, wheezing
      b. Unequal breath sounds, unequal percussion sounds
      c. Weight loss
      d. Hemoptysis
      e. Recurrent pneumonia
      f. Seizure
   3. Nursing interventions
      a. Provide support for patient and family
         (1) Hospice care, if appropriate
         (2) Medical equipment and supplies for the home
         (3) Psychotherapy, if additional support is needed
      b. Instruct patient and family on pain management
         (1) Medication administration
         (2) Reporting side effects or ineffectiveness
      c. Encourage use of support groups (provide access information)
   4. Nursing diagnoses
      a. Pain, alteration
      b. Grieving, anticipatory
      c. Gas exchange, impaired (actual or potential)
      d. Skin integrity, impaired (actual or potential)
      e. Fluid imbalance, risk for
      f. Knowledge deficit

VI. TUBERCULOSIS

A. Definition
   1. Disease caused by infection with mycobacterium *Tuberculosis hominis* (TB)
   2. May invade any organ of the body but usually develops in the apex of one or both lungs
B. Prevalence
   1. Cases in the United States in 1996 were 8 per 100,000 (lowest since 1953)
   2. 37% of cases were in persons born outside the United States
   3. Older adults (over age 65) have the highest case rate (16 per 100,000)
C. Classifications
   1. Primary TB: occurs in a person lacking previous contact with the tubercle bacillus (initial infection)

      2. Reactivation TB: type of infection most common in older adults as the result of reinoculation

        a. Endogenous: from an old infection

        b. Exogenous: from an active case

  D. Etiology

      1. Acquired by inhalation of droplet nuclei containing microorganisms aerosolized from untreated people

      2. Then goes to the alveolar surface of the lung

  E. Pathophysiology

      1. Stage one: infection process (individuals do not develop the disease unless the immune system is compromised)—positive skin test, normal chest x-ray, negative acid-fast bacilli (AFB) sputum smear and culture

      2. Stage two: disease process—positive skin test, abnormal chest x-ray (cavitation), positive AFB sputum smear and culture; sensitivity tests must be done on positive cultures to detect multi-drug resistant bacilli

  F. Typical clinical presentation

      1. Stage one is asymptomatic

      2. Prolonged productive cough

      3. Fever, night sweats

      4. Anorexia, weight loss

      5. Hemoptysis

      6. Dull chest ache

  G. Nursing management of the patient with tuberculosis

      1. Nursing assessment: subjective

        a. Anorexia, weight loss, and fatigue

        b. Dull chest ache, pleurisy, bronchitis (seen more commonly in older adults)

        c. History of cough over 3 weeks, wheezing, history of COPD, pneumonia

        d. Shortness of breath

        e. Recent contact with someone who has TB

        f. Change in behavior or mentation, depression

        g. History of illegal IV drug use, alcoholism, smoking

      2. Nursing assessment: objective

        a. Low-grade temperature

        b. Hepatomegaly, unexplained masses

        c. Adventitious sounds, sputum (green/yellow), hemoptysis

        d. Tenderness or enlargement of cervical, supraclavicular, axillary, epitrochlear, or inguinal lymph nodes

      3. Nursing interventions

        a. Accurately interpret TB skin test (Boxes 12-2 and 12-3)

        b. Report positive results to physician for further evaluation

---

BOX 12-2   Tuberculin Skin Testing Procedure

1. Patients with a history of prior positive testing should not be tested again
2. Test should be read at 48 to 72 hours; definition of a positive reaction varies with risk groups
3. Administration: five tuberculin units (intermediate strength) of purified protein derivative (PPD) in 0.1 ml of solution is injected intradermally on the forearm (demonstration form should have either left or right arm indicated for accurate reading)
4. Negative test may require a repeat test 1 week later for booster phenomenon*
5. Factors associated with false-negative tests are secondary to loss of cellular immunity

---

*Booster phenomenon refers to the fact that the second test can increase the effectiveness due to activation of the immune response in an elderly person.

Modified from Ferri FE, Fretwell MD, Wachtel TJ: *Practical guide to the care of the geriatric patient*, ed 2, St Louis, 1997, Mosby.

BOX 12-3   TB Skin Test Interpretive Guidelines

5 mm	10 mm	15 mm

5 or more mm induration is considered positive for the highest risk groups:

Immunosuppressed people who have any:
- HIV infection
- Immunosuppressive therapy
- Reticuloendothelial disease
- Cancer
- End-stage renal disease

Recent TB contacts

People with abnormal chest x-ray consistent with tuberculosis

A reaction of 2 mm is strongly suggestive of positive test for people with HIV infection

10 or more mm induration is considered positive for other high-risk groups:

Foreign-born people from high TB-prevalent countries

Low-income populations

Substance abusers

Residents of:
- Correctional institutions
- Nursing homes

People over age 70

Employees of:
- Hospitals
- Mycobacterial labs

People who provide service to high-risk groups

People with medical conditions known to increase TB risk:
- Diabetes mellitus
- Prolonged corticosteroid treatment
- Chronic malabsorption syndrome
- Silicosis
- Below ideal body weight by 10% or more

15 mm or more induration is considered positive for:

People who do not have any risk factors mentioned

---

    c. Report infection and/or active disease to health department for surveillance
    d. Place patient in proper isolation room
    e. Use appropriate protective equipment for staff and patient
    f. Ensure good nutrition and hydration
    g. Ensure close monitoring for drug side effects and interactions (risk of drug-induced hepatitis in older adults)
    h. Schedule and provide reminders for a liver function test every 3 months
  4. Nursing diagnoses
    a. Infection, risk for
    b. Anxiety
    c. Gas exchange, impaired
    d. Nutrition, altered: less than body requirements
    e. Social interaction, impaired
    f. Personal identity disturbance

VII. ALLERGIES (FOR ALLERGIC ASTHMA, SEE HEADING FOR COPD, THEN ASTHMA)

    A. Allergic alveolitis (also known as hypersensitivity pneumonitis) results from
        1. Exposure to inhaled organic dusts or related occupational antigens
        2. Tree bark, sawdust, animal dander
        3. Actinomycetes bacteria found in humidifiers, hot tubs, and swimming pools
    B. Inflammatory response follows within several hours of exposure to offending cause
    C. Typical clinical presentation
        1. Labored breathing
        2. Dry cough
        3. Chills and fever
        4. Headache and malaise
    D. Nursing management
        1. Identify the offending organisms/causes
        2. Discuss a mechanism for removal of offending source
    E. Nursing diagnoses
        1. Respiratory pattern, altered related to allergies
        2. Gas exchange, impaired
        3. Social interaction, impaired (when removal of offending source limits interactions)

REFERENCES

Black J, Matassarin-Jacobs E: *Medical-surgical nursing: clinical management for continuity of care,* ed 5, Philadelphia, 1997, WB Saunders.

Clark J, Queener S, Karb V: *Pharmacologic basis of nursing practice,* ed 5, St Louis, 1997, Mosby.

Ferri FE, Fretwell MD, Wachtel TJ: *Practical guide to the care of the geriatric patient,* ed 2, St Louis, 1997, Mosby.

Leidy N: Functional performance in people with chronic obstructive pulmonary disease, *Image J Nurs Scholar* 27(1):20-34, 1995.

Monahan FD, Neighbors M: *Medical-surgical nursing: foundation for clinical practice,* ed 2, Philadelphia, 1998, WB Saunders.

Porth CM: *Pathophysiology: concepts of altered health states,* ed 5, Philadelphia, 1998, JB Lippincott.

Stanley M, Beare PG: *Gerontological nursing,* ed 2, Philadelphia, 1999, FA Davis.

Wold GH: *Basic geriatric nursing,* ed 2, St Louis, 1999, Mosby.

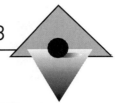

CHAPTER 13

GASTROINTESTINAL PROBLEMS

Sue E. Meiner

LEARNING OBJECTIVES

Upon completion of this chapter, the reader will be able to:

- Describe gastrointestinal changes in older adults
- Discuss the most common gastrointestinal (GI) disorders of older adults
- Identify nursing diagnoses appropriate to specific GI disorders of older adults

I. PRIMARY FUNCTION OF THE GI SYSTEM

A. Digestion and absorption of nutrients
B. Accomplished by secretions and motility

II. AGE CHANGES

A. Mouth and teeth
   1. Dentition is a major concern for older adults
   2. Many are edentulous or depend on dentures; many have dentures but do not wear them; others cannot afford to purchase dentures
   3. Saliva level may decline with age because of iatrogenic causes
B. Esophagus
   1. GI muscle strength and motility decrease with a resultant decrease in peristalsis
   2. Relaxation of the lower esophageal sphincter slows the emptying of the esophagus
   3. Lower end of esophagus dilates causing digestive discomfort (presbyesophagus)
   4. Hiatal hernias occur in about 60% of older adults over age 70
C. Stomach
   1. Cells responsible for production of hydrochloric acid and pepsin are reduced in numbers, reducing the amount of secretions made by those cells
   2. Alkaline protection of the stomach is lost with an increase in stomach pH
   3. Loss of smooth muscle causes a delayed emptying time
D. Liver, gallbladder, and pancreas
   1. Volume and weight of the liver decreases 17% to 28% after age 65
   2. Liver blood flow is decreased; protein is not as efficiently broken down
   3. Gallbladder function remains, so the potential for cholelithiasis and cholecystitis increases
   4. Decline in pancreatic secretions and enzyme output affecting fat digestion can lead to fatty food intolerance in older adults
E. Small intestine
   1. Decrease in smooth muscle, Peyer's patches, and lymphatic follicles
   2. Calcium use is affected by lack of adequate gastric acid and slow active transport in the body

3. Malabsorption of vitamins B_1, B_{12}, calcium, and iron can cause vitamin and mineral deficiencies in the older adult

F. Large intestine
   1. There is structural atrophy of the layers and glands and a decrease in mucous secretions
   2. Internal sphincter of the large intestine loses its muscle tone, which can lead to problems of bowel elimination
   3. Weakness of the intestinal wall can lead to diverticula

III. ORAL AND DENTAL CONDITIONS: PERIODONTAL DISEASE

A. Definition: degeneration of tissues supporting the teeth
B. Causes
   1. Malnutrition
   2. Poor absorption of vitamins (especially niacin, B_1, and B_{12})
   3. Poor dental hygiene
   4. Irritation by partial dentures
   5. Mouth-breathing (dryness)
   6. Faulty bridges
C. Incidence
   1. 86% of older adults have moderate periodontal disease
   2. 50% of adults over age 65 are edentulous from tooth decay or periodontal disease
D. Typical clinical presentation
   1. Pain
   2. Swelling
   3. Inflammation
   4. Bleeding gums
   5. Loose teeth
   6. Bad taste
   7. Halitosis
E. Nursing management: assessment
   1. White, scaly patches (leukoplakia), which may indicate early cancer
   2. Visual inspection of buccal cavity, including tongue (texture, moisture, color), palate, gingiva, teeth and/or dentures, lips, voice, and swallowing ability
F. Nursing diagnoses
   1. Knowledge deficit: related to the need for oral hygiene
   2. Nutrition, altered: less than body requirements, associated with gingivitis
G. Medical/dental interventions
   1. Properly fitting dental appliances
   2. Regular dental check-ups

IV. DYSPHAGIA

A. Definition: difficulty in swallowing
B. Swallowing impairment increases with age when some chronic conditions co-exist
   1. Dementia
   2. S/P CVA
   3. Parkinson's disease
   4. Sjogren's syndrome (decrease in salivary flow)
   5. Other musculoskeletal disorders
C. Incidence: approximately 50% of institutionalized older adults have oropharyngeal dysphagia
D. Typical clinical presentation
   1. Complaint of swallowing difficulty by patient or family
   2. Drooling or leakage of fluids or food from the mouth

3. Facial droop
4. Coughing before, during, or after swallowing fluids or food
5. Choking while drinking or eating
6. Recurrent pneumonia, upper respiratory infections, or chronic congestion
7. Retention of food in the oral cavity after placing it in the mouth

E. Nursing management
1. Position the patient in an upright position for all meals and oral fluids
2. Ensure that the consistency of all fluids and food is not so thin that it will splash into the pharynx and potentiate aspiration
3. Instruct anyone assisting with feeding to cut all food into manageable bites
4. Instruct anyone assisting with feeding to proceed slowly with meals
5. Make all caregivers aware of the condition during reports
6. Do not assist with eating when the patient is drowsy; proceed only when patient is fully awake
7. Interventions to facilitate eating
   a. Apply gentle downward pressure, of a spoonful of food, on the tongue when introducing food into the mouth
   b. Change the food texture as needed for thicker consistency
   c. Alternate cold and hot foods for sensory stimulus

F. Nursing diagnoses
1. Alteration in comfort, pain with swallowing
2. Aspiration, risk for: related to dysphagia
3. Nutrition, altered: less than body requirements

V. HIATAL HERNIA

A. Definition: protrusion of the stomach into the thoracic cavity through the esophageal opening in the diaphragm
B. Association
1. Commonly affects older adults over age 60
2. Commonly associated with gastroesophageal reflux
C. Typical clinical presentation
1. Epigastric distress
2. Heartburn
3. Dysphagia
4. Nausea
5. Vomiting
D. Nursing management
1. Instruct in diet modifications
2. Instruct in maintaining upright position following meals
3. Raise head of bed during sleep
4. Instruct in use of antacids, noting precautions associated with timing of administration of other medications
E. Nursing diagnoses
1. Pain, chronic: related to hiatal hernia
2. Nutrition, altered: more than body requirements
3. Swallowing, impaired: related to delayed swallowing mechanism

VI. GASTROESOPHAGEAL REFLUX DISEASE (GERD)

A. Definition: upward flow of gastric contents into the esophagus with a gradual breakdown of the esophageal mucosa
B. Association
1. Can be associated with a sliding hiatal hernia

    2. Cause is attributed to an inappropriate relaxation of the lower esophageal sphincter (LES); the exact cause of the relaxation is unknown; however, it happens more often in older adults

        a. An alteration in the innervation of the pressure zone in the region of the gastroesophageal sphincter

        b. Displacement of the angle of the gastroesophageal junction

        c. An incompetent LES

C. Typical clinical presentation

    1. Sudden or gradual onset of heartburn, odynophagia, dysphagia, acid regurgitation, or eructation

    2. Pain that can radiate to the back, neck, or jaw

    3. Intensity of pain increases when patient is lying supine or when stomach is distended

    4. Dysphagia is worse at the beginning of meals

    5. Differentiation between GERD and cardiac problems can be made with a nitroglycerin trial to relieve the pain; chest pain is relieved, GERD is not

D. Nursing management

    1. Instruct patient in the use of antacids; avoid taking with other prescription medications; time is important with 1 hour before or 2 to 3 hours after a meal

    2. Instruct patient to restrict diet to small, frequent meals (4 to 6/day), drink adequate fluids at meals to assist food passage

    3. Instruct patient to eat slowly and chew thoroughly to add saliva to the food

    4. Instruct patient to avoid extremely hot or cold foods, spices, fats, alcohol, coffee, chocolate, and citrus juices

    5. Instruct patient to avoid eating or drinking up to 3 hours before lying down

    6. Instruct patient and family to elevate the head of the bed on 6- to 8-inch high solid blocks to prevent reflux at night (pillows do not work)

    7. Monitor medications for appropriate actions; may include

- Bethanechol
- Cisapride
- Metoclopramide
- Omeprazole
- Misoprostol

    8. Monitor to avoid anticholinergic drugs, calcium channel blockers, and theophylline, which can decrease LES pressure or delay gastric emptying

E. Nursing diagnoses

    1. Pain, chronic: related to irritation of the esophagus associated with gastric reflux

    2. Injury, risk for: related to surgical procedure (e.g., Nissen fundoplication, Hill operation, Belsey operation)

VII. GASTRITIS AND ULCER DISEASE

A. Definition: associated with inflammatory change and erosion in the stomach's mucous membrane

B. Etiology

    1. Ulcers result from increased stomach acidity (common in older adults)

        a. Iron, aspirin, nonsteroidal antiinflammatory medications

        b. Alcohol intake

    2. Ulcers also arise from psychologic stress due to hospitalization or nursing home placement or from bacteria *(Helicobacter pylori)*

C. Incidence: gastric ulcers are more common in older adults, peptic ulcers more common in men

D. Typical clinical presentation

    1. Epigastric pain

    2. General malaise

    3. Anorexia and weight loss

    4. Vomiting, melena, and anemia

  E. Nursing management

    1. Check stools for occult blood, prepare patient for GI series

    2. Instruct patient in reduction or elimination of alcohol intake

    3. Instruct patient in use of antacids, giving precautions associated with timing the administration of other medications

    4. Report abnormal findings to the primary care provider

      a. Vital signs: decrease in blood pressure with increase in pulse rate

      b. Blood in vomitus or stool

      c. Epigastric pain that does not respond to medications prescribed

  F. Nursing diagnoses

    1. Pain, chronic: related to ulceration of stomach mucosa

    2. Knowledge deficit: related to self-care activities

VIII. HEPATIC DISEASES (HEPATITIS AND CIRRHOSIS)

  A. Hepatitis

    1. Hepatitis A: the most common type, spread by oral-fecal route, either through oral-anal sexual practices or by contaminated food, water, or shellfish

      a. Hepatitis A vaccine is available for persons planning foreign travel, day care workers, military personnel, persons living in endemic areas, anyone exposed to hepatitis A

    2. Hepatitis B: transmitted via blood but can also be transmitted by semen or saliva; perinatal infection from infected or carrier mothers

      a. Hepatitis B vaccine is now recommended by The American Academy of Pediatrics for all infants shortly after birth

    3. Hepatitis C: transmission includes IV drug use, blood transfusions, and other blood and blood-product exposure; sexual, family, and mother-to-infant transmission is rare

      a. Evaluation and treatment of patients acutely infected is still controversial

    4. Hepatitis D: (delta agent) occurs as a co-infection with hepatitis B or a super-infection that is imposed on chronic hepatitis B or hepatitis B carrier; when present can change a mild case of hepatitis B into fulminating hepatitis; can lead to chronic hepatitis or cirrhosis

    5. Hepatitis E: occurs primarily in developing countries such as India, other Southeast Asian countries, parts of Africa, and Mexico; spread by oral-fecal route, presents like hepatitis A, without causing chronic or carrier states of hepatitis

    6. Other forms of hepatitis: alcoholic hepatitis, drug-induced hepatitis, and autoimmune hepatitis

  B. Cirrhosis

    1. Definition: diffuse fibrous tissue serves to replace normal functioning liver tissue and form constrictive bands that disrupt flow of the vascular and biliary systems in the liver

    2. Types

      a. Laennec's (micronodular) cirrhosis or alcoholic cirrhosis: accounts for up to 50% of adult cirrhosis

      b. Immune-related bile duct injuries, including primary biliary cirrhosis and sclerosing cholangitis, primarily affect middle-aged women

      c. Postnecrotic cirrhosis caused by hepatic necrosis; may be related to hepatitis, liver diseases, exposure to industrial chemicals or hepatotoxins

  C. Typical clinical presentation

    1. Hepatitis

      a. Dark urine, pale stools

      b. Nausea, vomiting, anorexia, and abdominal pain

      c. Fever, headache, malaise

       d. Jaundice

       e. Hepatomegaly with tenderness, with less-seen splenomegaly, diffuse adenopathy, and rash

   2. Cirrhosis

       a. Weight loss with anorexia

       b. Abdominal pain

       c. Jaundice

       d. Easy bruising

D. Nursing management: assessment

   1. Hepatitis B

       a. Fatigue

       b. Jaundice, weight loss, enlarged liver on palpation

       c. Review laboratory data for liver function test results

   2. Cirrhosis

       a. Fatigue

       b. Jaundice, emaciation, ascites, gynecomastia, and lower leg edema

       c. Review laboratory data for liver function test results

E. Nursing management: interventions

   1. Hepatitis B

       a. Use universal precautions and impeccable care when giving blood or blood products and using skin-piercing instruments

       b. Instruct in personal hygiene behaviors (not sharing razors, manicure instruments, toothbrushes, or other personal items)

       c. Provide symptomatic measures for comfort when there is nausea/vomiting and malaise

       d. Follow laboratory data to monitor liver function

       e. Review and enforce precautions of transmission routes

       f. Encourage 1 to 2 weeks of rest from strenuous physical activity

       g. Elderly patients may need to be hospitalized for nutritionally balanced diet, IV hydration, electrolyte management, with potential vitamin K and fresh frozen plasma administration

       h. Instruct to avoid all alcohol and smoking

   2. Cirrhosis (Laennec's)

       a. Encourage taking vitamins and minerals, such as folate, thiamine, vitamin B_6, vitamin K, magnesium, and phosphate

       b. When hepatic encephalopathy is present, prepare to support the withholding of dietary protein

F. Nursing diagnoses

   1. Nutrition, altered: less than body requirements

   2. Activity intolerance

   3. Mobility, impaired physical

   4. Knowledge deficit: related to disease and long-term treatment

   5. Fatigue: related to decreased metabolic energy production

   6. Anxiety: related to uncertainty of the effects of the disease prognosis

IX. BOWEL OBSTRUCTION

A. Acquired causes of mechanical obstruction: polyps, tumors, post-operative adhesions, hernias

B. Neurogenic obstruction: no mechanical blockage; results from ineffective intestinal peristalsis

C. Paralytic ileus: post-operative impairment of peristalsis (reversible)

D. Intestinal pseudo-obstruction: associated with generalized visceral neuropathy; endocrine, neurological, or pharmacological causes

E. Typical clinical presentation
   1. Vomiting
   2. Abdominal distention
   3. Abdominal pain increasing with increased distention
   4. Post-operative absence of bowel sounds/flatus
   5. Cachexia
F. Nursing management: interventions (acute)
   1. Assess bowel elimination patterns
   2. Symptom control with analgesics as ordered
   3. Distention management by NG tube or rectal tube as ordered
   4. Preparation for surgical procedures as ordered
   5. Ongoing monitoring of fluid and electrolyte balance
G. Nursing management: interventions (home management)
   1. Encourage increasing physical activity
   2. Instruct to increase dietary fiber and fluids
   3. Encourage toileting at times when defecation urge is strongest
H. Nursing diagnoses
   1. Alterations in bowel elimination
   2. Alterations in comfort: related to bowel obstruction
   3. Nutrition, altered: related to insufficient fiber content in diet
   4. Knowledge deficit: related to disease process

X. DIVERTICULITIS/DIVERTICULOSIS

A. Definition: multiple pouches or sacs of intestinal mucosa in the weakened muscular wall of the colon, occurring in older adults
B. Causes include overeating, straining during bowel movement, alcohol, spicy foods (mucosal irritant), refined foods with low fiber, atrophy of musculature, and obesity
C. Older men have a higher incidence; 30% to 40% of all older adults have diverticula
D. Typical clinical presentation
   1. Left lower quadrant pain (LLQ)
   2. Nausea, vomiting, abdominal bloating
   3. Alternating constipation/diarrhea, painful defecation
   4. Low-grade fever
   5. Melena
   6. Mucus in the stool
E. Nursing management: assessment
   1. Left lower quadrant pain, distended abdomen
   2. Patterns of elimination and stool characteristics
   3. Patterns of diet, including fluid intake
   4. Weight
   5. Patterns of exercise
F. Nursing management: interventions
   1. Monitor NG tube placement and function during acute phase
   2. Support adequate fluid intake, monitor IV fluids in acute phase
   3. Instruct about disease process and prescribed medications
   4. Encourage daily fiber intake, unless bowel rest is ordered
   5. Instruct in bowel regimen to achieve routine elimination pattern
G. Nursing diagnoses
   1. Alteration in comfort, abdominal pain
   2. Nutrition, altered: related to insufficient fiber content in diet
   3. Knowledge deficit: related to disease process
   4. Fluid volume deficit, risk for: related to GI fluid and electrolyte losses

XI. CONSTIPATION

A. Definition: hard, dry stools that are difficult to pass; frequency differs from person to person
B. May have a different meaning to the patient; identification of meaning is necessary to understand; daily bowel movements to three times a week can be normal habits
C. Bowel changes with aging or chronic illness increase the risk for hard, dry stools
    1. Decreased abdominal muscle tone
    2. Inactivity, immobility
    3. Prescription medication side effect
D. Nursing management: assessment
    1. History of laxative use
    2. History of low-fiber diet
    3. Rectal pain when defecating
    4. Two or fewer bowel movements where 25% involve straining
    5. Abdominal distention
    6. Guaiac test of stool specimens (3 times)
E. Nursing management: interventions
    1. Encourage fluid intake of at least 2 quarts a day (unless contraindicated)
    2. Instruct to increase dietary fiber with bran and bulking agents
    3. Encourage participation in regular exercise
    4. Encourage patient to include at least 4 servings of fresh fruit and vegetables daily
    5. Instruct patient to develop a regular elimination schedule by attempting to have a bowel movement after a meal
    6. Instruct in taking stool softeners as prescribed
    7. Discuss the differences in antacids (aluminum-based may cause constipation)
    8. Instruct in reduction or elimination of the use of laxatives
F. Nursing diagnoses
    1. Nutrition, altered: related to insufficient fiber content in diet
    2. Constipation: related to (specific cause)
    3. Knowledge deficit: related to fluid balance

XII. DIARRHEA/FECAL INCONTINENCE

A. Definition: increased frequency of the passage of loose stools, increased bowel motility
B. Nursing management
    1. Maintain adequate hydration and nutrition
    2. Monitor for signs and symptoms of electrolyte imbalance
    3. Depending on causative factors, administration of antispasmodics/antidiarrheal medications as ordered
C. Nursing diagnoses
    1. Nutrition, altered: related to insufficient fiber content in diet
    2. Diarrhea: related to intestinal hypermotility, secondary to irritation
    3. Knowledge deficit: related to fluid balance
    4. Fluid volume deficit, risk for: related to GI fluid and electrolyte losses

XIII. FECAL IMPACTION

A. Definition: a mass of hardened feces trapped in the rectum that cannot be expelled, usually the result of unrelieved constipation
B. Typical clinical presentation
    1. Frequent oozing of thin or liquid discharge of feces from the rectum without evidence of passing solid stool
    2. Abdominal cramping or rectal pain
    3. Abdominal distention
    4. Anorexia

C. Nursing management
   1. Assess for bowel sounds
   2. Perform digital examination of the rectal vault for hardened mass(es)
   3. Determine the appropriateness of performing a manual evacuation of stool
   4. If appropriate, remove impaction as gently as possible
   5. Review all medications that may contribute to reduced peristalsis and consult with primary care provider as needed
   6. Initiate a nursing care plan that will prevent further impaction
      a. Increase mobility
      b. Increase dietary fiber with associated increase in fluids
      c. Record food and fluid intake and adjust before incurring a deficit
D. Nursing diagnoses
   1. Nutrition, altered: related to insufficient fiber content in diet
   2. Alterations in bowel elimination: fecal impaction
   3. Knowledge deficit: related to fluid balance

XIV. COLORECTAL CANCER

A. Highest percentage (90%) occurs in adults over age 50
B. Familial or hereditary factors may be present
   1. Familial polyposis
   2. Turcot syndrome
   3. Juvenile polyposis
   4. Gardner's syndrome
   5. Peutz-Jeghers syndrome
   6. Family cancer syndrome
   7. Crohn's disease
   8. Ulcerative colitis or other bowel disease
C. Typical clinical presentation
   1. Malaise, fatigue, anorexia, and weight loss
   2. Change in bowel patterns
      a. Diarrhea, constipation: early sign
      b. Small diameter stool: later sign
      c. Tenesmus
      d. Presence of blood in stools: next after the early signs
      e. Sense of incomplete bowel evacuation
   3. Pain: vague, dull, continuous ache and abdominal cramps
   4. Sense of fullness in the rectum
   5. Anemia and elevated liver enzymes may be present because of metastases
D. Nursing management
   1. Discuss self-care measures to reduce incidence and severity of side effects of treatment or surgical options
   2. Provide comfort measures specific to the patient's needs
   3. Provide emotional support for patient and family
   4. Monitor food and fluid intake and adjust as necessary to meet patient's needs
E. Nursing diagnoses
   1. Anxiety: related to cancer diagnosis
   2. Nutrition, altered: less than body requirements
   3. Fluid volume deficit, risk for: related to GI fluid and electrolyte losses

REFERENCES

Black JM, Matassarin-Jacobs E: *Medical-surgical nursing: clinical management for continuity of care,* ed 5, Philadelphia, 1997, WB Saunders.

Kayser-Jones J, Pengilly K: Dysphagia among nursing home residents, *Geriatr Nurs* 20(2):77-82, 1999.

Kim MJ, McFarland GK, McLane AM: *Pocket guide to nursing diagnoses,* ed 7, St Louis, 1997, Mosby.

Kosta JC, Mitchell CA: Current procedures for diagnosing dysphagia in elderly clients, *Geriatr Nurs* 19(4):195-199, 1998.

Lueckenotte AG: *Pocket guide series: gerontologic assessment,* ed 3, St Louis, 1998, Mosby.

Luggen AS: *NGNA core curriculum for gerontological nursing,* St Louis, 1996, Mosby.

Luggen AS, Travis SS, Meiner SE: *NGNA core curriculum for gerontological advanced practice nurses,* Thousand Oaks, CA, 1998, Sage.

Porth CM: *Pathophysiology: concepts of altered health states,* ed 5, Philadelphia, 1998, Lippincott-Raven.

Smithard DG, O'Neill PA, England RE, et al: The natural history of dysphagia following a stroke, *Dysphagia* 12:188-193, 1997.

Society of Gastroenterology Nurses and Associates: *Gastroenterology nursing: a core curriculum,* St Louis, 1998, Mosby.

Wold GH: *Basic geriatric nursing,* ed 2, St Louis, 1999, Mosby.

CHAPTER 14

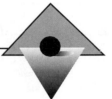

URINARY AND REPRODUCTIVE PROBLEMS

Beverly Reno

LEARNING OBJECTIVES

Upon completion of this chapter, the reader will be able to:

- Identify normal age-related changes in the genitourinary tract for the older male and female
- Implement a plan of care to alleviate problems and complications from disorders of the prostate in the older male
- Discuss nursing interventions for the older adult with sexual dysfunction
- Discuss nursing interventions for urinary incontinence in the older adult
- Discuss primary etiologies of urinary tract infections (UTI) in the older adult
- Identify various modalities in the prevention and treatment of UTIs
- Identify the causes of end-stage renal disease (ESRD) specific to the older adult
- Discuss a teaching plan for the treatment of vaginitis

I. NORMAL AGE-RELATED CHANGES

A. Female
1. Urgency and frequency because of thinning and fragility of the urethral mucosa from a decrease in estrogen production
2. Urgency and stress incontinence not uncommon and related to a decrease in perineal muscle tone
3. Increase in nocturia
4. Decrease in breast size; vagina narrows and shortens; acidity of vaginal secretions decrease
5. Uterus decreases in size; dryness of vaginal mucosa and uterine prolapse may occur

B. Male
1. Enlarged prostate, which may result in dribbling, urgency, nocturia, hesitancy, alterations in emptying the bladder and involuntary contractions of the bladder
2. Decreased production of testosterone, which results in prolonged refractory period and a sluggishness of the phases of intercourse
3. Testes become smaller and firmer, a diminished sperm count occurs, and viscosity of seminal fluid decreases

II. BENIGN PROSTATIC HYPERTROPHY (BPH)

A. Normal anatomy and function of prostate gland
1. Gland is located below the bladder and surrounds the urethra (Figure 14-1)

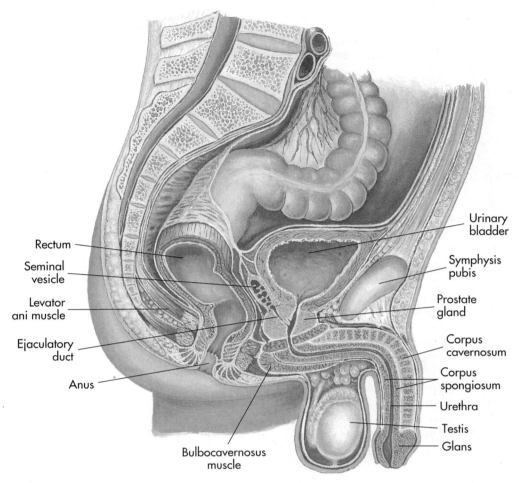

Figure 14-1 Male reproductive/urinary anatomy.
(From Seidel HM, et al: *Mosby's guide to physical examination*, ed 4, St Louis, 1999, Mosby.)

    2. Gland is smooth, regular in form, and rubbery on palpation

    3. Thin milky fluid is produced on ejaculation

B. Pathophysiology

    1. High incidence with alterations in testicular testosterone hormone and increased estrogen levels

    2. Hyperplasia of the periurethral gland (prostate)

    3. Hyperplasia of the periurethral gland; develops slowly and reduces the normal prostate, resulting in displacement of the normal tissue into the periphery of the prostate gland; hyperplasia leads to a gradual bladder outlet obstruction

    4. Urinary tract infections and urinary retention are the main result of BPH complications

C. Incidence

    1. BPH is one of the most common disorders in men

    2. 50% of men in their fifth decade have pathologic incidence of BPH; prevalence increases to 90% by the ninth decade

    3. African-American males have a high occurrence of BPH

    4. The second most common surgical intervention in males over the age of 65 is a transurethral prostatectomy (TURP)

5. Aging and the presence of functioning testes are two factors essential for the development of BPH

D. Risk factors
   1. Major risk factor is the aging process
   2. Diet, chronic inflammation, heredity, and race

E. Assessment
   1. Early BPH may go undetected
   2. Major early symptoms are urinary frequency, hesitancy, dribbling, decreased force of stream, nocturia, overflow incontinence and constipation; late signs/symptoms may be flank pain during voiding, nausea, and vomiting
   3. Physical assessment to detect bladder distention; dull sound over bladder upon percussion; rectal exam to determine size, contour, and symmetry of prostate gland
   4. Diagnostic studies to rule out or confirm the diagnosis
      a. Laboratory studies (CBC may indicate anemia in the presence of metastatic disease)
      b. WBCs, PSA (normal is <4 ng/ml), prostatic acid phosphatase (PAP); PAP and PSA are good indicators for monitoring the progression of prostate cancer
      c. X-rays (IVP [intravenous pyelogam] may disclose ureteral obstruction caused by metastasis to the lymph nodes)
      d. Cystoscopy, direct visualization of the bladder, KUB (direct visualization of the kidneys, ureters, and bladder)
      e. BUN and creatinine will be elevated if kidney function has been compromised
   5. Completion of a post-void residual (PVR)
   6. Ultrasound; useful in estimating the size of the cancerous or noncancerous enlargement
   7. Magnetic resonance imaging (MRI) and computed tomography (CT) are painless and show cross-sections of prostate

F. Interventions
   1. Focus on early detection and treatment
   2. Teach the patient to eat a diet low in fat and cholesterol and to include a lot of fruits and vegetables in daily intake
   3. Have patient limit fluid intake especially at night and avoid caffeine and alcohol
   4. Administer specific pharmacological agents as prescribed
      a. Antispasmodic agents (Ditropan and Probanthine)
      b. Testosterone-ablating drugs (Androcur and Zoladex), which decrease amount of circulating testosterone, resulting in slowed growth of prostatic tissue growth
      c. Alpha-reductase inhibitors, which block 5-alpha reductase enzyme that converts testosterone to dihydrotestosterone (Finasteride, Proscar)
      d. Alpha-adrenergic blocking agents (Hytrin, Minipress), which relax muscles and decrease the obstruction of the urinary outlet
   5. Inform patient about surgical procedure that is to be performed
      a. Transurethral resection of the prostate (TURP): advantages and disadvantages
         • Return to normal voiding pattern
         • Incontinence, bleeding, impotence
      b. Visual laser ablation (VLAP) is the newest form of surgery
         • Can be done as an outpatient
         • Local anesthesia
         • Usually done in 10 to 15 minutes and is bloodless
      c. Transurethral electrovaporization prostatectomy (TVP)
         • Bloodless, painless, cost-effective
         • Only partial relief from symptoms and infection

6. Nursing care post-operatively
   a. Monitor urinary output
   b. Maintain constant bladder irrigations (CBI) as prescribed to keep catheter free of clots
   c. Monitor for signs of water intoxication: confusion, agitation, nausea, and vomiting
   d. If not contraindicated, encourage fluid intake of 2500 to 3000 ml in 24 hours
   e. Monitor for signs of retention after catheter is removed
   f. Teach Kegel exercises
   g. Monitor for bladder spasms and medicate appropriately; ditropan is a drug of choice
   h. Monitor for signs and symptoms of infection
   i. Teach patient about activities after discharge
G. Nursing diagnosis
   1. Urinary elimination, altered: related to bladder obstruction outlet
H. Specific goal: patient will maintain schedule of complete bladder emptying every 2 to 4 hours during waking hours with two or fewer episodes of nocturia per night

III. PROSTATE CANCER

A. Pathophysiology
   1. Cells that don't look normal but haven't developed into cancerous cells
   2. Malignant cells usually develop in outer portion of prostate
   3. Early-stage tumors do not occlude the urethra so no symptoms may appear
   4. Cancer cells that are stimulated by testosterone may remain in the prostate or metastasize to bone, spine, or lymph nodes
   5. Slow progression of adenocarcinoma usually means it remains in the prostatic lobe
B. Incidence
   1. Is the second leading cause of death in males in the United States
   2. Incidence of prostate cancer increases with age
   3. Rare in men under age of 40 but tends to be aggressive
C. Risk factors
   1. Increased levels of serum testosterone
   2. Diet high in fat and low in beta-carotene
   3. Increases with age, especially in males >60
   4. Genetics, especially in first-line relatives
   5. African-American males
D. Assessment
   1. Digital rectal exam (DRE) that reveals a hard nonmovable nodule in the prostate gland is highly suspicious
   2. Evaluation of urinary patterns
      a. Early signs and symptoms: hesitancy, nocturia, urgency, frequency, difficulty maintaining a firm erection, and new onset of impotence
      b. Late signs and symptoms: edema in lower extremities, pain in lower back, rectal pressure or full feeling and aching in legs and hips
   3. Complete family history
   4. American Cancer Society recommends that men >50 request annual screening tests: DRE, prostate-specific antigen (PSA), a blood serum test that is unique to the prostate gland (>4 ng/ml may signify prostate cancer)
   5. A needle biopsy is often done if elevated PSA or abnormal rectal exam is found; a biopsy is often done with ultrasound and can determine if the tumor is malignant
   6. Bone scan to determine if bones of the pelvis have been damaged and if any repair has taken place, which may signify metastasis
   7. CT or MRI, which may be able to detect where cancerous tumors are located

      8. Cystoscopy or visualization of the bladder to determine if there is another cause for the patient's problem

      9. Five stages and grades of tumor

         a. Stage I: tumor in center and nonpalpable, cells symmetrical and tightly enclosed

         b. Stage II: tumor can be palpated and is on side of prostate, cells symmetrical and loosely enclosed

         c. Stage III: tumor can be palpated and is large, nonsymmetrical and separated cells

         d. Stage IV: tumor outside prostate, cells in groups with varying shapes

         e. Stage V: tumor metastasized, cells irregular in structure and form

     10. Diagnostic studies: see BPH

  E. Interventions

      1. See BPH on nursing care and teaching for patients who have undergone major surgery

      2. Recent studies have shown that a "wait and see approach" may be an effective treatment modality vs. surgery or some medical approach; the rationale is that tumors discovered in the older adult (whether they are treated or not) do not increase life expectancy; the tumor is usually slow growing and the older adult would be dead of "natural causes" before the cancer could kill him

      3. Assess the patient's readiness to discuss sexual concerns; assist the patient in identifying pertinent issues and solutions

      4. Discuss sexual problems with the patient, informing him of the causative factor; this will decrease anxiety and encourage nurse-patient communication

      5. Assess for the impact of sexual dysfunction between patient and significant other; this will allow the nurse to determine the degree of sexual problems between patient and significant other

      6. Inform physician of any potential or actual problems identified and seek out social services to identify appropriate community resources for counseling

      7. Explore with physician on informing patient of surgical and non-surgical treatments for erectile dysfunction

      8. Inform patient and family of support groups in community

      9. Discuss modalities to decrease the side effects of chemotherapy and radiation

  F. Nursing diagnosis

      1. Sexual dysfunction: related to surgical procedure

IV. SEXUAL DYSFUNCTION

  A. Age-related changes

      1. Older adults do not lose their interest in or capacity for sexual activity

      2. Since the 1990s, the term *erectile dysfunction* (ED) has become the preferred term to use as opposed to *impotence;* although ED is common among older men, it is not the result of normal age-related changes

      3. Male

         a. Degenerative changes in reproductive organs

         b. Response to sexual stimulation is slower, less intense, and of shorter duration

         c. Refractory time lengthens, may be 24 hours after orgasm before the older male can have another erection

      4. Female

         a. Atrophy of reproductive organs: thinning and drying of vaginal wall, decreased length and width of vagina, decreased lubrication of vagina; hormonal changes may result in contraction of the uterus, making intercourse painful; all these changes affect the response to intercourse

         b. The response to sexual stimulation is slower, less intense, and of shorter duration

  B. Pathophysiology

      1. Vascular insufficiency occurs in the male, affecting erectile functioning

    2. Health disorders in the male (see also section on BPH and cancer of the prostate)
      a. Erectile dysfunction is a common reversible condition
        (1) BPH does not generally affect sexual functioning, unless the hypertrophy becomes so severe that urinary retention becomes a problem
        (2) Prostatic cancer may not affect sexuality until the later stages
        (3) Surgery for these conditions may result in impotence and incontinence
        (4) Alzheimer's disease may impair cognitive functioning, which may contribute to sexual impairment
        (5) Diseases may affect the erectile tissue of the penis, including Peyronie's disease and priapism
    3. Health disorders in the female
      a. Osteoporosis, which is a loss of bone mass, may affect sexual functioning
      b. After intercourse, some females may experience burning and urinary frequency because of a decrease in vaginal lubrication and irritation from penile penetration
      c. Cystocele, prolapsed uterus, and rectocele
      d. Prominent symptom of decreased estrogen production is the "hot flash"; the brain triggers dilation of blood vessels near the surface of the skin, producing the sensation of heat
      e. Cancer of the cervix, uterus, fallopian tubes, or ovaries; the cancer itself does not affect sexuality directly until the later stages; the treatment of the cancer could affect sexuality; after a hysterectomy some females have reported a decrease in sexual desire and others have experienced no change
      f. Mastectomy, which may result in impaired body image
      g. Incontinence
      h. Obesity
      i. Older women are more susceptible to urethritis and vaginitis caused by thinning of the vaginal wall and decreased lubrication of vagina
      j. Alzheimer's and Parkinson's diseases may result in cognitive impairment that affects sexual functioning
      k. Systemic diseases, such as diabetes and arthritis
      l. Chronic illnesses (e.g., chronic obstructive pulmonary disease [COPD], cardiac disease)
C. Incidence
    1. Sexual frequency declines with age, but the desire and competence of older adults does not change unless there are physical, social, or psychological reasons
    2. Men are more sexually active than women throughout life
    3. Sexual activity of women is often more influenced by such factors as available partner, spousal death, and illness
    4. Life-long pattern of sexual interest, attitudes, and activity does not change significantly with the aging process
D. Risk factors
    1. Misunderstanding and myths about sexuality in the elderly
    2. Social misgivings (e.g., loss of a partner)
    3. Atrophy of genital organs because of disuse
    4. Relationship discord
    5. Fear of performance failure
    6. Psychological problems (e.g., depression, anxiety)
    7. Medications (e.g., antihypertensives)
    8. Illness of partner
    9. Use of alcohol
   10. Environmental factors, lack of privacy (e.g., nursing home)
E. Assessment
    1. Before a nurse completes a sexual history, he/she must first look at his/her own attitudes, myths, and biases about older adult sexual behavior

2. Complete a comprehensive nursing history and assessment to include
   a. Medication history
      (1) Alcohol use results in erectile problems, diminished libido, and delayed orgasm in women
      (2) Antidepressants reduce libido and delay ejaculation
         - Elavil (amitriptyline)
         - Aventyl (nortriptyline)
         - Tofranil (imipramine)
         - Zoloft (sertraline)
         - Serzone (nefazodone)
      (3) Antihistamines block parasympathetic nervous innervation of sex glands
         - Benadryl (diphenhydramine)
         - Phenergan (promethazine)
      (4) Anticholinergics inhibit parasympathetic innervation of sex glands and may result in decreased libido, impaired ejaculation, impotence, and retrograde ejaculation
         - Robinul (glycopyrrolate)
         - Lomotil (diphenoxylate hydrochloride)
         - Cogentin (benztropine)
         - Levodopa (L-dopa)
      (5) Diuretics may result in decreased potency, impaired ejaculation
         - Lasix (furosemide)
         - Edcrin (ethycrynic acid)
      (6) Phenothiazides/antipsychotics may result in impotence, erectile problems, and decreased libido
         - Thorazine (chlorpromazine HCl)
         - Risperdal (risperdone)
         - Haldol (haloperidol)
         - Compazine (prochlorpromazine)
         - Mellaril (thioridazine)
      (7) Sedative/hypnotics, when used regularly, cause decreased libido and potency
         - Barbiturates: nembutal, seconal, and phenobarbital
      (8) Benzodiazepines/tranquilizers block autonomic innervation of sex glands
         - Ativan (lorazepam)
         - Librium (chlordiazepoxide)
         - Tranxene (chlorazepate)
         - Valium (diazepam)
   b. Physical/social history
3. Assessment should be totally individualized
4. Questions should glean information about gynecological aspects of female sexual function and genitourinary aspects of male function
5. If the patient responds with an open-ended question, then the nurse should seek clarification and respond to the needs identified
6. Assessment should glean enough information so appropriate resources can be used
7. If risk factors are identified in interview, an in-depth assessment may not be needed
8. Assess for privacy
9. Assess for losses

F. Interventions
1. Assess the ability of the patient to communicate sexual concerns
2. Maintain a nonjudgmental demeanor and be a good listener during the interview
3. Provide the patient with information regarding age-related changes that affect sexual expression

4. Increase patient's knowledge base about sexuality and sexual functioning
5. Provide the patient with alternative ways to engage in sexual intercourse in lieu of the "missionary position"—reverse positions, side-to-side position, sitting positions, and rear entry position
6. Provide solutions if pain is experienced during sexual activity
7. Discuss alternative sexual activities that are compatible with lifestyle (e.g., massage, single or mutual masturbation, and sexual aids other than sexual intercourse)
8. Refer to therapist if appropriate
9. Discuss surgical and other medical interventions, including hormonal replacement for post-menopausal older women; hormone injections or oral testosterone; however, for men may lead to liver damage and enlargement of the prostate; Viagra is the newest treatment for ED; other alternatives are external vacuum therapy (EREC), penile injection therapy, penile implants, and vascular reconstructive surgery
10. If an older adult is institutionalized, provide for privacy if a significant other is available
G. Nursing diagnosis
1. Sexuality patterns, altered: related to medications (alternate rationales may include chronic illness, terminal illness, systemic diseases, psychosocial circumstances [loss of significant other])

V. URINARY INCONTINENCE

A. Urinary incontinence is not a result of normal age-related changes; it is the involuntary loss of urine sufficient to be a problem
B. Pathophysiology
1. The involuntary leakage of urine
2. Incontinence can be classified as urge, overflow, stress, functional, and psychological
3. Anatomical placement of the bladder and bladder neck in the older woman is altered because of perineal weakness and changes in the urethrovesical angle; this change in anatomical structure results in a downward pressure on the bladder, producing incontinence
4. The male has incontinence primarily because of BPH, which results in retention, stress incontinence, and overflow
5. Incontinence is often the result of surgery for BPH or cancer of the prostate
C. Incidence
1. Incontinence occurs in more than 10 million Americans
2. It is increased in the older adult population because of pathological, physiological, and functional contributing factors
3. Women over the age of 60 have twice the incidence as men
4. Without assessment, incontinence often leads to institutionalization
5. Social isolation and depression can accompany the embarrassment of urinary incontinence
6. An annual multi-billion dollar/year cost can be attributed to incontinence
7. Impact can be devastating and costly; increased falls because of wet floors result in fractures and immobilization, skin breaks down, decubitus ulcers require extensive and expensive treatment, and UTIs result in hospitalization
D. Risk factors
1. The most frequent cause of incontinence is an interference with sphincter control
2. Fecal impaction can be a factor
3. Physical, psychosocial, and pharmacological factors can also contribute to incontinence
   a. Inflammation, urethritis, atrophic vaginitis, polyuria, nocturia (secondary to poorly controlled diabetes), congestive heart failure, and hypercalcemia
   b. Drugs are also known to cause incontinence: sedative hypnotics, psychotropics, diuretics, anticholinergics, antispasmodics, and alpha-adrenergic agents
4. Alcohol is a major factor in incontinence

5. Anatomical damage to the detrusor muscle, urethra, or urethrovesical junction causes incontinence; common causes of damage to the urethrovesical junction are aging, difficult births, and abdominal surgery
6. Obesity can have an effect on abdominal and perineal muscles, resulting in incontinence

E. Assessment
1. Complete an interview using open-ended questions, followed by specific questions
2. Note that urinary incontinence is under-reported
3. Identify contributing factors
4. Perform a history, including duration, characteristics such as amount of urine lost, time of day, frequency, precipitating factors, nocturia, dysuria, hesitancy, hematuria, type and amount of incontinence products used
5. Stress maintenance of voiding pattern
6. Perform an environmental assessment
7. Perform a physical examination of the abdomen, genitalia, rectum, and, additionally in the female, a pelvic exam; other physical findings possibly affecting incontinence include edema, neurological deficits, decreased mobility and dexterity
8. Perform a urinalysis, PVR
9. Check sensory/motor function by means of uroflowmeter and cystometry; findings may suggest a mixed-type urinary incontinence

F. Interventions
1. Use behavioral, surgical, and pharmaceutical interventions
   a. Behavioral
      (1) Teach bladder training for urge and stress incontinence
      (2) Develop habit training or timed voiding for urge incontinence
      (3) Teach prompted voiding for the cognitively impaired and frail
      (4) Teach Kegel exercises for urge and stress incontinence
      (5) Use biofeedback as an adjunct treatment
      (6) Modify environment for functional incontinence, including adequate lighting, furniture that promotes ease of sitting and rising, toilet within easy reach, alteration of clothing with wide openings in slacks and velcro closure to provide easy removal, and proper adaptive equipment such as grab bars, elevated commode, and use of portable commode, if necessary
      (7) Encourage patient to maintain fluid intake at 1500 ml before evening hours; limit caffeine products to breakfast and lunch hours
      (8) Encourage patient to maintain good bowel pattern
   b. Medical/surgical
      (1) Artificial sphincter
      (2) Collagen injection
      (3) Penile implants
      (4) Intermittent catheterization
      (5) Insertion of pessaries; have been used for many years to treat cystocele in women
      (6) Foley catheters; but only for 2 to 4 weeks to prevent secondary problems
      (7) External urinary devices; but only for a short period of time because of increased risk of UTI
   c. Pharmaceutical
      (1) Anticholinergics: dicyclomine (Bentyl) relieves smooth muscle spasms in the bladder; urecholine is used in bladder atony
      (2) Alpha-adrenergic agonists: for incontinence due to urethral sphincter insufficiency; oxybutynin (Ditropan) increases sphincter resistance
      (3) Estrogen supplement: for postmenopausal women with incontinence secondary to atrophic vaginitis or urethritis

G. Nursing diagnoses
   1. Urinary elimination, altered: related to incontinence
   2. Knowledge deficit: related to normal urinary function

VI. URINARY TRACT INFECTIONS

A. Urinary incontinence may be the earliest and only sign of UTI
B. Pathophysiology
   1. Stasis of urine as a result of incomplete emptying of the bladder, often associated with cystocele, uterine prolapse, or loss of pelvic muscle tone
      a. Loss of vaginal lactobacilli, an organism that inhibits infection; this loss of bacteria is the result of a decrease in estrogen
      b. Changes in vaginal microflora
      c. Diabetes changes the pH of the urine; bacteria grow best in an alkaline environment
      d. Altered immune status
C. Incidence
   1. Postmenopausal women may experience a greater number of UTIs than younger women
   2. Female anatomy contributes to the increased susceptibility to UTIs
   3. Approximately 6 to 7 million office visits a year can be attributed to UTIs
   4. The rate of UTIs among women per year is 20%
   5. UTI is the most common infection in the older adult
   6. Persons over the age of 65 are at increased risk for bacteruria
   7. UTIs in men <50 years old are rare
   8. 5% to 8% of UTIs are the result of nosocomial infections
D. Risk factors
   1. Aging
   2. Atrophic vaginitis and urethritis
   3. Fecal incontinence
   4. Catheterization and cystoscopy
   5. Diabetes mellitus
   6. BPH
   7. Urinary obstructions (e.g., urinary calculi)
   8. Urinary stasis
   9. Improper perineal cleansing; *Escherichia coli (EC),* a bacterium, causes the majority of UTIs
   10. Hospitalization and institutionalization
   11. Dehydration
   12. Estrogen use for more than a year
E. Assessment
   1. Lower tract UTI
      a. Urethritis: inflammation of the urethra
      b. Prostatitis: inflammation of the prostrate
      c. Cystitis: inflammation of the bladder
   2. Upper tract UTI
      a. Pyelonephritis: inflammation of the kidney and renal pelvis
   3. Complete nursing history and physical assessment
      a. Objective data
         (1) Urine culture and sensitivity depicting 100,000 colonies/ml in a midstream specimen or 1000 colonies/ml in a catheterized specimen
         (2) Increased glucose levels in urine
         (3) Low-grade fever
         (4) Change in mental status
         (5) Confusion

      (6) Patient asymptomatic until high bacterial count
      (7) Upper tract infection may result in nausea and vomiting
      (8) Hematuria
      (9) Reduced amount of urine voided; check for residual
   b. Subjective data
      (1) Burning on urination
      (2) Urgency and frequency
      (3) Tenderness in the suprapubic region
      (4) Dull, aching pain in the flank area occurs in pyelonephritis
      (5) Urinary meatus may be irritated or have drainage
      (6) Chills
      (7) Dysuria

F. Interventions
1. Focus on early detection, education, and treatment
2. Instruct patient on importance of follow-up treatment after the medication regimen has been completed
3. Teach patient to avoid fluids that irritate the bladder (e.g., alcohol, coffee, tea, colas, citrus and carbonated drinks)
4. Instruct patients to drink at least eight, 8-ounce glasses of fluid a day; if patient is taking a sulfa drug, fluids are even more important to prevent the forming of crystals in the urine; encourage the consumption of cranberry juice or eating blueberries, which reduces the occurrence of UTIs; these two fruits contain tannins, called proanthocyanidins, which inhibit E. coli from adhering to the lining of the urinary tract
5. Instruct patient to void when urgency occurs; a good habit is to void every 2 to 3 hours
6. Teach patient who is experiencing pain to take warm baths
7. Teach patient proper perineal cleansing
8. Instruct patient to abstain from douching
9. Instruct patient to wear cotton and white underwear and avoid tight-fitting clothing (e.g., panty hose)
10. Instruct patient to void 10 to 15 minutes after coitus
11. Instruct patient to change protective padding at least every 2 to 3 hours
12. Teach handwashing techniques
13. Instruct patient about early signs and symptoms of UTI and the need to take antibiotics immediately
14. Instruct patient to take all antibiotics until gone; do not save any even if symptoms have subsided
15. Pharmacological interventions
   a. Antimicrobials
      (1) Amoxicillin, Augmentin, and Geocillin
      (2) Cephalosporins: Ceclor, Cefobid, and Rocephin
      (3) Quinolones: Cipro, Noroxin, and Floxin
      (4) Sulfonamides: Gantanol, Bactrim, Bactrim DS, Trimpex, and Proloprim
   b. Antiseptics
      (1) Furadantin and Furalan
      (2) Urised and Hiprex
   c. Antispasmodics
      (1) Hyoscyamine
      (2) Ditropan
      (3) Urecholine
   d. Analgesics
      (1) Pyridium
      (2) Pyridiate

G. Goals
   1. Patient will be compliant with drug regimen
   2. Patient will be responsible in follow-up care
   3. Patient will be free of UTIs
   4. Patient will verbalize signs and symptoms of early UTI
   5. Family will participate in care, if appropriate
H. Nursing diagnosis
   1. Urinary elimination, altered: related to urinary tract infection

VII. END-STAGE RENAL DISEASE (ESRD, RENAL INSUFFICIENCY)

A. Normal age-related changes
   1. Decreased ability to regulate the H^+ ion
   2. Inability of kidney to concentrate urine
   3. Nephron degeneration, resulting in a decrease in the glomerular filtration rate (GFR); by the age of 70, there is a 33% to 50% decrease
   4. More difficulty maintaining homeostasis and fluid balance
   5. Glomerular filtration rates decrease 6.5 ml/min each decade of life
B. Pathophysiology
   1. Progressive loss of renal function because of the destruction and wasting away of the nephrons
   2. Changes result in inability of the kidney to concentrate urine; the tubules cannot reabsorb electrolytes, which results in salt-wasting and polyuria
   3. Even with monitored treatment of chronic renal failure (CRF), it can progress to end-stage renal disease
   4. Uremia and death are the consequences of CRF; dialysis and kidney transplant remain the only treatments
C. Incidence
   1. Older adults are at an increased risk because of their compromised cardiovascular system
   2. Because of other age-related changes and BPH, the likelihood of renal pathology is increased
   3. The major cardiovascular problem of hypertension results in at least 50% to 60% of deaths due to CRF
D. Risk factors
   1. Diabetes mellitus (DM) and hypertension (HTN) are the two main risk factors for patients requiring dialysis; these factors account for >60% of dialysis patients
   2. Chronic illnesses, infections, and inflammatory processes all contribute to the development of CRF, often leading to ESRD; diseases include pyelonephritis, HTN, renal calculi, and DM; nephrotoxic factors (drug overdose and medication toxicity) are also major risk factors
E. Assessment
   1. Complete a comprehensive nursing history and physical exam
   2. Subjective data
      a. Severe and intractable pruritis
      b. Vomiting
      c. Nausea
      d. Loss of appetite
      e. Fatigue
   3. Objective data
      a. Peripheral neuropathy
      b. Decrease in creatinine clearance
      c. Hypocalcemia but can be hypercalcemia because of overstimulation of the parathyroid
      d. Elevated BUN (blood urea nitrogen)

      e. Decreased osmolarity of urine indicates severe pyelonephritis and renal tubular necrosis

      f. Hyperlipidemia

      g. Metabolic acidosis

      h. Oliguria to anuria

      i. Anemia

      j. Skin dryness

      k. Constipation

      l. Edema

      m. Altered mental status

      n. Depression with possible suicidal ideation

F. Interventions

1. Assist the patient in selecting and managing a diet low in protein, sodium, and potassium
2. Teach the patient about his/her medications: purpose, dosage, administration, side effects, and toxic effects
3. Teach the signs and symptoms of infection on a graft for dialysis and how to manage and report
4. Educate the patient on how to remain compliant with all treatment regimens: fluid restrictions, diet, medications, and managing blood pressure within normal limits for the individual patient
5. Monitor all laboratory values and report and treat appropriately
6. Selected pharmacotherapeutics
   a. Diuretics: Lasix
   b. Cardiac glycoside: Digoxin
   c. ACE inhibitor: Vasotec
7. Psychosocial issues
   a. Teach patient and family effective coping skills
   b. Assist patient and family in selecting support groups in the community
   c. Provide an open and trusting relationship
   d. Assess for patient safety and refer the patient and/or family to appropriate source
   e. Assess patient and family for spirituality and use appropriately in planning care

G. Nursing diagnoses

1. Nutrition, altered: less than body requirements, related to anorexia and nausea
2. Skin integrity, impaired: related to itching, edema, and dryness of skin
3. Knowledge deficit: related to disease process and treatment
4. Coping, ineffective individual: depression with suicidal ideation, related to extreme stress from chronic life-threatening disease
5. Coping, ineffective family: related to chronic illness, feelings of hopelessness about patient's destiny, and role reversal

VIII. VAGINITIS AND URETHRITIS

A. Normal age-related changes

1. Estrogen levels decrease
2. Vaginal wall thins and becomes drier
3. Vaginal epithelium becomes less elastic and loss of subcutaneous fat is common after menopause
4. Labia majora and minora flatten out
5. Shortening of the urethra may occur

B. Pathophysiology

1. Because of the changes in the vaginal wall, the susceptibility to infection increases in the older adult woman
2. Atrophy of urethra may result in increased urethritis and vaginitis
3. Vaginal secretions become watery and alkaline, which is conducive for bacterial growth

C. Incidence
    1. No data to reflect the exact number of older adults affected
D. Risk factors
    1. Most common cause of urethritis in the male is sexually transmitted diseases (STDs), gonorrheal and chlamydial
    2. Contributing factors for female urethritis are feminine hygiene sprays, perfumed toilet paper, wearing sanitary pads or Attends too long
    3. Factors that can cause vaginitis are all related to normal age-related changes in the vagina
    4. Vaginitis can be the result of prolonged steroid therapy and antibiotics
    5. Congestion of the pelvic organs
E. Assessment
    1. Complete a comprehensive nursing history and physical assessment, focusing on sexual activity, urinary patterns, and appearance of genitals
    2. Urethritis in the male presents with a urethral discharge
    3. Urethritis in the female presents with inflammation of the urethral lining, pyuria, edema of the meatus
    4. In the male and female, dysuria, frequency, and nocturia are common
    5. Assess for lower abdominal pain or perineal pain and discomfort in the female
    6. Perform diagnostic studies (CBC, UA, and cultures for STDs)
    7. Complete a medication history; determine steroid and antibiotic use when ruling out factors for vaginitis
    8. Complete a pelvic exam in diagnosing vaginitis
    9. Assess for profuse, pungent odor and purulent drainage with vaginitis
    10. Assess for pruritis of vulva area, dyspareunia, and vaginal burning
    11. Vulval excoriation can occur if a secondary infection is present
F. Interventions
    1. Urethritis
      a. Remove the cause
      b. Apply topical antibiotics
      c. Administer antibiotics
      d. Order baking soda sitz baths
      e. Recommend fluid intake of at least 2500 to 3000 ml/day, if not contraindicated
      f. Recommend use of condoms for vaginal intercourse and anal intercourse
      g. Teach patient that STDs can be transmitted anally, orally, and vaginally
      h. Instruct patient to avoid intercourse until symptoms have subsided
    2. Vaginitis
      a. Instruct diabetic patient about the importance of having blood sugar under control; hyperglycemia affects vaginal secretions
      b. Instruct the patient to refrain from douching and using perfumed, scented sanitary pads or powders
      c. Instruct the patient to cleanse the perineum from front to back and wash hands after elimination and changing of pads
      d. Advise patient to change perineal pads and/or Attends when soiled
      e. Inform patient that tight-fitting clothing and nylon panty hose increase susceptibility to vaginitis; instruct patient to wear panties that have a cotton liner
      f. Instruct patient that early detection is imperative; report any signs or symptoms of vaginitis
G. Nursing diagnoses
    1. Alteration in comfort: related to inflammation of urethral lining, genitals, and presence of STD
    2. Knowledge deficit: related to medications, disease process, and perineal hygiene

REFERENCES

Agency for Health Care Policy and Research: *Clinical practice guidelines: benign prostatic hypertrophy,* Rockville, MD, 1992, (PHS) (Publication No 94-0582), US Department of Health and Human Services.

Black J, Jacobs E: *Medical-surgical nursing: clinical management for the continuity of care,* ed 5, Philadelphia, 1997, WB Saunders.

Ebersole P, Hess P: *Toward healthy aging: human needs and nursing response,* ed 5, St Louis, 1998, Mosby.

Eliopoulos C: *Gerontological nursing,* ed 3, Philadelphia, 1997, JB Lippincott.

Evans E: Indwelling catheter care: dispelling the misconceptions, *Geriatr Nurs* 20(2):85-89, 1999.

Frizzel J: The PSA test, *AJN* 98(4):14-15, 1998.

Hollander J, Diokno A: Prostatism: benign prostatic hyperplasia, *Urol Clin North Am* 23(2):75, 1996.

Howell A, Vorsa N: Scientists solve the mystery behind cranberry juice, *RN* 62(2):69, 1999.

Kaplan S, Te A: Transurethral electrovaporization of the prostate: a novel method of treating men with benign prostatic hyperplasia, *Urology* 45(4):566-572, 1995.

Kerton C: Assessing for bladder distention, *Nursing* 97(4):64, 1997.

Krames Communication: *Living with prostate cancer: AK-III Education Company,* San Bruno, CA, 1996, The Company.

Lueckenotte A: *Pocket guide to gerontologic assessment,* St. Louis, 1994, Mosby.

Marchiondo K: A new look at urinary tract infection, *AJN* 98(3):34-39, 1998.

Merril J, Enoch A: Prostatic cancer detection, *NGNA: New Horizons,* March-April, 1996.

Miller C: *Nursing care of older adults: theory and practice,* ed 3, Philadelphia, 1997, JB Lippincott.

O'Hanlon Nichols T: Lower urinary tract infections: treatment and prevention, *J Urol Nurs* 14(3):1120, 1995.

Reno B, Batchelor N: Genitourinary problems. In Luggen AS, Travis SS, Meiner SE, editors: *NGNA core curriculum for gerontological advanced practice nurses,* Thousand Oaks, CA, 1998, Sage.

Stanley M, Blair K: *Gerontological nursing: a health promotion/protection approach,* ed 2, 1999, Philadelphia, FA Davis.

Stockert P: Getting UTI patients back on track, *RN* 62(3):49-52, 1999.

Strong B, Devault C: *Human sexuality,* ed 5, New York, 1994, McGraw-Hill.

Tuttle J: VLAP is quicker, less painful, and cheaper than a TURP, *Clin Laser Month* 12:187-189, 1993.

Willis D: Taming the overgrown prostate, *AJN* 92(2):34-40, 1992.

Zaccagnini M: Prostatic cancer, *AJN* 99(4):34-35, 1999.

CHAPTER 15

HEMATOLOGICAL PROBLEMS

Ann Schmidt Luggen

LEARNING OBJECTIVES

Upon completion of this chapter, the reader will be able to:

- List the most common forms of anemias among older adults
- Discuss the nursing management of older adults with anemias
- Name the stages of the disease course of chronic lymphocytic leukemia
- Describe the nursing management of chronic lymphocytic leukemia

I. ANEMIAS

A. Definition: anemia is a decrease in circulating red blood cell mass
   1. There is a decrease in hemoglobin (hb) with aging
   2. If patient is greater than 65 years old, evaluate if Hb <14, hematocrit (Hct) <42
B. Iron-deficiency anemia
   1. Can result from slow gastrointestinal bleeding, esophageal varices, hemorrhoids, diverticulosis, or cancer
   2. Also a result of poor dietary intake of foods with iron content, defective absorption
   3. Pathophysiology
      a. Chronic, microcytic-hypochromic anemia
      b. Erythrocytes are small and pale with low hemoglobin levels
      c. Develops slowly with three identifiable stages
         (1) Stage I: body's stores of iron are depleted
         (2) Stage II: insufficient iron is transported to bone marrow
         (3) Stage III: small, hemoglobin-deficient cells enter the circulation in large numbers, replacing normal erythrocytes as they age; hemoglobin production is diminished
   4. Typical clinical presentation
      a. Attention is not sought until hemoglobin level is about 7 to 8 g/dl
      b. Shortness of breath
      c. Weakness, fatigue
      d. Fingertips, earlobes, palms, and conjunctival pallor
      e. Nails become thin, brittle, and spoon shaped or concave
      f. Sore tongue with redness and burning
      g. Soreness and dryness at the corners of the mouth, cracking may occur
   5. Nursing management: interventions
      a. Assess for sensory and motor function, mental status, cardiovascular and respiratory function, and gastrointestinal function
      b. Provide a safe environment to prevent injury
      c. Assist with ambulation during weakness or fatigue periods

       d. Maintain a warm environment

       e. Monitor vital signs for reportable changes

       f. Assist with frequent gentle mouth care

       g. Instruct in dietary changes that will increase intake of iron sources

   6. Nursing diagnoses

       a. Fatigue: related to decreased tissue oxygenation

       b. Sensory/perceptual alterations: related to tissue hypoxia

       c. Skin integrity, impaired

       d. Nutrition, altered: less than body requirements

C. Pernicious anemia

   1. Chronic, progressive, macrocytic (megaloblastic) anemia caused by a deficiency of intrinsic factor

   2. Pathophysiology

       a. Atrophy of the glandular mucosa of the gastric fundus leads to a lack of intrinsic factor

       b. Prolonged iron-deficiency anemia can lead to gastric atrophy and then to pernicious anemia

       c. Shilling test: distinguishes between B_{12} deficiency because of lack of intrinsic factor and malabsorption

       d. Treatment: cyanocobalamin injections

   3. Typical clinical presentation remains the same as with iron-deficiency anemia (see Section I, B4)

   4. Nursing management: interventions

       a. Monitor vital signs and report abnormal findings

       b. Prepare the patient for administration of vitamin B_{12} injections monthly for the rest of his/her life

       c. Maintain bedrest and assist with ambulation during the acute phase

       d. Use a bed cradle to prevent pressure on lower extremities

       e. Encourage patient to eat a diet high in vitamins, iron, and protein

       f. See other nursing interventions under iron-deficiency anemia

   5. Nursing diagnoses

       a. Injury, risk for: related to sensory and motor losses; alteration in mental status

       b. Skin integrity impaired, risk for: related to capillary fragility

       c. Gas exchange, impaired: related to inadequate number and impaired function of erythrocytes

D. Posthemorrhagic anemia (can follow any type of surgery in the older adult)

   1. Rapid loss of a smaller volume is more dangerous than a slower loss of more blood

       a. Loss of 20% of total blood volume can result in vascular insufficiency

       b. Loss of 30% of total blood volume can cause circulatory failure, shock, and coma

       c. Loss of 40% of total blood volume leads to death unless STAT blood replacement is performed

   2. Pathophysiology

       a. Within 24 hours, the reduced blood volume moves fluids from the interstitium into the blood vessels and plasma volume expands

       b. A decrease in viscosity of the blood causes the flow to be faster and with greater turbulence than normal blood

       c. Response can be ventricular dysfunction, cardiac dilation, and heart valve insufficiency

       d. Hypoxia causes arterioles, capillaries, and venules to dilate, speeding blood flow

       e. Congestive heart failure may result when the heart must pump harder and faster to prevent congestion from the rapid venous return

   3. Typical clinical presentation

       a. Signs and symptoms of hypovolemia and hypoxemia

         • Tachycardia

         • Hypotension

- Cold skin, may be moist, with pallor
- Weakness, lethargy
- Decreased urinary output

b. Changes specific to the aging process
- Skin may not be moist
- Confusion, irritability, or stupor
- Rapid deep respirations that later become shallow

4. Nursing management: interventions
   a. Prepare to administer blood and fluid replacement
      (1) Observe for blood reaction during replacement infusion; flank pain, chills, fever, and hematuria
      (2) Observe for fluid overload when high volumes are administered
   b. Monitor apical pulse, heart sounds, orthostatic BP, and respirations
   c. Measure intake and output (urinary output of >30 ml/hr needed)
   d. Prepare to administer oxygen and monitor blood gases
   e. Provide rest and anticipate patient's needs
   f. Instruct patient to avoid stress (e.g., nonproductive coughing, straining at stool)
   g. Once the crisis has passed, instruct in dietary and pharmacological measures to increase iron intake

5. Nursing diagnoses
   a. Cardiac output, decreased: related to decreased circulating blood volume
   b. Tissue perfusion, altered: peripheral
   c. Fluid volume deficit: related to loss of blood volume

II. CHRONIC LYMPHOCYTIC LEUKEMIA

A. Disease of older adults, often discovered as an incidental finding on routine CBC; life span normal, 5 years; median survival, 9 years
B. Symptoms: weakness, fatigue, weight loss, cardiovascular disease, abdominal pain, lymphadenopathy, infection, splenomegaly; 25% of patients are symptomatic
C. Laboratory: CBC (complete blood count) with high lymphocyte count >15,000, small mature lymphocytes
D. Disease course
   1. Stage 0: asymptomatic; 60% at diagnosis; >10 years life expectancy
   2. Stage 1: lymphocytosis >50,000
   3. Stage 2: lymphocytosis + hepatomegaly or splenomegaly
   4. Stage 3: lymphocytosis + hgb <11
   5. Stage 4: lymphocytosis + thrombocytopenia
E. Treatment
   1. No cure, treat symptomatically
   2. Palliative therapy
      a. Radiation
      b. Chemotherapy for bone marrow failure
         - For bulky symptomatic disease
         - For increased lymphocytosis >100,000
         - Chlorambucil
      c. Surgery: splenectomy
F. Nursing management
   1. Pain: because of tumor growth, infection, chemotherapy side effects
      a. Assess frequently, administer analgesics, monitor side effects
      b. Teach relaxation techniques, distraction, imagery
   2. Activity intolerance because of anemia, side effects of chemotherapy
      a. Encourage frequent rest periods

     b. Light activity as tolerated

     c. Nutritional supplements as needed

     d. Energy conservation techniques

  3. Teach patient to minimize risk of infection

  4. Avoid aspirin, NSAIDs, which may interfere with platelet function

REFERENCES

Belcher AE: *Blood disorders: Mosby's clinical nursing series,* St Louis, 1993, Mosby.

Bialor B: Hematology. In Ferri F, Fretwell M, Wachtel T: *The care of the geriatric patient,* ed 2, St Louis, 1997, Mosby.

Duffy E, Meiner S: Hematology/anemias. In Luggen AS, Travis SS, Meiner SE: *NGNA core curriculum for gerontological advanced practice nurses,* Thousand Oaks, CA, 1998, Sage.

Ferri F: Vitamin B_{12} deficiency. In Ferri F, Fretwell M, Wachtel T: *The care of the geriatric patient,* ed 2, St Louis, 1997, Mosby.

Lippincott JB: *Lippincott manual of nursing practice,* ed 6, CD-ROM, Philadelphia, 1996, JB Lippincott.

Miller CA: *Nursing care of older adults,* ed 3, Philadelphia, 1999, JB Lippincott.

Tyson SR: *Gerontological nursing care,* Philadelphia, 1999, WB Saunders.

Wachtel TJ: Hematologic malignancies. In Ferri F, Fretwell M, Wachtel T: *The care of the geriatric patient,* ed 2, St Louis, 1997, Mosby.

Wold GH: *Basic geriatric nursing,* ed 2, St Louis, 1999, Mosby.

CHAPTER 16

MUSCULOSKELETAL PROBLEMS

Ann Schmidt Luggen

LEARNING OBJECTIVES

Upon completion of this chapter, the reader will be able to:

- Describe the mobility problems of older adults
- Discuss the role of nursing in the management of falls
- Define types of osteoporosis and the extent of the problem
- Differentiate different types of arthritis and the management of each type

I. MOBILITY PROBLEMS, FALLS, AND FRACTURES

A. Definitions
   1. Impairment: loss or abnormality of anatomical, physiological, or psychological structure or function
   2. Disability: restriction or lack of ability to perform a normal activity, resulting from impairment
   3. Handicap: disadvantage resulting from impairment or disability that limits or prevents the fulfillment of a role normal to the individual
B. Theory: functional elements needed for mobility
   1. Cognition and motivation: needed to think through steps that need to be initiated for self-movement and the motivation to undertake the energy expenditure to accomplish tasks of mobility
   2. Skeletal system: intact and capable of supporting body weight to perform logical and critical steps of mobility
   3. Muscular system: strong and functional to propel the body in activities such as walking, running
   4. Neurological system: allows interaction with musculoskeletal system
C. Anatomy and physiology of normal structure and function
   1. Skeletal bones
      a. Give shape to musculoskeletal system; continual processes of formation and reabsorption throughout the lifespan; bone growth regulated by physical activity, weight-bearing, and genetic factors
      b. Trabecular bone forms majority of bone in vertebral body and flat bones
      c. Cortical bone forms most of long bones
      d. Bone composed of 95% collagen fiber and bone salts, including calcium, phosphate, and other minerals
   2. Ligaments, muscles, tendons, joints, and bursae
      a. Ligaments are flexible bands of strong connective tissue connecting articular bone; allow freedom of movement

      b. Tendons are fibrous cords of connective tissue that connect muscles to bone

      c. Joints are points of articulation between bone structures

      d. Bursae are small, fluid-filled sacs that surround joints and prevent friction

   3. Muscular/neurological system

      a. Muscles interact with the neurological system to produce body movements

         (1) Flexion is the movement in which both ends of any part are pulled together (bending)

         (2) Extension is the movement in which both ends of a part are pulled apart (straightening)

         (3) Abduction is the lateral movement of the limb away from the medial plane of the body

         (4) Adduction is the movement of a limb toward the medial plane of the body

         (5) Pronation is the act of turning, such as palm of the hand downward

         (6) Supination is the act of turning, such as palm of the hand upward

         (7) External and internal rotation is a muscle revolving a part on its axis

         (8) Atrophy occurs if muscles are not used; it leads to decrease in muscle size and strength

D. Mobility changes that occur with aging

   1. Loss of bone mass: after age 40-50 there is incremental process of bone absorption without successful new bone formation, leading to gradual loss of bone; this loss is greater in women, especially following cessation of menses; initial loss occurs in trabecular bone, leading to compression fractures in the vertebral column; later, cortical bone loss occurs, leading to femoral bone fractures

   2. Loss of muscle strength: muscle cells decrease with aging; degree of muscle strength loss varies among muscle groups and among people, depending on exercise

   3. Decrease in reaction time: with decline in the neurological system, reaction time and speed of movement declines, ultimately affecting muscle strength

   4. Decreased speed of movement: lack of exercise causes loss of muscle strength and speed of recovery following exercise

E. Common health problems affecting mobility in older adults

   1. Osteoporosis (see Section II, pp. 106-107)

   2. Osteomalacia

      a. Inadequate supply of calcium and phosphorus in bone tissue matrix, often caused by vitamin D deficiency, lack of sunshine, dietary deficiency, inability to absorb nutrients because of digestive disorders

      b. Women lose bone mass more rapidly than men

      c. With bone loss, bone strength decreases and thinning of the vertebral body of the spine occurs

   3. Arthritis: osteoarthritis, rheumatoid arthritis, gout (see Sections III, IV, V)

   4. Polymyalgia rheumatica

      a. Chronic common inflammatory disease of older adults >65, characterized by pain and stiffness of neck, shoulders, and hips

      b. Females to males: ratio 2:1

      c. Seen most often in Caucasians in North America

      d. Related to giant cell arteritis

      e. Abrupt onset, difficulty getting out of bed, symmetrical symptoms

      f. Tenderness and limitation of movement, elevated ESR (40 to >100)

      g. Treat with prednisone medically for 1 to 2 years; can recur

      h. Nursing care focuses on pain relief, education about prednisone, and activity-rest patterns

   5. Fibromyalgia

      a. Rheumatic condition characterized by chronic aching, stiffness, pain, and tenderness of musculoskeletal system

      b. Widespread pain of 3 months' duration with multiple tender points, sleep disturbances, morning fatigue, emotional stress

      c. Normal laboratory studies

      d. Treatment centers on alleviation of emotional distress, hot showers, moderate activity, rest, massage of affected areas, local heat, avoidance of cold and wet weather, and analgesics for pain

   6. Foot disorders

      a. Congenital and non-congenital foot disorders may alter the foot's basic structure and interfere with gait by shortening tendons and debilitating foot muscles and ligaments

      b. Corns, hammertoe, and bunions (hallux valgus) affect ability to walk and cause pain

      c. Assess feet: cleanliness, skin condition (dry, scaly, edema, color)

      d. Assess toes: infection, fungus, nails ingrown and thickened

      e. Treatment involves podiatry, physical therapy, medicine, nursing

      f. Treatment may involve special footwear or surgical procedures

F. Falls

   1. Important health problem of those >75 years of age, especially women

   2. Causes: physical frailty, visual impairment, psychological stress, polypharmacy, environmental hazards, physical illness, tranquilizers and sleeping pills, urinary bladder dysfunction

   3. Environmental hazards include inadequate lighting, absence of rails on stairs and bathtubs, slippery floors, obstructions in pathways (pets, piles of objects, cords), uneven surfaces

   4. Most falls occur during the day; but most falls from bed occur at night

   5. A previous fall is a predictor for future falls

   6. Precipitating factors

      a. Physical activities: rising from a chair, bending, walking, running, using stairs

      b. Physical conditions: dizziness, medications, sensory deficits, weakness, arthritis/stiffness

      c. Environment: furniture, floor surfaces, walkers, canes, wheelchairs, vehicles, poor-fitting shoes

   7. Falls are the leading cause of injury in institutionalized elders >75 years

   8. Falls are the second leading cause of all accidental deaths

   9. Falls account for 90% of all reported hospital incidents

  10. Nursing management

      a. Diagnoses

        • Injury, risk for: related to falls

        • Mobility, impaired physical

      b. Goals: prevent injury, promote optimum mobility, prevent deformity

      c. Interventions: use assistive devices and techniques to facilitate mobility safely; maintain adequate nutrition and fluid intake; maintain normal elimination

      d. Consult with physical therapy, occupational therapy

      e. Provide environmental assessment and intervention

      f. Conduct assessment of musculoskeletal, neurological systems

      g. Educate about need for exercise, proper use of assistive devices, problems of immobility, risk reduction

G. Fractures

   1. Hip fractures have high morbidity and mortality; 15% to 20% of patients die as a result of complications each year; complications include immobility, pneumonia, sepsis/urinary tract infection, pressure ulcers

      a. X-ray the hip if there is pain and difficulty ambulating with weight-bearing

      b. Surgical management will include a pin or prosthesis

      c. Physical therapy usually begins within days following surgery

      d. Post-surgical complications include deep vein thrombosis, infection from Foley catheter, delirium/confusion, constipation/impaction, pressure ulcers

      e. Multidisciplinary rehabilitation program necessary

      f. Discharge planning should include assistance because of impaired mobility and potential for social isolation

      g. Outcome is self-care and independence

  2. Vertebral compression fractures are common and present as back pain

      a. May present as acute pain in the middle to low thoracic vertebrae during routine daily activities such as opening a window, making the bed

      b. Treatment is symptomatic relief and bed rest (however comfort can be attained)

      c. Pain treatment with muscle relaxants, heat, analgesics, as needed

      d. Moving from the bed slowly and with support

      e. Supervised exercises to increase tone; swimming maintains flexibility

      f. Educate to prevent back strain; to avoid twisting, forceful movements and bending; teach how to lift and carry heavy objects

  3. Pelvic fractures occur often after a fall

      a. Pelvic fractures represent only 3% of fractures but 5% to 20% of cases of mortality in older adults with fractures

      b. May cause intra-abdominal injury, such as lacerated colon

      c. Cause dysfunctional walking; often patients require a walker, cane; patients may fear walking and falling after occurrence

II. OSTEOPOROSIS

  A. Definition

    1. Type I, postmenopausal osteoporosis: results from rapid drop of estrogen production; estrogen is important for calcium absorption into bone; a contributing factor is a diet deficient in calcium and vitamin D

    2. Type II, age-related or "senile" osteoporosis: occurs in both men and women over age 70; results from the steady decline of bone mass over time; age-related changes in renal function that slow down conversion of vitamin D may also contribute to the problem

  B. Incidence: 10 million Americans have osteoporosis; 18 million are at risk; about 30% of women over 60 have clinical osteoporosis; bone mass declines about 2% to 3% per year after menopause; 1:2 women and 1:5 men are likely to experience osteoporotic fractures/year; 700,000 per year occur in the United States; for patients experiencing hip fractures, 15% to 20% die from complications each year

  C. Risk factors: age; sex; Caucasian or Asian race; heredity; decreased estrogen and testosterone; drug use, such as steroids, thyroid, and heparin; lifelong calcium deficiency; low weight (obesity is protective); immobilization; tobacco use; and heavy alcohol intake

  D. Disease characteristics: loss of height because of compression fractures, stooped posture (kyphosis), protruding abdomen (ribcage drops because compression fractures of vertebrae in spine)

  E. Lab: bone scans (DEXA) estimate risk for fracture, comparing patient with 30-year-old female normal value

  F. Therapy

    1. ERT: estrogen replacement therapy slows rate of bone loss; usually given with calcium supplements and vitamin D

    2. Alendronate (Fosamax): given with 6 to 8 oz water on empty stomach; advise patient to sit up for 30 minutes after, without other medications or food, to avoid common esophageal irritation side effect

    3. Calcitonin (Miacalcin) nasal spray: increases spinal bone mass; it irritates nasal passages, so advise alternating nostrils, storing in refrigerator

    4. Raloxifene (Evista): prevents osteoporosis, is a selective estrogen receptor modulator; prevents bone loss without risk of uterine cancer as may occur with estrogen; can cause venous thrombosis

G. Nursing management
   1. Educate on high risk for injury from fractures
   2. Educate on fall prevention, fall awareness, assess environment; assess vision, mobility, muscle strength, flexibility
   3. Manage pain from compression fractures, inflammation, bleeding; may take 1 to 2 months to subside; use cool packs, ice packs for 24 to 48 hours with analgesics and limited periods of bedrest
   4. Advise to avoid recliners, which increase weight on the spine
   5. Advise to avoid activities such as raising garage door and windows, lifting heavy bags, pushing vacuum
   6. Medicare (7/1/98) now provides coverage for bone density measurement

III. Osteoarthritis (OA)

A. Definition: localized disease of cartilage in which there is degeneration and loss of cartilage and new formation of bone and cartilage at the joint margins (osteophytes); there may be a secondary synovitis in the joint lining; 80% of people >70 have x-ray evidence of OA
B. Classification: primary and secondary osteoarthritis
   1. Primary osteoarthritis: idiopathic, of unknown cause, in three or more joints; examples are Heberden's and Bouchard's nodes (osteophytes) in interphalangeal joints of hands or feet; occurs most often in women
   2. Secondary osteoarthritis: caused by trauma, congenital abnormalities such as congenital hip displacement, endocrine abnormalities such as obesity, and other bone and joint disorders such as Charcot's arthropathy
C. Risk factors: increased age, female gender, genetic predisposition, congenital abnormalities, joint stress and trauma such as occurs through repetitive use (housemaid's knee), and obesity
D. Clinical features: pain, stiffness, loss of mobility, bony enlargement, crepitus (crunching sound on movement), synovial effusion (fluid); no lab abnormalities; x-ray abnormalities do not correlate well with clinical severity
E. Pain characteristics: worse with use; improves with rest (does not improve with rest with severe OA); stiffness is worst with rest, improves with activity
F. Joint examination: knee is most commonly affected joint; also hip joint and fingers commonly involved; physical findings: swelling, tenderness, pain on movement, muscle wasting, deformity (enlargement), decreased range of motion, crepitus, occasional warmth with effusion
G. Nursing diagnoses: pain, chronic; mobility, impaired physical; self-care deficit
H. Nursing management: includes goals of pain management, preservation of function and mobility, and patient education
I. Interventions
   1. Weight reduction
   2. Protection of joints from overuse, especially weight-bearing joints; use cane for knee OA—use in hand opposite affected joint
   3. Physical therapy to reduce spasm, relieve pain, increase range of motion
   4. Use of around-the-clock acetaminophen unless pain is episodic (<4000 mg/qd); monitor liver function; new Cox-2 inhibitor drugs may be useful for older adults with history of GI bleeding
   5. Use narcotics for acute joint flares or end-stage severe disease
   6. Patient may receive intra-articular injections of corticosteroids for flares

IV. Rheumatoid Arthritis (RA)

A. Definition: systemic autoimmune disorder, cause unknown, characterized by chronic, symmetrical erosive synovitis of peripheral joints; joint destruction and deformity commonly occurs

B. Incidence/prevalence: occurs in about 10% of those >65; female to male ratio is 2.5:1; the prevalence increases with age

C. Classification: seropositive and seronegative RA
   1. Seropositive RA: 80% have positive rheumatoid factor, an autoantibody; this is associated with severe, progressive disease with diminished life expectancy
   2. Seronegative RA: less severe disease course; may become positive for rheumatoid factor after a number of years

D. Clinical manifestations: major finding at diagnosis is symmetrical polyarthritis with inflammation; onset of disease in older adults usually more abrupt compared to younger adults; more systemic features such as weight loss, shoulder involvement, less hand and foot involvement, positive rheumatoid factor; affected shoulder difficult to detect on physical exam and "frozen" shoulder may occur without preventative exercises; patients may have muscle spasms, pain, tenderness, swelling, erythema, morning stiffness, depression, fever (low grade)

E. Specific joints commonly affected
   1. Hands: common deformities are the 'swan-neck' deformity of fingers with flexion of proximal and hyper-extension of the distal joints
   2. Wrist: carpal tunnel syndrome common from nerve compression
   3. Foot and ankle: RA affects metatarsophalangeal joint most commonly; when these joints are affected, function of the individual is greatly affected
   4. Hip: common; symptoms occur in groin, thigh, lower back, or knee
   5. Knee: effusions easily observed; assess for Baker's cyst, which can rupture and mimics thrombophlebitis
   6. Cervical spine: common involvement in cervical spine, rare in thoracic, lumbar
   7. Shoulder: see preceding discussion

F. Extra-articular problems
   1. Rheumatoid nodules in 25% to 50% of RA, occurring in acute flares; they are subcutaneous on tendons and bursae and in the heart on valves; also occur in the lung
   2. Pleuritis and interstitial lung disease: difficult to diagnose; seen at autopsy
   3. Pericarditis: rarely diagnosed but often found at autopsy (50%)
   4. Neurological problems: cervical myelopathy, nerve entrapment with synovitis

G. Management: rest, activity modification, patient education, physical therapy, joint protection, NSAIDs, DMARDs, pain control

H. Pharmacological: pyramid approach of increasingly more potent drugs
   1. NSAIDs (nonsteroidal antiinflammatory drugs)
      a. GI bleeding problems common
      b. Include naproxen, ibuprofen
      c. Cox-2 inhibitors said to cause fewer bleeding complications
   2. DMARDs (disease-modifying antirheumatic drugs)
      a. Require frequent lab monitoring
      b. Include gold, azathioprine, hydroxychloroquine, methotrexate
      c. May be used in conjunction with NSAIDs or prior to NSAIDs
   3. Glucocorticoids
      a. Antiinflammatory, immunosuppressive
      b. Used for acute flares; tapered and discontinued quickly or given as intra-articular injection

I. Nursing diagnoses: pain, acute and chronic; mobility, impaired physical; self-care deficit; depression; fatigue: social isolation; home maintenance management, impaired; body image disturbance

J. Nursing management
   1. Education: cornerstone of management of chronic illnesses; focus areas
      a. Maintenance or improvement of function, psychosocial status
      b. Self-management of pain
      c. Self-management of other symptoms

2. Pain management (see Pain, Chapter 25)
   a. Warm baths usually helpful in morning for stiffness and pain
3. Rest and exercise
   a. Program of rest and activity essential; fatigue common
   b. Exercise needed via physical therapy program to maintain flexibility and exercises to maintain strength
   c. Arthritis Foundation has aquatic programs for non–weight-bearing exercises
4. Impaired mobility
   a. Assess ADLs and follow over time
   b. Identify need for adaptive, assistive equipment, which is available (e.g., jar openers, large-handled spoons and pencils)
   c. Occupational therapists can help with splints to rest specific joints

V. GOUT

A. Definition: genetic defect of purine metabolism, which causes excess uric acid crystal accumulation in joints; acute inflammation reaction in and around joint secondary to deposition of crystals; gout is caused by overproduction and/or under-excretion of uric acid; may be family history of gout
B. Clinical presentation: sudden onset of pain and swelling and limitation of mobility in a distal joint, often the foot, great toe (50% of first attacks); joint is warm, dusky red, very sensitive to touch; more common in women; often occurs around Heberden's nodes
C. Characteristics: hyperuricemia (>7 mg/dl); monoarticular (one joint) arthritis attacks with tophaceous deposits of uric acid crystals in and around joints and kidneys; acute attacks are less frequent in older adults; treated as chronic gout after several acute episodes
D. Diagnosis: aspiration urate crystals from joint
E. Prevention: hyperuricemia does not equate to gout; diet: avoid high purine foods, such as red and organ meats, shellfish, game, lunch meats, meat gravy; also alcohol
F. Management: education, pain control, medications, prevention
   1. Acute gout management
      a. NSAIDs (nonsteroidal antiinflammatory drugs): tolerated better than colchicine (indomethacin not tolerated by older adults)
      b. Colchicine: poorly tolerated especially in older adults; causes GI distress, including nausea, vomiting, diarrhea if taken by mouth; can be given IV after surgery but toxic; so give 50% of dose to older adults; extravasation is a problem; give slowly, carefully
      c. Joint aspiration: for a single inflammatory joint can give relief
      d. Intra-articular steroids
      e. Bedrest and joint immobilization
      f. Ice packs or heat may be useful for pain
   2. Chronic gout management
      a. Long-term use of medications may cause toxicity in older adults
      b. Allopurinol given for uric acid over-producers; usually given concomitantly with colchicine to avoid induction of an acute attack; side effects include rash, GI upset, headache, alopecia, fever
      c. Probenicid given for uric acid under-excretors; monitor renal status

REFERENCES

Burrage RL, Sutter CA: Arthritis. In Stone J, Wyman J, Salisbury S, editors: *Clinical gerontological nursing,* ed 2, Philadelphia, 1999, WB Saunders.

Dennis C: Maintaining wellness of bones and muscles. In Tyson SR, editor: *Gerontological nursing care,* Philadelphia, 1999, WB Saunders.

Dowd R, Cavalieri RJ: Help your patient live with osteoporosis, *AJN* 99(4):55-60, 1999.

Luggen A, Luggen M: Arthritis and musculoskeletal/immunological disorders: osteoporosis, mobility issues, pain and comfort. In Luggen AS, Travis SS, Meiner SE, editors: *NGNA core curriculum for gerontological advanced practice nurses,* Thousand Oaks, CA, 1998, Sage.

Miller CA: *Nursing care of older adults,* ed 3, Philadelphia, 1999, JB Lippincott.

Patillo MM, Stanley M: The aging musculoskeletal system. In Stanley M, Beare PG, editors: *Gerontological nursing,* ed 2, Philadelphia, 1999, FA Davis.

Sanders RG: Arthritis in the elderly, *Audio Digest Intern Med* 45(09), 1999, California Medical Association.

Solomon J: Osteoporosis—when supports weaken, *RN* 61(5):37-40, 1998.

CHAPTER 17

METABOLIC AND ENDOCRINE PROBLEMS

Sue E. Meiner

LEARNING OBJECTIVES

Upon completion of this chapter, the reader will be able to:

- Identify disorders of temperature regulation that are extremes of hot and cold experiences
- Name and describe the type of diabetes most commonly diagnosed in older adults
- Describe the most common form and nursing management of hypothyroidism/hyperthyroidism
- Discuss the metabolic deviations that can lead to imbalances in the older adult
- List the postmenopausal changes that occur in women

I. HYPOTHERMIA/HYPERTHERMIA

A. Definition: thermoregulation is the hypothalamic control and maintenance of core body temperature (97° to 99° F) in a range of environmental temperatures; hypothermia is less than normal core body temperature; hyperthermia is higher than normal core body temperature

B. Age-related changes
 1. Inefficient vasoconstriction
 2. Decreased cardiac output
 3. Decreased subcutaneous tissue
 4. Diminished shivering
 5. Diminished sensory perception of temperatures
 6. Diminished thirst perception

C. External factors affecting thermoregulation: age-related decrease in febrile response

D. Hypothermia: core body temperature 95° F or below
 1. Physiological changes
  - Muscle contraction
  - Increased heart rate
  - Peripheral vasoconstriction
  - Shivering (produces heat, causes vasodilatation)
  - Pituitary activity, resulting in thyroxine and corticosteroid secretion
 2. Risk factors
  - Increased age (>75)
  - Inactivity/immobility
  - Infection
  - Alcohol
  - Antidepressants

- Electrolyte imbalance
- Dehydration
- Diabetes
- Hypothyroidism
- Cardiovascular disease
- Cerebrovascular disease
- Cold exposure

3. Stages of hypothermia
   a. Early: no signs or symptoms; no feeling of cold; temperature lower than usual baseline
   b. Mid: mental functioning impaired, slurred speech, slowed or irregular pulse, diminished tendon reflexes, slowed and shallow respiration
   c. Late: hypothermia progresses rapidly after the core body temperature falls to 93° F; muscular rigidity occurs; diminished urinary output; stupor; coma; skin cool and pink

4. Intra-postoperative hypothermia
   a. Causative factors
      - Cold operating rooms
      - Intravenous infusions at room temperature
      - Peripheral vasodilatation from medications
      - Skin exposure, thin draping materials
   b. Nursing actions
      - Temperature monitoring
      - Warming blanket
      - Warmed intravenous solutions
      - Cardiac monitoring
      - Core rewarming (late stage) by cardiac bypass technique

E. Hyperthermia: core body temperature 99° F or above

1. Physiological changes
   - Diminished sweating
   - Diminished sensory perception of heat

2. Risk factors
   - Increased age (>75)
   - Sustained muscle activity
   - Infection
   - Alcohol
   - Medications: diuretics, neuroleptics, anticholinergics
   - Electrolyte imbalance
   - Dehydration
   - Diabetes
   - Hyperthyroidism
   - Cardiovascular disease
   - Cerebrovascular disease
   - Heat exposure

3. Forms of hyperthermia
   a. Heat cramps
      (1) Characterized by painful musculoskeletal cramps and spasms, usually caused by sodium depletion; associated with tender muscles and moist skin; body temperature may be normal or slightly elevated
      (2) Treatment consists of oral intake of a saline solution while resting in a cool place, and avoiding salt tablets because of gastric irritation
   b. Heat syncope
      (1) Characterized by a sudden episode of unconsciousness, resulting from cutaneous vasodilatation and subsequent hypotension (<100 mm/Hg), weak pulse; skin is cool and moist

(2) Treatment consists of recumbency and rest in a cool place and the intake of fluids (orally or intravenously)

c. Heat exhaustion

(1) Related to a gradual loss of salt and water in the presence of a hot environment

(2) Characterized by thirst, fatigue, nausea, oliguria, giddiness, and delirium; gastrointestinal flu-like symptoms are common

(3) Treatment consists of rest in a cool environment, intake of adequate fluids with salt replacement, intravenous fluids if needed

d. Heat stroke

(1) Severe life-threatening failure of thermoregulatory mechanisms, resulting in an excessive rise in body temperature (>104° F); most common in persons over >65, with a mortality as high as 80%; U.S. mortality from heat stroke is 5000 annually, with two thirds over age 60

(2) Characterized by absence of sweating, loss of consciousness, death, resulting from a failure to perceive environmental temperatures as the body temperature rises

(3) Treatment consists of removing excess clothing, rapid cooling of the core temperature (without producing shivering, which can produce a feedback elevation in temperature); methods include submersion in cold water and use of ice packs and spraying the body with tepid water with a fan blowing across the body to remove heat by convection

F. Nursing diagnoses

1. Thermoregulation, ineffective: hypothermia/hyperthermia

2. Fluid volume deficit: related to loss of fluids from heat

3. Knowledge deficit: related to cold (or heat) tolerance

4. Adaptive capacity, decreased: related to aging changes associated with hypothermia/hyperthermia

G. Nursing management

1. Patient education to eliminate risk factors associated with thermoregulation disorders (including financial considerations during extreme weather conditions, which may lead to decreased use of utilities to save money)

2. Instruct patient to select the proper clothing: layers during cold weather and lighter garments during hot weather

3. Check on older adults at risk for thermoregulation disorders

a. During heat alerts

b. In homes without air conditioning in hot weather

c. During electrical outages or interruptions of service

II. DIABETES MELLITUS (DM)

A. Definition: diabetes mellitus is a disorder of carbohydrate, protein, and fat metabolism, resulting from an imbalance between insulin availability and insulin need; it can be an absolute insulin deficiency, impaired release of insulin by the pancreatic beta cells, inadequate or defective insulin receptors, or the production of inactive insulin or insulin that is destroyed before it can be effective; the cause remains undecided, with autoimmunity, genetics, obesity, viruses, or lifestyle as possibilities

1. Female diabetic patients account for 19% of individuals over >65

2. Non-insulin-dependent diabetes mellitus (Type II) is the most common form of DM in older adults

B. Physiological changes associated with DM

1. Basal metabolic rate (BMR) diminishes with increased age

2. Diminished sensitivity to negative feedback control in hypothalamus and pituitary glands

3. Increased levels of circulating antidiuretic hormone (ADH)

4. Diminished secretion of sex hormones

5. Diminished thyroid hormonal balance (TSH and T_4)

      6. Decreased adrenal hormone secretion

      7. Decreased glucose tolerance with increasing age

      8. Increased renal threshold for glucose

C. Pathophysiology associated with DM

      1. Inadequate insulin production results in hyperglycemia, increased blood glucose

      2. Inadequate insulin production and hyperglycemia result in glycosuria (increased glucose in the urine)

      3. Use of protein stores and fat stores in DM (gluconeogenesis) causes ketoacidosis, with free fatty acids, ketones, and triglycerides in blood plasma

      4. Abnormal tissue changes with DM affect a number of body systems and organs

        a. Cardiovascular

        b. Renal

        c. Central nervous system

        d. Retina

D. Typical clinical presentation

      1. Assessment: subjective

        a. Fatigue

        b. Polydipsia, polyuria, polyphagia (classical symptom triad) may be missing in some older adults with DM

        c. Constipation or diarrhea

        d. Numbness and tingling in peripheral extremities

        e. Impotence: penile neuropathy with erectile failure affects at least 50% of men with DM over the age of 60

        f. Vaginal mucosa dryness: vaginal lubrication diminished and delayed

        g. Headache

      2. Assessment: objective

        a. Cardiovascular: angina, coronary heart disease, systolic hypertension, diminished peripheral pulses

        b. Integument: rashes, changes in oral mucosa, dry vaginal mucosa, breaks in skin that heal slowly, angiopathy from vascular and neurological changes, slowed healing, increased infection

        c. Eye: microvascular disease of retina, cataracts

        d. Renal: impaired renal function with proteinuria evident, diminished creatinine clearance

        e. Neurological: central—confusion, mental status alterations, arteriosclerosis, atherosclerosis; peripheral—diminished nerve function, slowed nerve conduction, loss of deep tendon reflexes (DTRs), burning, tingling, numbness, pain, weakness (neuropathy)

      3. Laboratory or diagnostic tests

        a. DM: fasting plasma glucose 126 mg/dl on one occasion

        b. Glucose tolerance test (GTT): preparation includes 8 to 12 hours NPO

        c. Impaired glucose tolerance test (IGT)

          (1) Fasting plasma glucose <140 mg/dl

          (2) Two-hour plasma glucose >140 and <200 with one intervening value >200 after a 75-g glucose load

        d. Baseline data to obtain

          (1) Fasting cholesterol and triglycerides

          (2) ECG

          (3) Urine culture and sensitivity, protein

          (4) Blood urea nitrogen (BUN), creatinine

          (5) Fasting blood sugar, random blood glucose

          (6) 24-hour collection for urine glucose (rarely done because of age-related changes in renal threshold)

E. Nursing management: interventions
   1. Teaching prevention of emergent or life-threatening events
      a. Hyperglycemia
         (1) Nutritional education and/or referral to registered dietitian (RD)
         (2) Exercise regimen
         (3) Blood glucose testing by finger stick method
      b. Hypoglycemia
         (1) Evaluation of need for or self-administration of oral hypoglycemic agents or insulin
         (2) Blood glucose testing by finger stick method
      c. Sepsis
   2. General patient education
      a. Medication administration and side effects/adverse reactions
      b. Pathophysiology of DM
      c. Monitoring of blood glucose and urine ketones
      d. Signs and symptoms of hyperglycemia and hypoglycemia
      e. Sick-day management
      f. Foot care, eye care, and potential complications
      g. Using the food exchange lists to prepare the diabetic diet
      h. Identification of emergency needs
      i. Need for regular, planned exercise
F. Nursing diagnoses
   1. Injury, risk for: related to decreased sensitivity in extremities
   2. Self-care deficit: related to inability to prepare insulin injections
   3. Health maintenance, altered
   4. Activity intolerance, risk for: related to maintaining a balance between diet, activity, and blood glucose levels
   5. Knowledge deficit: related to management of sick days
   6. Skin integrity, impaired: related to reduced sensitivity to injury
   7. Tissue perfusion, altered: related to complications of long-term hyperglycemia
   8. Pain: altered perception, related to decreased sensitivty in extremities

III. THYROID DISEASES

A. Hypothyroidism: alterations in immune function, taking specific medications, and mismanagement of hyperthyroidism contribute to the high incidence of hypothyroidism
   1. Incidence
      a. 15% of all clinical hypothyroidism occurs in patients >60
      b. Females outnumber males by 9:1 ratio
   2. Pathophysiology
      a. Increased fibrosis, lymphocyte infiltration, and nodularity
      b. Decreased T_4 production but normal serum T_4 and free T_4 because of decreased tissue utilization rate of T_4
      c. Decreased T_3 and free T_3 because of decreased T_3 production and conversion rate of T_4 to T_3
      d. Increased average TSH serum levels, partly caused by increased titers of antithyroid antibodies
      e. Despite the previous changes, overall thyroid gland function is adequately maintained throughout life
   3. Types of hypothyroidism
      a. Primary hypothyroidism: most common form of thyroid disease
         (1) Autoimmune disease (Hashimoto's thyroiditis)
         (2) Use of radioactive iodine for hyperthyroidism

          (3) Destruction, suppression, or removal of all or some of the thyroid tissue by thyroidectomy

          (4) Dietary iodide deficiency

          (5) Subacute thyroiditis

          (6) Lithium therapy

          (7) Over-treatment with antithyroid drugs

    b. Secondary hypothyroidism: inadequate secretion of TSH caused by disease of the pituitary gland (i.e., tumor, necrosis)

          (1) Inadequate secretion of thyroid hormone leads to a general slowing of all physical and mental processes

          (2) General depression of most cellular enzyme systems and oxidative processes

          (3) Metabolic activity of all cells of the body decreases; producing less body heat

  3. Nursing management of hypothyroidism: assessment

    a. Typical clinical presentation

          (1) General: fatigue and lethargy, social withdrawal, weight gain or loss, confusion

          (2) Neurological: depression, seizures, altered cerebellar functioning, dementia, mild psychotic disturbance

          (3) Gastrointestinal: constipation, fecal impaction

          (4) Musculoskeletal: myalgia, decreased mobility, falls

          (5) Genitourinary: incontinence

          (6) Cardiovascular: syncope, angina, congestive heart failure

          (7) Sensory: cold intolerance, complaints of cold hands and feet, reduced aural acuity

          (8) Integument: dry skin, coarse and dry thick hair, eyebrows sparse with loss of outer third margins, pitting or non-pitting edema of face and legs

    b. Interventions

          (1) Monitor vital signs frequently to detect changes in cardiovascular status

          (2) Monitor ECG tracing to detect arrhythmias

          (3) Prevent chilling to reduce strain on the heart

          (4) Avoid rapid rewarming techniques because of cardiovascular strain (CHF)

          (5) Assess for increase in episodes of angina and report findings

          (6) Instruct patient/family regarding medications that will need to be taken for the remainder of the patient's life

          (7) Instruct patient and family in nutritional and fluid balance needs—to limit calories and reduce weight (if needed)

  4. Laboratory/diagnostic tests

    a. Elevated plasma cholesterol

    b. Elevated triglycerides

    c. Thyroxine (T_4) levels low

    d. TSH elevated

  5. Nursing diagnoses for hypothyroidism

    a. Cardiac output, decreased: related to decreased metabolic rate

    b. Cardiac output, decreased: related to decreased cardiac conduction

    c. Nutrition, altered: related to lack of iodine in diet

    d. Knowledge deficit: related to signs and symptoms of hypothyroidism

    e. Activity intolerance: related to persistent lack of energy

B. Hyperthyroidism

  1. Pathophysiology: an excess delivery of thyroid hormone to the peripheral tissue

  2. Types: Graves' disease and thyroid storm

  3. Nursing management of hyperthyroidism: assessment

    a. Typical clinical presentation

          (1) General: sullen lethargy, anorexia, weight loss, may or may not have a goiter

          (2) Neurological: confusion, nervousness, agitation, irritability, with a fine muscle tremor

       (3) Gastrointestinal: constipation

       (4) Musculoskeletal: muscle weakness

       (5) Cardiovascular: palpitations, increased angina, tachycardia, arrhythmias, congestive heart failure

       (6) Sensory: decreased heat tolerance, excessive sweating, exophthalmos (may or may not be present)

       (7) Integument: moist, flushed skin, fine smooth hair

  b. Interventions

       (1) Offer patient support during administration of radioactive iodine or other medications and treatments

       (2) Encourage food intake to balance energy expenditures

       (3) Instruct in fall prevention

       (4) Instruct patient/family regarding medications that will need to be taken for the remainder of the patient's life

  4. Laboratory/diagnostic tests

    a. Thyroxine (T_4) elevated

    b. Triiodothyronine (T_3) elevated

  5. Nursing diagnoses

    a. Knowledge deficit: related to signs and symptoms of hyperthyroidism

    b. Anxiety: related to disease process

    c. Thought processes, altered: related to irritability and nervousness

IV. ELECTROLYTE IMBALANCES

A. Potassium

  1. Physiology and pathophysiology

    a. Vital role in maintaining resting membrane potential

       (1) Cardiac rhythm

       (2) Normal transmission/conduction of nerve impulses

       (3) Skeletal and muscle contraction

    b. Potassium not preserved in the body

    c. Sudden changes in potassium levels can be fatal

    d. Older adults are at risk when nutritional intake is poor

  2. Typical clinical presentation for potassium imbalances

    a. Hyperkalemia (blood level >5.5 mEq/L)

       (1) ECG changes: peaked T-wave, widened QRS, absent P-wave, depressed ST segment

       (2) Cardiac dysrhythmias

       (3) Abdominal cramping and diarrhea

       (4) Muscle irritability, progressing to weakness

       (5) Numbness or tingling

    b. Hypokalemia (blood level <3.5 mEq/L)

       (1) ECG changes: premature ventricular contractions, ST depression, depressed and inverted T-wave and prominent U-wave

       (2) Constipation and paralytic ileus

       (3) Muscle weakness and cramping

  3. Nursing management: interventions

    a. Hyperkalemia

       (1) Correct underlying problem after beginning IV fluids; may require glucose and insulin and calcium gluconate to prevent cardiac arrest

       (2) Monitor ECG patterns and report abnormal findings immediately

       (3) Prepare to administer Kayexalate to reduce potassium level

       (4) Monitor for signs of congestive heart failure

       (5) Perform peritoneal or hemodialysis

      (6) Instruct on food selection; foods high in potassium
- Fruits: bananas, cantaloupe, honeydew melon, oranges
- Vegetables: potatoes, broccoli, cabbage
- Canned white beans with/without pork and tomato sauce

  b. Hypokalemia
    (1) ECG monitoring
    (2) Prepare to administer oral potassium with water or juice (irritating to gastric mucosa if not diluted)
    (3) Assess for knowledge deficits concerning potassium-enriched foods

B. Sodium
  1. Physiology and pathophysiology
    a. Most powerful cation in extracellular fluid (ECF)
    b. Imbalances occur with alterations in body water volume
    c. Regulates osmolality and acid-base balance through sodium bicarbonate and sodium phosphate
    d. Increased excretion in the aging kidney
    e. Causes of hypernatremia
      (1) Failure to drink sufficient water; older adults commonly have a blunted thirst response
      (2) Diabetes insipidus, diarrhea, polyuria, diabetes mellitus, renal disease
      (3) Cushing's syndrome
      (4) High-sodium diet, over-use of saline IV fluids or hypertonic feedings
    f. Causes of hyponatremia
      (1) Sodium loss from vomiting, diarrhea, or GI suctioning
      (2) Burns and Addison's disease
      (3) Inadequate sodium intake because of low sodium diets and diuretics, water intoxication (drinking too much water)
      (4) IV fluid replacement with D5W without sodium replacement
      (5) Syndrome of inappropriate antidiuretic hormone (SIADH)
      (6) Comorbidity with hyperlipidemia, hyperproteinemia, and hyperglycemia
  2. Typical clinical presentation for sodium imbalances
    a. Hypernatremia (blood level >145 mEq/L)
      (1) Edema, weight gain, neurological changes because of cellular dehydration
      (2) Restlessness, agitation, lethargy, confusion
      (3) Decreased blood pressure, tachycardia, pulmonary edema, dry skin and mucous membranes
    b. Hyponatremia (blood level <136 mEq/L)
      (1) Confusion, apprehension, muscle weakness, lethargy, seizures, and coma
      (2) Dilutional hyponatremia presents as weight gain, edema, ascites, and jugular venous distention
  3. Nursing management: interventions
    a. Hypernatremia
      (1) Administer hypotonic IV and oral fluids slowly
      (2) Monitor for reduction of serum sodium at not greater than 2 mEq/L per hour for the first 48 hours
      (3) Assess for knowledge deficit regarding foods that are high in sodium (pizza, potato chips, cheeses, luncheon meats, soups, etc.)
      (4) Instruct patient to avoid caffeine products and alcohol because they promote diuresis; avoid taking OTC medications that are high in sodium
    b. Hyponatremia
      (1) Correct the underlying problem
      (2) Prepare to administer hypertonic saline IV if symptoms are severe
      (3) Restrict fluid as ordered

(4) Administer diuretics as ordered

(5) Assess for knowledge deficit regarding fluid restriction if condition is the result of excess fluid intake

C. Calcium

1. Physiology and pathophysiology

a. Found in bone tissue, 50% bound to protein in the blood, 40% free or ionized (physiologically most important)

b. Major cation for bones and teeth

c. Cofactor for blood clotting

d. Needed for transmission of nerve impulses and for muscle contractions

e. When calcium levels are increased, phosphate levels decrease (inverse relationship)

f. Controlled by parathyroid hormone, vitamin D, and calcitonin

g. Causes of hypercalcemia

(1) Hyperparathyroidism

(2) Bone metastases from breast, prostate, or cervical cancer

(3) Hypophosphatemia

(4) Excess vitamin D levels

(5) Excess use of calcium-containing antacids

h. Causes of hypocalcemia

(1) Decreased calcium intake (nutritional deficiency)

(2) Vitamin D deficiency

(3) Multiple blood transfusions (citrate binds with calcium)

(4) Pancreatitis

(5) Osteomalacia

(6) Parathyroid gland removal (hypoparathyroidism)

(7) Malabsorption

(8) High phosphorus due to renal failure

2. Typical clinical presentation for calcium imbalances

a. Hypercalcemia (blood level >10.5 mg/dl)

(1) Weakness, lethargy, fatigue, anorexia, nausea, constipation, and kidney stones

(2) ECG changes, shortened QT segment and depressed T-wave

b. Hypocalcemia (blood level <8.5 mg/dl)

(1) Confusion, paresthesia around the mouth

(2) Chvostek's sign (twitching of the mouth when the facial nerve below the temple is tapped)

(3) Trousseau's sign (carpopedal spasm when the BP cuff is inflated above the systolic pressure for 3 minutes)

(4) Intestinal cramping and hyperactive bowel sounds

(5) ECG changes, prolonged QT interval

(6) Convulsions and tetany

3. Nursing management: interventions

a. Hypercalcemia

(1) Correct the underlying problem

(2) Prepare to administer oral phosphate, normal saline, and diuretics to enhance renal excretion

(3) Assess for knowledge deficit regarding foods high in calcium (dairy products, oatmeal, spinach)

(4) Assess the use of calcium-containing antacids

b. Hypocalcemia

(1) Correct the underlying problem

(2) Prepare to treat acute hypocalcemia with calcium gluconate or calcium chloride given slowly

(3) Monitor ECG patterns and report abnormalities

(4) Prepare to treat chronic hypocalcemia with oral calcium and vitamin D supplements
- Instruct to take 30 minutes before meals with milk

(5) Prepare to instruct on self-administration of phosphate binders (aluminum hydroxide) to lower phosphate levels, inversely raising calcium levels

(6) Instruct to avoid carbonated beverages that are high in phosphate

(7) Assess for knowledge deficit regarding foods high in calcium

D. Phosphate
  1. Physiology and pathophysiology
    a. Found primarily in bone
    b. Provides energy for muscle contraction (ATP)
    c. Has an inverse relationship with calcium (see previous discussion)
    d. Balance controlled by parathyroid hormone, vitamin D, and calcitonin
    e. Causes for hyperphosphatemia
      (1) Renal failure
      (2) Cathartic abuse, especially phosphate-containing enemas or laxatives
      (3) Hyperparathyroidism
    f. Causes for hypophosphatemia
      (1) Malabsorption syndrome, chronic diarrhea, diuretic therapy
      (2) Chronic alcohol abuse, vitamin D deficiency
      (3) Use of magnesium and aluminum-containing antacids
      (4) Hyperparathyroidism
  2. Typical clinical presentation for phosphate imbalances
    a. Hyperphosphatemia (blood level >4.5 mg/dl)
      (1) Confusion, paresthesia around the mouth
      (2) Chvostek's sign (twitching of the mouth when the facial nerve below the temple is tapped)
      (3) Trousseau's sign (carpopedal spasm when the BP cuff is inflated above the systolic pressure for 3 minutes)
      (4) Convulsions and tetany
      (5) ECG changes, prolonged QT interval
      (6) Intestinal cramping and hyperactive bowel sounds
    b. Hypophosphatemia (blood level <3.0 mg/dl)
      (1) Muscle weakness, confusion
      (2) Tachycardia
      (3) Hypercalcemia
  3. Nursing management: interventions
    a. Hyperphosphatemia
      (1) Correct the underlying problem
      (2) Prepare to administer aluminum hydroxide to bind phosphate in the GI tract and eliminate in feces
      (3) Prepare patient for peritoneal or hemodialysis when ordered
      (4) Assess for knowledge deficit regarding foods high in phosphate (e.g., beef liver, sole, lentils, canned clams, soybeans)
    b. Hypophosphatemia
      (1) Correct the underlying problem
      (2) Use extreme caution when IV phosphate is given (monitor for hypocalcemia)
      (3) Prepare to administer oral phosphates as ordered
      (4) Assess for knowledge deficit regarding use of antacids and laxatives
E. Magnesium
  1. Physiology and pathophysiology
    a. Major intracellular cation with similar action of potassium

       b. Absorbed from the small intestines with calcium
       c. Assists with the transmission and conduction of nerve impulses and the contraction of skeletal, smooth, and cardiac muscles
       d. Increased calcium or phosphorus intake can decrease magnesium absorption from the intestines
       e. Causes of hypermagnesemia (blood level >2.5 mEq/L)
          (1) Renal failure
          (2) Overuse of magnesium-containing antacids
          (3) Severe dehydration
       f. Causes of hypomagnesemia (blood level <1.5 mEq/L)
          (1) Malnutrition, malabsorption syndrome
          (2) Alcoholism
          (3) Renal disease or thiazide diuretics
          (4) Total parenteral nutrition (TPN) without appropriate magnesium replacement

   2. Typical clinical presentation for magnesium imbalances
       a. Hypermagnesemia
          (1) Nausea, vomiting
          (2) Muscle weakness
          (3) Hypotension, bradycardia
          (4) Respiratory depression
       b. Hypomagnesemia
          (1) Irritability, muscle weakness, tetany, convulsions
          (2) Cardiac dysrhythmias
          (3) Abdominal distention

   3. Nursing management: interventions
       a. Hypermagnesemia
          (1) Correct the underlying problem
          (2) Prepare patient for peritoneal or hemodialysis
          (3) Assess for knowledge deficit regarding constipation problems
             • Avoid laxatives
             • Eat foods high in fiber
             • Intake adequate amounts of fluid daily
             • Avoid foods high in magnesium (cashews, chili, and halibut)
       b. Hypomagnesemia
          (1) Correct the underlying problem
          (2) Prepare to administer IM or slow infusion of IV magnesium sulfate or oral magnesium
          (3) Assess for knowledge deficit regarding foods high in magnesium

 F. Nursing diagnoses
   1. Knowledge deficit: related to (specific electrolyte imbalance)
   2. Oral mucous membranes, altered: related to inadequate volume of oral fluids
   3. Injury, risk for: related to muscle weakness; hypotension; seizures (or other causes)
   4. Nutrition, altered: more or less than body requirements (according to disorder)
   5. Cardiac output, decreased: related to hyperkalemia (or other disorder)

V. POSTMENOPAUSAL CONDITIONS

 A. Physiological changes at menopause
   1. Cessation of menstruation: transition from fertility to non–reproductive state
   2. Gradual decrease in the number of maturing ovarian follicles and a decline in ovarian estrogen
   3. Ovaries become unresponsive to pituitary hormones and atrophy
   4. Vaginal lubrication declines and dryness becomes the norm (atrophic vaginitis)

     5. Other signs and symptoms vary with the individual older woman
        a. Vasomotor instability can be mild, moderate, or severe
- Hot flashes
- Night sweats
- Palpitations and dizziness

        b. Loss of subcutaneous fat in the breast tissue
        c. Waist size (abdominal fat) increases
        d. Emotional symptoms or depressive reaction

B. Typical clinical presentation
    1. Atrophic vaginitis
        a. Vaginal epithelium loses its elasticity and subcutaneous fat
        b. Epidermal layer thins, labia majora and minora flatten
        c. Urethra may atrophy with increase in cystitis and urethritis
        d. Pubococcygeus muscles tend to lose tone, leading to urinary incontinence (UI)
    2. Osteoporosis (see Chapter 16 for additional information)

C. Nursing management: interventions
    1. Instruct in self-care advice
        a. Vaginal dryness control: water–soluble vaginal lubricants
        b. Prevention of osteoporosis
        c. Prevention of urinary tract infection
            (1) Void every 2 to 3 hours during the daytime
            (2) Increase fluid intake
            (3) Wear cotton panties or panties with a cotton crotch
            (4) Perform perineal hygiene
            (5) Perform pelvic muscle exercises daily
    2. Encourage physical activity to maintain muscle mass and bone health
    3. Instruct in healthy nutrition that includes foods with calcium and vitamin D

D. Nursing diagnoses
    1. Activity intolerance: related to decreased energy levels
    2. Body image disturbance: related to postmenopausal changes
    3. Coping, ineffective individual: related to reproductive cessation
    4. Urinary elimination, altered: related to pelvic muscle relaxation
    5. Sleep pattern disturbance: related to night sweats

REFERENCES

Black JM, Matassarin-Jacobs E: *Medical-surgical nursing: clinical management for continuity of care,* ed 5, Philadelphia, 1997, WB Saunders.

Braxmeyer D, Keyes J: The pathophysiology of potassium balance, *Crit Care Nurs* 16(5):59-71, 1996.

Ebersole P, Hess P: *Toward healthy aging: human needs and nursing response,* St Louis, 1998, Mosby.

Innerarity SA, Stark JL: *Fluids and electrolytes,* ed 2, Springhouse, PA, 1994, Springhouse Publishing.

Kim MJ, McFarland GK, McLane AM: *Pocket guide to nursing diagnoses,* ed 7, St Louis, 1997, Mosby.

Lewis SM, Collier IC, Heitkemper MM: *Medical surgical nursing: assessment and management of clinical problems,* ed 4, St Louis, 1996, Mosby.

Lueckenotte A: *Gerontologic nursing,* St Louis, 1996, Mosby.

Monahan FD, Neighbors M: *Medical surgical nursing: foundations for clinical practice,* ed 2, Philadelphia, 1998, WB Saunders.

Paradiso C: *Lippincott's review series: fluids and electrolytes,* Philadelphia, 1995, JB Lippincott.

Porth CM: *Pathophysiology: concepts of altered health states,* ed 5, Philadelphia, 1998, JB Lippincott.

Stanley M, Beare PG: *Gerontological nursing,* ed 2, Philadelphia, 1999, FA Davis.

Williams SR: *Essentials of nutrition and diet therapy,* ed 7, St Louis, 1999, Mosby.

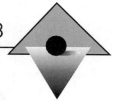

CHAPTER 18

IMMUNOLOGICAL PROBLEMS

Anita C. All ● *LaRae I. Huycke*

LEARNING OBJECTIVES

Upon completion of this chapter, the reader will be able to:

- Discuss issues associated with immunosuppression in older adults
- Describe the factors associated with immunological problems and infections
- Define terminology used with HIV/AIDS
- Describe the prevalence of HIV/AIDS in older adults
- Discuss issues associated with older adults and HIV/AIDS
- List three risk factors for HIV/AIDS in older adults
- Describe HIV/AIDS prevention/education strategies for older adults

I. TERMINOLOGY

A. *Acquired immunity:* the protection developed following an encounter with an antigen

B. *Antibody:* a protein produced by the immune system in response to specific antigens

C. *Antigen:* a substance capable of producing a specific immune response

D. *Acute or primary HIV infection phase:* the period of time immediately after the virus enters the body; during this phase the virus replicates in large numbers, depression of the immune system occurs, and there is an increase in the p24 antigen levels

E. *AIDS (acquired immunodeficiency syndrome):* the most severe manifestation of infection with the virus known as HIV; it includes all HIV-infected persons with a CD4+ T-cell count <200 cells/mm^3 or a CD4 lymphocyte percentage below 14% in the presence of HIV infection; in 1993, the Centers for Disease Control and Prevention (CDC) expanded this definition to include 23 opportunistic infections and neoplasms that can occur in the presence of HIV infection

F. *AIDS dementia complex:* a neurological complication that may include encephalitis, meningitis, spinal cord tumors, nerve damage, behavioral changes, and difficulty in thinking

G. *Antiretroviral:* a substance that either destroys a specific type of virus or suppresses its replication

H. *Asymptomatic:* a term used in the AIDS literature to describe persons infected with HIV who show no clinical signs or symptoms of the disease

I. *CD4 T-lymphocytes:* the white blood cells killed or disabled during HIV infection; these cells are also known as T helper cells

J. *HIV-1 (human immunodeficiency virus type 1):* the virus that causes AIDS

K. *HIV-2 (human immunodeficiency virus type 2):* a virus closely related to HIV-1 that also causes immune suppression; this virus is the most common cause of AIDS in Africa

L. *Immunity:* the collection of physiologic mechanisms with the capacity to recognize and destroy foreign or non-self materials

M. *Immune response:* the physiological reaction of immunity

N. *Immunology:* the study of the responses, activities, interactions, and outcomes (both desirable and undesirable) of the cells, tissues, organs, and body fluids of the immune system
O. *Older persons:* in this chapter, refers to males and females over the age of 50 years
P. *Primary response:* the body's initial response to an antigen; marked by production of antibodies
Q. *Secondary response:* the body's reaction to a subsequent encounter with the antigen; this response occurs after antibodies are no longer detected in the serum
R. *Opportunistic infection:* an illness (caused by an organism) that generally would not occur in a person with a normal immune system; the pathogen is capable of causing disease only when a person's defense mechanisms are weakened

II. IMMUNOSUPPRESSION IN OLDER ADULTS

A. Definition: decline in immune function that reduces spontaneous and induced immunity in older adults; the decline reflects a generalized decrease in the immune system's response to antigens
B. Age-related changes in the immune system
   1. Decreased resistance to bacterial, fungal, and viral infections
   2. Increased risk of reactivating latent infections
   3. Absence of the classic signs and symptoms of infection
   4. Many older adults are unable to mount a delayed cutaneous hypersensitivity response and may have less vigorous and/or delayed hypersensitivity reactions
   5. Older adults have a diminished response to vaccines
   6. Older adults at risk for diseases associated with impaired immune function are those who are nutritionally compromised or immunosuppressed
   7. Older adults with chronic disease, debility, and those living in institutions are at increased risk for infectious processes
   8. Older adults have an increased incidence of autoimmune disorders

III. INFECTIONS IN OLDER ADULTS

A. Usual symptoms of infection may be absent or diminished in older adults
B. Older adults have an increased risk of mortality from infections
C. Older adults have an increased incidence of infection
D. Age-related changes that increase one's susceptibility to infections
   1. Changes in the skin and mucous membranes
   2. Decreased ciliary action in the respiratory tract
   3. Decreased stomach acid

IV. GENERAL ISSUES FOR OLDER ADULTS WITH HIV/AIDS

A. Educational campaigns fail to target the unique needs of older persons, particularly in relation to HIV/AIDS prevention; these messages have been almost exclusively focused on the younger at-risk population
B. Health care professionals frequently do not take a sexual history from older persons and often do not screen them for HIV or other sexually transmitted diseases
C. Other age-related diseases mimic the signs and symptoms of HIV/AIDS
D. Older persons may hesitate discussing sexual or other risk behaviors
   1. They may be willing to discuss their sex lives when they understand it is for their health and the health of those they love
E. Older persons generally are more misinformed and know less about HIV/AIDS than younger persons
F. Older persons with HIV/AIDS are less likely to receive treatment even when diagnosed
G. Persons over 50 are the most rapidly growing HIV-infected population, with an increase of 138% since 1993
   1. Ten percent of persons with HIV/AIDS are age 50 or older
   2. Five percent of all newly reported cases of HIV occur in persons age 50 or older

H. Support systems for older persons with HIV/AIDS often lack health care providers capable or willing to provide the complex and intense care needed

I. The belief that HIV/AIDS-infected older persons contracted the virus from a blood transfusion is a myth
   1. Forty-seven percent of older persons with HIV/AIDS have acquired the disease through sexual contact
   2. The number of AIDS cases attributed to heterosexual transmission is presently greater among Americans age 50 and older than in any other age group

J. The normal CD4+ count may differ in older persons and complicate tracking of HIV/AIDS progression

K. The use of protective devices, such as condoms, declines with age
   1. May be related to a reduced risk of pregnancy in this age group
   2. Failure of older persons to see themselves at risk for sexually transmitted diseases
   3. Older persons report embarrassment about purchasing condoms
   4. Conflicts with condom use and personal values
   5. Perception that condoms hinder physical comfort

L. When older persons are made aware of their risk for HIV and are shown specific ways to avoid infection, they can and do reduce their risk

M. The period between infection and the onset of AIDS-related symptoms is shorter and death may occur earlier in older persons with HIV/AIDS; this may be the result of a weakened immune system in this age group

N. Health care professionals and the public often do not acknowledge that aging does not necessarily mean the end of sexual activity; persons in their 80s may remain sexually active and seldom use condoms

V. PSYCHOSOCIAL ISSUES OF OLDER ADULTS WITH HIV/AIDS

A. Issues of testing, starting or not starting drug therapy, opportunistic infections, disease progression, and death are faced by all persons with HIV/AIDS, regardless of age

B. Prejudice and the stigma of HIV/AIDS persist in American society

C. Disclosure of HIV status and the manner in which it was acquired to older persons' adult children may be difficult; this disclosure may force children to confront parents' sexuality

D. This age group often experiences the death of partners, friends, and loved ones from causes other than HIV/AIDS
   1. Many believe they have had a full life and feel sorrow for younger persons with HIV/AIDS
   2. Older persons may express the view that death is less tragic at 55 than at 35

VI. SPECIFIC ISSUES OF OLDER WOMEN WITH HIV/AIDS

A. Mid-life and older women are frequently not diagnosed until late in the disease process, sometimes only after death

B. Facts about women over the age of 50 with AIDS
   1. 43% of women over age 65 die within 1 month after being diagnosed
   2. Women aged 50 to 64 account for 39% of patients with short survival rates

C. Clinical trials often exclude older women because they have more than one specific disease

D. Older women are frequently family caregivers and tend to neglect their own health care

E. Older women may be more physiologically susceptible to HIV and other STDs
   1. Reduced lubrication and friability of the vagina
   2. Tendency toward microabrasion can facilitate viral entry

F. Postmenopausal women are less likely to receive gynecological care and are generally more susceptible to all types of infections

VII. SPECIFIC ISSUES OF OLDER MEN WITH HIV/AIDS

A. After the death of an uninfected long-term partner, older gay men may turn to younger men; younger men are more likely to be infected

B. Homosexuality and bisexuality are not limited to younger adults

C. Older homosexual men are less likely to have "come out" and do not openly live gay lifestyles

D. Older gay men may feel more isolated than their younger counterparts

E. About one half of older adults with HIV are men having sex with men; this group confronts a triple stigma

1. Homosexuality
2. HIV status
3. Stereotypes associated with aging

VIII. NURSING ASSESSMENT OF OLDER ADULTS WITH HIV/AIDS

A. AIDS-associated dementia is particularly difficult to differentiate, but peripheral neuropathies such as paresthesias and weakness should raise the index of suspicion

B. Comprehensive history-taking, particularly regarding sexual activity, drug use, and blood transfusions, is crucial

C. Certain symptoms in older persons may be related to HIV/AIDS just as in younger individuals

1. Weight loss, anorexia
2. Fatigue
3. Night sweats
4. Dry cough
5. Fever

D. HIV/AIDS may be hard to distinguish from other diseases common in older persons, such as pneumonia, dementia, and malnutrition

E. Older persons with HIV/AIDS frequently have other diagnoses

1. *Pneumocystis carinii* pneumonia
2. Extra-pulmonary tuberculosis
3. Disseminated herpes zoster

F. Older persons should be encouraged to ask for HIV testing if they believe they are at risk or suspect they might be infected

G. Rapid vision changes, development of thrush, and unusually severe or multi-dermatomal herpes zoster should suggest HIV testing

H. Rapid memory decline unlike slow loss of cognition in Alzheimer's disease may be caused by HIV/AIDS (aphasia, common with Alzheimer's disease, rarely occurs in HIV/AIDS)

I. Nurses should be sensitive to risk factors in older persons who have undergone lifestyle changes, such as death of a spouse or long-term significant other and divorce

IX. ELEMENTS OF NURSING CARE OF OLDER ADULTS WITH HIV/AIDS

A. The older adult is more likely to present with AIDS at time of diagnosis

B. Actual nursing care for patients with AIDS does not differ to any great degree from care provided for younger persons

C. Nursing care, however, may involve functional assistance earlier in the course of the disease

D. Problems commonly encountered in older persons with AIDS that respond to nursing interventions

1. Pain
2. Gastrointestinal symptoms
3. Fever
4. Skin breakdown
5. Falls
6. Drug reactions

E. Renal and hepatic function must be monitored closely in the older person with AIDS as antiretroviral therapy may further compromise these systems

F. Nursing care needs to include the involvement of resources for meals and social support

X. Prevention/Risk Reduction in the Older Population

A. Direct education is needed to focus on the fact that persons over age 50 are not immune from HIV/AIDS
   1. Organizations affiliated with older persons
   2. Professionals working with older persons
   3. At sites where older people congregate
B. Encourage healthy lifestyles
   1. Sound nutritional practice
   2. Avoidance of exposure to infections
   3. Regular exercise
   4. Methods to enhance functional coping in older adults
C. Special attention in educational programs should be directed toward all older adults who may fall into the following groups
   1. Persons who received blood transfusions before 1985
   2. Gay and bisexual persons not a part of active gay communities
   3. The sexual partners of these persons who may not be aware of their partners' infection
   4. Educators also need to remember that different groups, depending on knowledge and need, will require different teaching strategies and methods
D. Focus education on safe sexual practices, including how to use a condom

REFERENCES

American Association of Retired Persons: *HIV/AIDS and older adults,* October 1, 1998, (news release posted on the World Wide Web). Retrieved May 16, 1999 from the World Wide Web: http://ww.aarp.org/press/1998/nr100198.htlm.

Anonymous: *AIDS scourge hits the elderly hard as the young fall victim,* March 29, 1999, [Bangkok Post, on line]. Retrieved May 16, 1999 from the World Wide Web: http://www.hivdent.org/publicp/ppashteh0399.htlm.

Anonymous: Providers not diagnosing HIV in older women, *AIDS Alert* 10(6):77-79, 1995.

Anonymous: *Recognizing and responding to the many faces of AIDS in the USA,* 1999, [on line]. Retrieved May 16, 1999 from the World Wide Web: http://www.gbgm-umc.org/mission/resolution/aidsusa.html.

Bartlett JA: Antiretroviral. In Bartlett JA, editor: *Care and management of patients with HIV infection,* Durham, NC, 1996, GlaxoWellcome Inc.

El-Sadr W, Gettler J: Unrecognized human immunodeficiency virus infection in the elderly, *Arch Internal Med* 155(2):184-186, 1995.

Feldman MD: Sex, AIDS, and the elderly, *Arch Internal Med* 154(1):19-20, 1994.

Flannery JC: Immunology. In Burrell LO, Gerlach MJ, Pless BS, editors: *Adult nursing: acute and community care,* ed 2, Stamford, CT, 1997, Appleton & Lange.

Flaskerud JH, Ungvarski PJ: Overview and update of HIV Disease. In Ungvarski PJ, Flaskerud JH, editors: *HIV/AIDS: a guide to primary care management,* ed 4, Philadelphia, 1999, WB Saunders.

Fletcher KR: Physical and laboratory assessment. In Stone JT, Wyman JF, Salisbury SA, editors: *Clinical gerontological nursing: a guide to advanced practice,* ed 2, Philadelphia, 1999, WB Saunders.

Garvey C: AIDS care for the elderly: a community-based approach, *AIDS Patient Care* 8(3):118-120, 1994.

Gordon SM, Thompson S: The changing epidemiology of the human immunodeficiency virus infection in older persons, *J Am Geriatr Soc* 43(1):7-9, 1995.

Grossman AH: The needs of special population. In Ungvarski PJ, Flaskerud JH, editors: *HIV/AIDS: a guide to primary care management,* ed 4, Philadelphia, 1999, WB Saunders.

Gueldner SH: The elderly: the silent population, *J Assoc Nurs AIDS Care* 6(5):9-10, 1995.

Gutheil IA, Chichin ER: AIDS, older people, and social work, *Health Social Work* 16(4):237-244, 1991.

Martin JN, Colford JM, Ngo L, et al: Effect of older age on survival in human immunodeficiency virus (HIV) disease, *Am J Epidemiol* 142(11):1221-1230, 1995.

Riley MW, Ory MG, Zablotsky D, editors: *AIDS in an aging society: what we need to know,* New York, 1989, Springer Publishing.

Schuerman DA: Clinical concerns: AIDS in the elderly, *J Gerontol Nurs* 20(7):11-17, 1994.

Scura KW, Whipple B: HIV infection and AIDS in the elderly. In Stanley M, Beare PG, editors: *Gerontological nursing,* Philadelphia, 1995, FA Davis.

Stall R, Catania J: AIDS risk behaviors among late middle-aged and elderly Americans: the national AIDS behavioral surveys, *Arch Inter Med* 154(1):57-63, 1994.

Stone JT, Steinbach C: Iatrogenesis. In Stone JT, Steinbach C, editors: *Clinical gerontological nursing. a guide to advanced practice,* ed 2, Philadelphia, 1999, WB Saunders.

Streit LA: Infections. In Burrell LO, Gerlach MJ, Pless BS, editors: *Adult nursing: acute and community care,* ed 2, Stamford, CT, 1997, Appleton & Lange.

Wallace JI, Paauw DS, Spach DH: HIV infection in older patients: when to suspect the unexpected, *Geriatrics* 48(6):61-64, 69-70, 1993.

Whipple B, Scura KW: The overlooked epidemic: HIV in older adults, *AJN* 96(2):22-29, 1996.

Wiersema LA: The integumentary system and its problems in the elderly. In Stanley M, Beare PG, editors: *Gerontological nursing,* Philadelphia, 1995, FA Davis.

Wutoh AK, Hidalgo J, Rhee W, et al: A characterization of older AIDS patients in Maryland, *J Nation Med Assoc* 90(6):369-373, 1998.

CHAPTER 19

NEUROLOGICAL PROBLEMS

Ann Schmidt Luggen • *Sue E. Meiner*

LEARNING OBJECTIVES

Upon completion of this chapter, the reader will be able to:

- Define Alzheimer's disease (AD)
- Differentiate dementia from delirium
- Name the classifications of stroke
- Discuss nursing management of stroke
- Describe the characteristics of Parkinson's disease (PD)
- Discuss the nursing management of PD
- Identify developmental disabilities in the older adult

I. NORMAL AGE-ASSOCIATED CHANGES: NEUROLOGICAL SYSTEM

A. The brain undergoes neurochemical, structural, and neuropsychological alterations with aging
   1. There is a small decrease in brain weight and volume (7% to 8%) with widening of cerebral cortical sulci and enlargement of the lateral ventricles
   2. Loss of large neurons in selective cortical and subcortical structures with an accumulation of lipofuscin and microscopic findings of neuritic plaques and neurofibrillary tangles
   3. Neurochemical changes include decreased activity of catecholamine synthesis, enzymes, and increased activity of monoamine oxidase
   4. Decreased amounts of neurotransmitter serotonin, noradrenaline, and dopamine
B. Age-associated memory changes
   1. Forgetting of specific details and names of people but remembering these later
   2. Able to learn new material but may have difficulty with information retrieval
   3. General awareness of memory impairment
   4. Memory impairment does not impair daily functioning
C. No clinically significant changes in behavior or personality

II. DISORDERS OF THE NEUROLOGICAL SYSTEM

A. Alzheimer's disease (AD)
   1. Non-reversible and progressive form of a dementing disease process that reduces the ability to think, remember, reason, judge, and concentrate and eventually prevents the performance of activities of daily living (ADL); personality and language abilities decline; approximately 66% of all dementias are of the Alzheimer's type
   2. Prevalence, incidence, and risk factors
      a. Four million Americans have been diagnosed with Alzheimer's type dementia
      b. Ten percent of people over 75 years of age are affected and 47% of people over 85 years of age are affected

c. Risk factors include advanced age and familial history of first-degree relatives diagnosed with AD

3. Pathophysiology of AD
   a. Neurofibrillary tangles and neuritic plaques are hallmarks of AD
   b. Amyloid protein is found in neuritic plaques on autopsy
   c. Cholinergic projection neurons degenerate
   d. Cerebral cortex and hippocampus are the most common area affected

4. Selected theories of causation of AD
   a. Amyloid precursor protein (APP) is found in AD brain tissue in excessive amounts with a genetic influence suspected
   b. Apolipoprotein E (APOE) is found in the neurofibrillary tangles; causes intercellular metabolism processes to be slowly destroyed
   c. Genetic connection is associated with defects on chromosomes 19 and 21 where, respectively, links to heart disease or Down syndrome are located
   d. Exogenous toxin exposure to elements such as zinc, aluminum, and mercury may play an interactive role in AD
   e. Infectious process, immune malfunction, and other causes have been hypothesized

5. Typical clinical presentation (AD may last from 3 to 20 years with an average of 8)
   a. Progression of symptoms and time of appearance is unique to the individual
   b. Three stages or phases of AD reflect early (mild), middle (moderate), or late (severe) symptoms
   c. Very early stage, usually considered questionable dementia
      (1) Forgets names, events, phone numbers, has difficulty telling time
      (2) Gets lost in familiar surroundings
      (3) Is easily angered, irritable, and lacks spontaneity
      (4) Has difficulty making decisions
      (5) Is aware of losses
   d. Early stage or mild phase
      (1) Suffers loss of recent memory: forgets to pay bills, has difficulty shopping for needed items, misplaces items, forgets messages
      (2) Has problems finding words or following a story line
      (3) Has impaired judgment: gets lost while driving, makes poor decisions, has trouble handling money, planning, or problem-solving
      (4) Forgets routine tasks, poor hygiene habits, inability to do ADLs
      (5) Overly anxious, complains of neglect by others, has personality and behavioral changes (restlessness, impatience, uses denial to cope)
   e. Middle stage or moderate phase
      (1) Increased memory loss, difficulty in recognizing family or friends
      (2) Confabulates or makes up stories to compensate
      (3) Perseverates or has preoccupation with certain thoughts, feelings, verbalizations
      (4) Wandering, hyperorality, immodesty, actively resists help with ADLs, intolerance to cold
      (5) Gait changes to small steps with halting gait and rigidity
      (6) Bowel and bladder incontinence
      (7) Decreased ability to read, do math, understand or express language, recognize objects, or demonstrate purposeful movement
      (8) Hallucinations, delusions, violent behavior, suspicious and paranoid behavior with a flat affect
   f. Late stage or severe phase (can last from 1 to 3 years [terminal stage])
      (1) Inability to perform any ADLs; must be dressed, fed, bathed, kept dry, turned, transferred
      (2) Little response to stimuli, may grunt or use agitation to communicate, loss of verbal abilities
      (3) Loss of body weight

       (4) Seizures, myoclonic jerking

       (5) Loss of bodily functions

       (6) Susceptible to infections

6. Nursing assessment

   a. The goal of the nursing assessment is to determine the individual's strengths (assets) and weaknesses (limitations) in each of the six following dimensions

       (1) Physical: oral health—nutrition, chewing, swallowing; weight—sleep/rest; bowel and bladder function; gait/balance; ADLs; instrumental activities of daily living (IADLs)

       (2) Cognitive (sensation): hearing, vision, task, smell, touch, perception/illusions/hallucinations, motor behavior, orientation/"sundowners syndrome," memory, communication abilities

       (3) Social: interactions, coping patterns, exercise

       (4) Emotional: anxiety, depression, agitated behavior, aggressive behavior, catastrophic reactions

       (5) Environmental: ability to access environment and self, ability to respond to cues (physical and social), safety

       (6) Behavioral: wandering, hiding/misplacing things, pacing

7. Nursing assessment (family, caregiver(s), and caregiving environment)

   a. Type and quality of prior relationship between caregiver and patient

       (1) Parent/child, marital, assumption of roles/role obligations

   b. Initiation and maintenance of caregiving relationship, caregiver physical and mental health

   c. Impact of caregiving and patient characteristics on caregiving relationship

       (1) Caregiver characteristics: family, work, social roles

       (2) Patient characteristics: premorbid personality, problematic behaviors

   d. Caregiver environment

       (1) Social supports

       (2) Community service

       (3) Financial conditions

   e. Impact of caregiving on caregiver's physical and mental health

       (1) Level of depression, stress, burden, strain

       (2) Physical health changes

8. Nursing management: interventions

   a. Goals are to help the resident feel safe, comfortable, in control, pleased, satisfied, and able to experience the highest possible physical, emotional, intellectual, and social functioning for as long as possible

   b. Interventions should be applied in a therapeutic milieu, which provides dementia care that is safe and supportive, offering structure, involvement, and validation

       (1) Attempt to communicate with verbal and nonverbal strategies appropriate for stage of illness

       (2) Support sensory function: glasses, hearing aids, dentures

       (3) Offer reassurance, convey warmth

       (4) Provide a routine with consistency, yet allow flexibility

       (5) Provide activities and exercise

       (6) Provide for nutritional and fluid needs

       (7) Avoid physical and chemical restraints

       (8) Keep things simple

       (9) Use appropriate environmental cues

   c. Nursing interventions: patient/caregiver education

       (1) Disease and stage

       (2) Behavioral management and communication strategies

       (3) Locating community resources

       (4) Legal/financial issues

(5) Advanced directives

(6) Long-term care options: home, community-based care management, respite, residential or nursing home, special Alzheimer's units

(7) Family and social support

(8) Monitoring for acute illnesses and effects of medications

(9) Monitoring for depression

(10) Drug therapies

B. Non-Alzheimer dementias (development of multiple cognitive impairments, including the loss of memory)

1. Short and long-term memory impairment: evidenced in early stages of dementias by an inability to learn new skills

2. Aphasia: difficulty with the use of language; can lead to confusion and withdrawal

3. Apraxia: difficulty performing motor skills; can lead to accidents or a tendency to avoid activities that previously were interesting

4. Agnosia: difficulty recognizing objects

5. Decrease in abstract thinking; lack of ability to plan and organize simple tasks

6. Classifications of dementias

    a. According to reversibility; majority of dementias are not reversible; not to be confused with treatable dementias

    b. According to etiology

        (1) Metabolic diseases: thyroid, hypoglycemia, hypercalcemia, renal failure, liver failure, Cushing's, Addison's, or Wilson's diseases

        (2) Toxins: heavy metals and organic poisons

        (3) Infections and neoplasms

        (4) Side effects of drugs: iatrogenic

        (5) Nutritional deficiencies

        (6) Degenerative neurological diseases

        (7) Cerebral vascular injuries, ischemia, or traumas

7. Nursing assessment

    a. Screening with standardized mental ability tests and focused history

        (1) Agency for Health Care Policy and Research (AHCPR) 1996, Clinical Practice Guideline # 19

        (2) Folstein MiniMental State Assessment Tool

        (3) Blessed Information-Memory-Concentration Test

    b. Physical assessment to focus on potential elements of etiologies

    c. Medication history over the past 5 years (prescription, OTC, etc.)

8. Nursing management: interventions

    a. Promote general health and personal independence

    b. Provide close supervision as the dementia progresses

    c. Monitor medications for effectiveness and adverse reactions

    d. Provide and monitor the environment for potential safety issues

    e. Support patient and caregivers

C. Delirium (also known as acute confusional state, acute brain syndrome, toxic psychosis, etc.)

1. Transient cognitive disorder with a rapid onset and brief duration; an acute organic mental disorder, commonly reversible within 7 days to 1 month

2. Typical clinical presentations

    a. Reduced ability to maintain attention to external stimuli

    b. Disorganized thinking with rambling, irrelevant, incoherent speech

    c. Difficulty in shifting, focusing, and sustaining attention to external and internal stimuli

    d. Sensory misperception and disordered thought patterns

    e. Reverses upon initiation of treatment to remove the underlying cause

3. Severity is based on the level of physiologic disturbance and the degree of cerebral edema

4. Nursing assessment
    a. Determine psychological elements under typical clinical presentations
    b. Identify physical elements of the acute disorder
       (1) Elevated pulse and respiratory rates
       (2) Temperature fluctuations
       (3) Tremors of hands, fingers, facial muscles, and lips
       (4) Headache and generalized weakness
5. Nursing interventions
    a. Offer immediate attention to prevent confusion from exacerbating
    b. Provide supportive and symptomatic care
    c. Guarantee continuity of caregiving personnel
    d. Correct sensory deficits through providing glasses, hearing aids, etc.
    e. Orient stimuli on an ongoing basis during the acute stage
    f. Encourage family visitation during hospitalization
    g. Provide ongoing presence and reassurance of a familiar person
D. Stroke (brain attack, cerebral vascular accident [CVA])
  1. Incidence/prevalence
    a. Third leading cause of disability; 700,000 suffer stroke each year in the United States
    b. 3 million people live with residual effects of stroke
    c. 75% of stroke patients are >65
    d. 40% of survivors have significant dysfunction
    e. 40% have mild dysfunction
    f. 10% recover completely
    g. 10% are institutionalized
  2. Classification
    a. Transient ischemic attack (TIA)
       (1) Acute focal neurological signs and symptoms lasting <24 hours
       (2) Brief stroke-like event, resulting from transitional block of blood flow to brain; neurological deficits resolve in <24 hours and most last 30 minutes or less
       (3) Precedes stroke in 50% to 70% of cases
    b. Intracerebral hemorrhage
       (1) Accounts for 20% of strokes
       (2) Blood vessel supplying the brain bursts
       (3) Nontraumatic, sudden-onset, severe headache, altered consciousness, and/or focal neurological deficits
       (4) Focal collection of blood
    c. Ischemic stroke
       (1) Accounts for 80% of strokes
       (2) Blood vessel of brain obstructed by blood clot
       (3) Rapid onset of focal neurological deficits with signs and symptoms lasting >24 hours
       (4) May be caused by cardiac source of emboli
       (5) Or be caused by significant atherosclerotic or arterial disease in carotid, vertebral, or basilar artery
       (6) There may be cerebral infarction of small arteries or arterioles
       (7) Clinical findings: hemiparesis, hemiplegia, hemisensory loss, dysarthria (clumsy hand syndrome)
  3. Course
    a. One third of TIA patients will have a stroke in 5 years
    b. Strokes often occur at night during sleep
    c. Patients awaken with deficit that then progresses

4. Symptoms: focal neurological deficits
   a. Difficulty speaking, slurred speech, difficulty swallowing
   b. Difficulty understanding speech
   c. Weakness, especially one side of the body
   d. Numbness
   e. Double vision, blindness, hearing difficulty, or other sensory problems
   f. Difficulty with balance
   g. Altered consciousness
   h. Terrible headache
5. Physiology
   a. Left brain: controls motor and sensory function on right side of body
   b. Right brain: controls motor and sensory function on left side of body
   c. Left brain: language area
   d. Right brain: perceptual, spatial areas
6. Stroke symptoms: CT and MRI scans (computed tomography, magnetic resonance imaging) determine location and cause of stroke
   a. One-sided weakness (hemiparesis)
   b. One limb weak (monoparesis)
   c. *Terrible* headache
   d. Diminished level of consciousness
   e. Sudden difficulty speaking (dysarthria)
   f. Sudden language difficulty (dysphasia)
   g. Sudden loss of vision in one or both eyes
   h. Double vision
   i. Loss of balance (ataxia)
   j. Weakness of extremity
   k. Sensation loss on one side of the body
7. Risk factors
   a. Modifiable: hypertension, smoking, diabetes mellitus, high cholesterol, cardiovascular disease
   b. Nonmodifiable: age (most important risk factor), family history of stroke, race (African Americans 2.5 times more likely to have a stroke than Caucasians)
8. Medical management: acute
   a. TPA (tissue plasminogen activator): relatively new drug called "clot-buster" that dissolves clots if given within 3 hours of onset of symptoms; one third of patients given TPA return home without functional impairment
   b. Any TIA that lasts 5 to 10 minutes should be treated as a stroke—call 911
   c. Evaluate ABC per resuscitation: airway, breathing, circulation
   d. Check BP
   e. Note seizure activity
9. Nursing management: chronic
   a. Educate patients and families about signs and symptoms and acute management of stroke, TIA
   b. Long-term management will depend on a rehabilitation team
   c. Right hemisphere stroke problems
      (1) Patient will neglect the left side of the body; is unaware of problems with the left side of the body; may walk, unaware of left leg paralysis
      (2) Patient will forget to groom the left side of the face, hair
      (3) Patient will not eat from the left side of the plate
      (4) Impaired judgment, poor judgment; needs protection
      (5) Impulsive behavior; needs protection
      (6) Rigid thinking

(7) Distortion of time

(8) Affect is labile

(9) Feelings of persecution

(10) Irritable, confused

(11) May appear lethargic

(12) Has difficulty retaining information

d. Left hemisphere stroke problems

(1) Language is affected

(2) No comprehension of speech or written language

(3) Difficulty expressing self verbally or in writing

(4) Difficulty initiating any task

(5) Slow processing

(6) Low frustration

(7) Verbal perseveration (repetition)

(8) Rapid performance of movements

(9) Compulsive behavior

(10) Easily distractable

e. Stroke complications

(1) Dysphagia (difficulty swallowing) 30%

(2) Urine incontinence 60%

(3) Pressure sores 60%

(4) Depression 60%

(5) Deep vein thrombosis 30%; leads to pulmonary emboli in 3%

10. Rehabilitation

a. Principles

(1) Restore function

(2) Improve quality of life

(3) Perform evaluation using team approach: geriatrician, nurse, physical therapist, occupational therapist, social worker, speech therapist, physiatrist, nutritionist, psychologist

(4) Set realistic, individual goals for each patient

(5) Reinforce that rehabilitation is a learning process

(6) Age of patient, relationship factors influence rehabilitation

- Social issues, financial support: Medicare conditions for reimbursement must be met; must document improvements
- Concurrent illnesses (dementias, depression)
- Impaired mobility (arthritis, Parkinson's disease)
- Frequent adverse drug reactions
- Impaired equilibrium, balance

(7) Rehabilitation begins at hospital and continues in

- Skilled nursing facility daily therapy, 1 hour/day
- Home therapy
- Outpatient therapy: Medicare Part B

(8) 80% of adaptive, assistive equipment covered by Medicare if well documented by health care provider

(9) Medicaid varies by state

11. Assistive devices

a. Canes: useful with unilateral deficit

(1) Use on unaffected side in hemiplegia

(2) Hold in hand of preference for foot, ankle, knee injuries

(3) Tripod or 4-pod provides increased support

(4) Pistol grip better than round handle

     b. Walker
       (1) 2-wheel, 4-wheel, pickup
       (2) Front wheel requires less strength and balance than pickup, best for Parkinson's disease patients
     c. Wheelchair: two types
       (1) Indoor: large wheels in the rear
       (2) Outdoor: large wheels in the front
       (3) Patients fitted and measured for wheelchairs
       (4) Clearance of doorways should be 2 inches on each side
       (5) One-arm drive wheelchair useful for hemiplegia
       (6) Motor wheelchair for very selected patients with neurological disorders
     d. Transfers
       (1) Need adequate equipment for safety
       (2) Toilet seats 20 inches from floor
       (3) Handrails on hemiplegia-unaffected side
       (4) Tub transfers need transfer bench

12. Nursing management
     a. Identify pre-illness functional state, capabilities; identify abnormal health patterns, severity of comorbid diseases
     b. Begin activity ASAP and when feasible: early mobilization will prevent skin breakdown, avoid contractures, maintain strength, reduce depression
     c. Keep skin dry, clean, without friction or pressure
     d. Do range of motion exercises frequently
     e. Prevent deep vein thrombosis: low-dose heparin, warfarin, elastic stockings
     f. Expect delayed mobility when there is
       (1) Coma
       (2) Progression of neurological signs
       (3) Cerebral hemorrhage
       (4) Orthostatic hypotension
       (5) Acute myocardial infarction
       (6) Acute deep vein thrombosis
     g. Monitor nutrition and hydration
     h. Evaluate bladder and bowel
       (1) Avoid indwelling catheter to prevent urinary tract infections
       (2) Begin incontinence programs
     i. Prevent complications
       (1) Evaluate sleep disturbances; keep patient active during daytime hours
       (2) Dysphagia: provide swallowing exercises, relearning swallowing, change the texture of food
       (3) Seizures: begin anticonvulsant therapy
       (4) Falls (high risk): increase supervision, provide wheelchair modification, chair modification, put call systems in place, provide regular toileting
       (5) Remember one stroke is risk factor for another stroke
       (6) One fall is risk factor for another fall

13. Interdisciplinary rehabilitation candidacy
     a. Referral criteria
       (1) Disability in two areas: mobility, ADLs, bowel or bladder control, cognition, emotional functioning, pain management, swallowing, communication
       (2) Moderately stable medically
       (3) Able to learn
       (4) Physical endurance to sit supported for 1 hour
       (5) Can participate actively in rehabilitation

E. Parkinson's disease
1. Definition: degenerative brain disorder of substantia nigra (midbrain), resulting in death of nerve cells whose role is motor function; there is a reduction in the neurotransmitter, dopamine, which facilitates transfer of electrical signals between nerve cells
2. Incidence/prevalence: 1.5 million people in the United States have PD
   a. Overall lifetime risk is 2%
   b. Present in 1% of those 65 to 74 years of age
   c. 3.1% of those 75 to 84
   d. 4.3% of 85 to 94
3. Cause: unknown—chemicals, pesticides, diet (?)
   a. Believed environmental in patients 50+ years of age
   b. Believed to be a genetic link in those <50
4. Pathophysiology
   a. Decreased dopamine results in motor deficits, tremor, muscle rigidity, bradykinesia (slow movement), gait and balance problems
   b. Other symptoms may occur in areas where dopamine acts, resulting in depression, dementia, and anxiety
   c. Autonomic disorders include
      (1) Slowed gastric emptying
      (2) Increased colon transit time
      (3) Altered swallowing
      (4) Dysregulation of blood pressure
      (5) Bladder dysfunction: neurogenic bladder
      (6) Increased secretion of sebaceous glands: seborrheic dermatitis
      (7) Increased perspiration
5. Diagnosis: no laboratory tests or scans assist in diagnosis; neurologist diagnoses based on characteristic symptoms
6. Disease course
   a. Early stage PD
      (1) First symptoms: mild, slight tremor in hand at rest, decreasing with purposeful movements and sleep (75%); purposeful movements such as brushing teeth become slow and difficult
      (2) First treatments
         • Amantadine (Symmetrol)
         • Selegiline (Eldepryl)
         • Bromocriptine (Parlodel)
         • Pergolide (Permax)
   b. Mid-stage PD
      (1) Increasing symptoms (months to 3 years)
      (2) Decreasing effect of medications
      (3) Add levodopa (Sinemet), a dopamine precursor (80% improvement of symptoms)
      (4) Add carbidopa, decreases side effects of levodopa, increases effect of levodopa
      (5) Side effects of levodopa are nausea, involuntary movements of mouth, face, limbs
   c. Late-stage PD
      (1) Decreasing effect of medications
      (2) Increasing difficulty with balance, increased muscle contractions, problems initiating movement, involuntary abnormal posture, nightmares, orthostatic hypotension, constipation, infrequent blinking, rigid face, depression, dementia; few patients experience all the symptoms
7. Newer therapies
   a. Dopamine agonists: ropinirole (Requip) or pramipexole (Mirapex) decrease motor dysfunction when given with lowered doses of levodopa/carbidopa

b. COMT (catechol-o-methyltransferase) inhibitors: tolcarpone (Tasmar) or entacapone (Cotess) are given with levodopa/carbidopa; a COMT inhibitor is given to block COMT, a chemical, and this allows dopamine to stay longer in the brain

c. Surgery: deep brain stimulation via implanted electrode in subthalamic nucleus; a wire is attached to the electrode and imbedded just below the skin in the shoulder; the electrode neutralizes inhibitory messages to the brain, allowing excitatory messages to predominate; the result is diminished shaking, fluid movements, increased speed

d. Future: gene therapy with genetically engineered virus administered in the brain to stimulate dopamine production

8. Nursing management

a. Medications need constant monitoring

b. Patient education: potential side effects of drugs, drug interactions, dietary modifications

c. Drug toxicity of levodopa and anticholinergics leads to confusion, decreased effect of the drugs, hallucinations, nightmares, dyskinesias, dystonia, reversed sleep–wake patterns

   (1) Decreasing the dosage may alleviate symptoms

   (2) Clozapine may increase the psychiatric side effects (hallucinations, delusions, paranoia)

d. Diet: anorexia, nausea, and vomiting are common side effects of levodopa; watch for weight loss

   (1) A high-protein diet blocks the effect of levodopa

   (2) Alkaline products (milk, antacids) slow drug absorption

   (3) Take levodopa on an empty stomach for best effect

   (4) Take protein in the diet at the last meal of the day

e. Exercise: physical therapy

   (1) Helps prevent immobility

   (2) Decreases tone abnormalities

   (3) Maintains or increases muscle ability, strength, speed

f. Specialists

   (1) Speech therapy can help swallowing abnormalities and decrease the incidence of pneumonia and silent aspirations

g. Functional assessment

   (1) Unified Parkinson's Disease Rating Scale (Fahn, 1987) is used to assess overall functional status of patients with PD

     • I: mentation, behavior, mood

     • II: ADLs—patients with PD may do ADLs but over a prolonged period of time

     • III: motor function

     • IV: therapy complications

     • V: disease assessment

h. Psychological/cognitive assessment

   (1) Symptoms, such as drooling, tremor, lost facial expression, shuffling gait, can cause embarrassment and discourage social activities; patients need emotional support, a supportive network

     • Encourage socialization

     • Plan activities for 'on' (energetic) periods; patients with PD have 'on-off' times of the day

i. Promotion of autonomy

   (1) Promote self-care as long as possible, as much as possible

   (2) Allow extended periods of time to accomplish minor tasks, ADLs

   (3) Support physical activity and fitness to prevent muscle atrophy, contractures, improve morale

   (4) Obtain clothes with velcro closures

   (5) Provide raised toilet seats

      j. Preventing complications

        (1) Upper respiratory infections are dangerous; pneumonia is second leading cause of death in advanced PD

        (2) Aspiration of foods because of dysphagia, poor muscle tone in pharyngeal muscles results in pneumonia; if tube feeding is needed, gastrostomy preferable

        (3) Soft and semisoft foods are less difficult to swallow

        (4) Urinary tract infections are common because of use of anticholinergics and occurrence of urine stasis; encourage fluids

        (5) Falls occur in 25% of patients with PD

        (6) Serious injury occurs in 15%; encourage canes, tripods, walkers, assistive devices, rubber mats in tubs, avoidance of throw rugs and telephone and other cords

F. Developmental disabilities with mental retardation (DD/MR)

  1. Pathological condition that develops before the age of 18 years and persists throughout the individual's lifespan

  2. Majority of life experience is limited to institutional living with limited community interactions

  3. Characteristics of the DD/MR older adult

    a. Multiple physical incapacities that include poor vision, hearing, and strength

    b. Education limitations because of a lack of educational opportunities during the older person's youth

    c. Physically and mentally impaired

    d. Physically and socially dependent

  4. Nursing interventions

    a. Promote personal ties through interactions with other older adults

    b. Substitute playing with toys or with pets when appropriate

    c. Patiently promote a sense of modesty, which may not have been developed during earlier years

    d. Encourage participation in programs of art, music, and physical movement in a setting of acceptance

REFERENCES

Black JM, Matassarin-Jacobs E: *Medical-surgical nursing: clinical management for continuity of care,* ed 5, Philadelphia, 1997, WB Saunders.

Ebersole P, Hess P: *Toward healthy aging: human needs and nursing response,* ed 5, St Louis, 1998, Mosby.

Eliopoulos C: *Gerontological nursing,* ed 4, Philadelphia, 1997, JB Lippincott.

Ferri F, Fretwell MD, Wachtel TJ: *The care of the geriatric patient,* ed 2, St Louis, 1997, Mosby.

Miller RM, Woo D: Stroke, current concepts of care, *Geriatr Nurs* 20(2):66-69, 1999.

Monahan FD, Neighbors M: *Medical surgical nursing: foundations for clinical practice,* ed 2, Philadelphia, 1998, WB Saunders.

Porth CM: *Pathophysiology: concepts of altered health states,* ed 5, Philadelphia, 1998, JB Lippincott.

Stanley M, Beare PG: *Gerontological nursing,* ed 2, Philadelphia, 1999, FA Davis.

Williams SR: *Essentials of nutrition and diet therapy,* ed 7, St Louis, 1999, Mosby.

CHAPTER 20

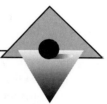

SLEEP ISSUES/DISORDERS

Ann Schmidt Luggen

LEARNING OBJECTIVES

Upon completion of this chapter, the reader will be able to:

- Describe the changes in sleep patterns that occur with aging
- Discuss the pathological sleep disorders more common in older adults
- List some of the interventions in the nursing management of sleep disorders

I. SLEEP

A. Definition: cyclic, rhythmic behavior occurring in 5 stages
   1. Four non-rapid eye movement stages
   2. One rapid eye movement stage, which decreases with aging

II. INSOMNIA

A. Definition: inability to sleep despite the desire to sleep
   1. Transitory: occasional restless nights because of environment (house), change (jet lag), anxiety
   2. Short-term: caused by temporary stresses such as loss of loved one, work pressures
   3. Chronic: greater than 3 weeks; caused by poor habits, alcohol, naps, psychological problems, sleep medications, health problems; 40% the result of sleep apnea, restless leg syndrome, chronic pain (arthritis)
B. Incidence of insomnia: affects 50% of older adults >65 years and 90% of those living in long-term care facilities; occurs less in healthy elders, more in those with health problems, especially those who are depressed or who have Alzheimer's disease, cardiovascular disease, pulmonary disease, or pain syndromes such as arthritis, prostate disease, and endocrine disorders
C. Changes in sleep patterns occurring with age
   1. Early morning awakening
   2. Daytime naps
   3. Diminished deep sleep
   4. Increased awakening from sleep
   5. Increased awake time at night
   6. Average 70-year-old sleeps 6 hours/night, 1.5 hours less than young adults
D. Common sleep complaints of older adults
   1. Trouble initiating sleep and maintaining sleep
   2. Daytime fatigue
   3. Loss of concentration, memory
E. Consequences of sleeplessness
   1. Less alert
   2. Decreased work performance

3. Decreased activity level
4. Polypharmacy
5. Increased mortality
6. In patients with Alzheimer's disease: increased agitation, wandering, restlessness, ("sundowners syndrome")
7. Diminished quality of life

III. HYPERSOMNIA

A. Characteristics: sleep more than 8 to 9/24 hours with complaint of excessive sleep
B. Cause: unclear—inactivity, depression (?)
C. Complaints of fatigue, weakness, memory problems

IV. SLEEP APNEA

A. Characteristics: cessation of breathing during sleep; snoring, interrupted breathing of >10 seconds, >5 to 8 episodes/hour; apnea may last 10 to 90 seconds
B. Cause: occurs more frequently in aged; associated with snoring, obesity, dementia, depression, hypothyroidism, nicotine use, alcohol and respiratory depressant medications
C. Risk: adult men, long history of snoring, obese, short thick necks
D. Symptoms: loud periodic snoring; unusual bedtime activities such as sleepwalking, falling from bed; broken sleep; frequent waking; memory changes; depression; daytime sleepiness; nocturia; morning headache
E. Sleep apnea treatment: surgical removal of redundant tissue in pharynx; avoidance of alcohol and drugs that interfere with arousal; sleeping in a chair

V. PROMOTING SLEEP

A. Prevention of sleep disturbances
   1. Regular exercise, especially afternoons
   2. Treatment of depression
   3. Limit sleeping to amount needed
   4. Regular rising time
   5. Light evening snack
   6. Cool room <75° F
   7. Avoidance of caffeine in the evening
   8. Avoidance of alcohol at night
   9. Avoid naps >2 hours
   10. Good mattress
B. Medications for sleeplessness
   1. L-tryptophan
   2. Sherry, wine
   3. Benadryl antihistamine (diphenhydramine)
   4. Vistaril (hydroxyzine)
   5. Chloral hydrate
   6. Benzodiazepines: triazolam (Halcion), oxazepam (Serax)
C. Nursing management
   1. Provide attention and education related to environmental factors, bedtime rituals
   2. Promote relaxation at bedtime, massage, snacks
   3. Position body for comfort
   4. Provide pain relief
   5. Provide blankets for warmth
   6. Do not give caffeine in the afternoon, evening
   7. Provide soft music (patient's preference)
   8. Offer warm milk

9. Offer nightcap of sherry, wine if relaxation a problem
10. Offer warm bath
11. Provide nature sound tapes or patient's preference

REFERENCES

Bahr RT: Sleep disturbances. In Stanley M, Beare PG, editors: *Gerontological nursing,* ed 2, Philadelphia, 1999, WB Saunders.

Ferri FF, Fretwell MD, Wachtel TJ: *Care of the geriatric patient,* ed 2, St Louis, 1997, Mosby.

Gershman K, McCullough DM: *The little black book of geriatrics,* Malden, MA, 1998, Blackwell Science.

Miller CA: *Nursing care of older adults,* ed 3, Philadelphia, 1999, JB Lippincott.

Wold GH: *Basic geriatric nursing,* ed 2, St Louis, 1999, Mosby.

CHAPTER 21

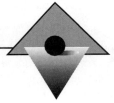

PSYCHIATRIC AND PSYCHOLOGICAL PROBLEMS

Robert Brautigan ● *Beverly Reno*

LEARNING OBJECTIVES

Upon completion of this chapter, the reader will be able to:

- Recognize the events that can precipitate psychological disequilibrium in the older adult
- Identify interventions that will meet the needs of older adults experiencing psychological and psychosocial issues
- Evaluate the effectiveness of the interventions used to reestablish the psychological equilibrium of the older adult
- Describe educational needs of the family who are caring for the older adult with psychological and psychosocial issues
- Assist the family in selecting available and appropriate support resources in the community

I. CRISIS

A. Definition: inability of an individual to cope effectively with either a traumatic or an advantageous event

B. General information
1. Crisis occurs throughout life
2. Older adults have less adaptive capacity and fewer available supports that may result in devastating effects
3. Crisis events always create stress
4. Perception of the event is the critical factor in response to a crisis

C. Causes
1. Translocation
2. Death of a roommate in institutions
3. Major physical disability
4. Multiple losses (i.e., financial, home, independence, and loved ones)

D. Assessment
1. Assess for stability of balancing factors
   a. Realistic perception of the precipitant event
   b. Effective coping mechanisms
   c. Available support systems
2. Assess for feelings of helplessness, hopelessness, anger, and fear
3. Assess for risk of self-destructive and/or socially inappropriate behavior

E. Nursing diagnoses
   1. Coping, ineffective individual: related to situational crises
   2. Role performance, altered: related to decline in adaptation
   3. Hopelessness and powerlessness: related to self-imposed social isolation
   4. Loneliness, risk for: related to social isolation
F. Interventions
   1. Provide a consistent and stable environment
   2. Facilitate the stabilization of balancing factors
   3. Use reminiscence therapy to assess self-esteem and coping mechanisms
   4. Re-establish a sense of patient control

II. CONFUSION/DISORIENTATION

A. Definition: multidimensional state involving changes in both cognition and behavior; confusion is also characterized by the patient's disorientation to person, place, and time; disorientation is a sensory inability to accurately relate to person, place, and time; it does allow the patient to experience accurate sensory perceptions
B. General information
   1. Confusion and disorientation are frequently used synonymously
   2. Disorientation is often associated with an organic disorder
C. Causes
   1. Can be the result of sensory overload or deprivation
   2. May result from systemic/physiological disorders
   3. Environmental factors can cause confusion and disorientation
   4. Response to crisis events/panic attacks
   5. Response to selected medications (i.e., anticholingerics)
D. Assessment
   1. Perform a complete nursing history and physical exam (laboratory studies. urinalysis, with an emphasis on auditory and visual screenings)
   2. Administer the Folstein MiniMental State Assessment Tool (see Chapter 10)
   3. Assess for changes in patient's environment
   4. Assess for recent changes or losses in the patient's life within the last year
   5. Perform a complete medication history, including OTC drugs, alcohol usage, homeopathic and herbal medications, (i.e., Saint John's Wort), antidepressants
E. Nursing diagnoses
   1. Coping, ineffective individual: related to misinterpretation of the environment
   2. Social interaction, impaired: related to disturbance in perception of the environment
   3. Injury, high risk for: related to confusion/disorientation
   4. Coping, ineffective family: related to patient's confusion/disorientation
F. Interventions
   1. Decrease environmental stimuli
   2. Engage in daily reality-focused activities
   3. Promote rest by active daily schedule and avoidance of hypnotics
   4. Maintain nutritional and fluid and electrolyte balance
   5. Monitor medications and their interactions
   6. Monitor elimination patterns
   7. Assist families in expressing effective coping skills when dealing with a confused significant other

III. WANDERING

A. Definition: moving aimlessly from place to place with no permanent residence, meandering; wandering may indicate parietal lobe pathology

B. General information
1. Wandering is nonverbal behavior
2. Wandering can be a form of communication
3. Wandering behavior can be a serious problem in acute- and long-term care settings
4. Wanderers have a higher level of global cognitive impairment than non-wanderers
5. Wandering outside the home/care setting may result in anything from becoming a victim of crime to exposure to the elements
6. Wandering in the home setting may result in injury and become problematic
7. Institutionalization is often the result of wandering

C. Causes
1. Environmental stimuli or lack of stimuli
2. Feelings of being lost, lonely, or separated
3. Situational insecurity, environmental changes, and psychological conflict
4. Feelings of boredom and fear
5. Sleep disorder and anxiety
6. Confusion from organic causes or pharmacological delirium
7. Unmet physical needs, such as pain, hunger, toileting, and exercise

D. Assessment
1. Assess for clinical manifestations according to Klebanoff (1993)
   a. Overtly goal-directed, exit-seeking
   b. Modeling from someone else who is ambulating
   c. Goal-directed behaviors to produce auditory or tactile stimulation
2. Assess for clinical manifestations according to Burke (1992)
   a. Expression of intent: "I'm going home now"
   b. Expression of loss of valued adult role: "The children need me now"
3. Assess for clinical manifestations according to Philipose (1999)
   a. Personality changes may be gradual
   b. Decrease in spontaneity and laughter
   c. Decreased interest in social life and participation in environment
4. Perform complete history and physical exam, including social history
5. Assess cognitive functioning, including memory, mentation, and sensory perception

E. Nursing diagnoses
1. Thought processes, altered: related to confusion and isolation
2. Injury, risk for: related to lack of awareness of environmental hazards
3. Knowledge deficit: family educational needs and/or problem management strategies

F. Interventions
1. Administer the Folstein MiniMental State Assessment Tool
2. Complete a functional assessment (i.e., ADL Scale, IADL Scale)
3. Modify environment to provide safety, rest, and sleep
4. Evaluate the patient's response to medications (some medications may increase the risk of injury because of potential for falls)
5. Avoid physical and pharmacological restraints
6. Secure identification onto patient and use Medic-Alert bracelets
7. Provide information to all staff members that patient is a wanderer; develop mechanism for identification
8. Provide patient with essential sensory aides (glasses, hearing aids, and walker)
9. Schedule toileting
10. Maintain a calm attitude toward wandering
11. Use grid-like markings in front of doorways
12. Use validation therapy
13. Develop a plan to follow if wanderer is missing
14. Provide community and social service referrals, including support groups

IV. SCREAMING

   A. Definition: loud unintelligible shrieking sound or a loud repetition of single words or phrases

   B. General information
     1. Usually unintentional
     2. Patient usually unaware of screaming
     3. Screaming is a form of communication

   C. Causes
     1. Manifestation of agitation, occasionally seen in a patient with dementia

   D. Assessment
     1. Obtain accurate baseline data
     2. Evaluate patient's environment and needs in relation to screaming behavior (tiredness, hunger, toileting)
     3. Focus on the unmet needs vs. the screaming behavior

   E. Nursing diagnoses
     1. Communication, impaired verbal: related to inappropriate verbalizations
     2. Self-care deficit: related to inability to coherently express needs

   F. Interventions
     1. Maintain consistency in staff assignments
     2. Identify needs that are not being met when screaming occurs
     3. Develop a plan that anticipates and fulfills patient's needs
     4. Assess family for special words different from the norm that the patient uses to express needs
     5. Encourage reminiscing and talk to the patient about familiar things
     6. Engage patient in simple group activities to increase socialization
     7. Play soft music and remain with patient when screaming occurs

V. ANXIETY

   A. Definition: perceived threat or danger to the self; the actual source is unknown; the fear is generalized and is defined as an emotional pain

   B. General information
     1. Experiences eliciting anxiety begin in infancy and continue throughout the lifespan
     2. Anxiety is a subjective experience
     3. Can be contagious in that anxiety can spread from one person to another
     4. It is part of a process and can occur at different levels of severity
     5. Between 10% to 25% of the U.S. population experience some form of anxiety disorder

   C. Causes
     1. Result of psychodynamic, biochemical, or existential factors
       a. Psychodynamic: Freud defines anxiety as involving the id, superego, and the ego; it originates in the ego and then attempts to find a balancing force between the "id" and "superego" demands; interpersonal theory defines anxiety as a reaction that results from interactions with others; a strongly developed self-system is needed to protect and adapt to anxiety and give a sense of security
       b. Biochemical: Hans Selye's general adaptation syndrome (GAS) describes the total body's response to stress; physiological changes occur in three stages: fight, flight, or adaptation response
       c. Existential: result of ageism, cultural prejudices, multiple losses, including physical and psychological

   D. Assessment
     1. Assess according to the DSM-IV (APA, 1994)
       a. Axis IV rates the severity of the psychosocial stressors as part of the multiaxial system for diagnosing mental illness

b. Types of anxiety
   (1) Generalized anxiety disorder: persistent anxiety for at least a month in which an individual spends most of his/her time worrying and experiencing motor tension, autonomic hyperactivity, scanning, and vigilance
   (2) Panic disorder: result of panic attacks; it can be anticipatory or phobic
   (3) Obsessive-compulsive disorder: involves uncontrolled recurring thoughts, images, or desires that are disturbing the individual; repetitive behaviors are used by the person to attempt to maintain control of the anxiety
   (4) Phobic disorder: a result of being unreasonably fearful of an object or situation
   (5) Post-traumatic stress disorder (PTS): hastened by a traumatic event; the individual experiences unresponsiveness to the external world; there are alterations in sleep pattern, memory loss, and repetitive mental reviewing of the event
   (6) Somatoform disorder: occurs when the patient presents with multiple physical complaints but no physical findings to validate the symptoms
   (7) Hypochondriasis: exaggerated concern for one's own health; overreaction and misinterpretation of physical feelings, resulting in the belief that a serious illness exists
2. Assess for affective, cognitive, behavioral and physical signs
   a. Sense of impending doom,★ excessive worry,★ and high levels of anxiety
   b. Cognitive manifestations include increased anxiety about normal everyday stresses; decreased creativity; errors in judgment; impaired attention, concentration, and recent memory★
   c. Behaviors that may be exhibited are hypermobility, hypochondriases, somatotization,★ inability to stay asleep, withdrawl,★ regression or putting others in role of parent, wanting to be cared for
   d. Physically the patient exhibits signs of autonomic nervous system hyperactivity as described by the "fight" syndrome in GAS; there are multiple somatic complaints and an increase in blood sugar, adrenal function, and a decrease in oxygen level and calcium
3. Assess for level of anxiety
   a. Mild: the patient is alert, has a broad perception, and is able to learn
   b. Moderate: the patient is alert but perception is diminished and concentration occurs with effort
   c. Severe: the patient is unable to learn, has distorted perception, and is unable to relate things
   d. Panic: results in dissociative disorder; the environment is distorted; patient is unable to communicate coherently, memory is impaired, personality is disorganized
   e. Evaluate for risk of suicide if panic attacks are evident
E. Nursing diagnoses
   1. Anxiety: related to recent loss of significant other
   2. Coping, ineffective individual: related to loss of financial resources
   3. Fear: related to loss of memory
   4. Powerlessness: related to translocation
F. Interventions
   1. Maintain safety (place on periodic safety checks)
   2. Do not interrupt ritualistic behaviors but substitute with activities such as brisk walking and other gross motor activities
   3. Encourage patient to participate in groups and activities
   4. Arrange for consistent caregiver if possible to establish trust
   5. Teach effective coping skills to deal with stressors; use cognitive behavior modification, relaxation training, stress management, and assertiveness training

★Most common in older adults.

6. Provide one-on-one caregiving each shift to encourage patient to vent feelings
7. Keep environment calm and quiet at first; stay with patient during anxiety attacks
8. Use the Beck Depression Scale and Hamilton Anxiety Rating Scale to differentiate levels of anxiety and depression
9. Assist patient and family in individual, group, and partial hospital programs
10. Use pharmacological therapy as appropriate
    a. Antianxiety (anxiolytic) drugs: Ativan (lorezepam),★ Xanax (alprazolam), Buspar (buspirone),★ Serax (oxazepam)
    b. Tricyclic antidepressants with anxiolytic effects: Tofranil (imipramine),★ Anafraril (chlomipramine)
    c. Antihistamines: Benadryl (diphenhydramine)★

VI. DEPRESSION

A. Definition: syndrome known as a mood or affective disorder characterized by severe debilitating sadness, impaired cognitive reasoning, and somatic changes precipitating feelings of loss and/or guilt (see the DSM-IV for specific categories of depression)
B. General information
   1. Most common mental health disorder in older adults
   2. Estimates of prevalence in older adults range from 5% to 40%
   3. 33% of people >60 have some depressive symptoms
   4. Depression prevalent in early dementia
   5. 45% of new admissions to mental hospitals are adults >65
   6. Potential for suicide is high, especially in older adult males
C. Causes
   1. Psychodynamic theory: depression is the result of experiencing significant losses in the early child-parent relationship; the feelings of anger and hate are internalized causing impaired self-esteem and depression
   2. Genetic theory: there is a higher incidence of depression in twins
   3. Biochemical theory: impairment in neurotransmitters results in changes in mood
   4. Cognitive theory: distortions in thinking result in negative attitudes and expectations of self and others
D. Assessment
   1. Perform complete physiological, psychosocial, and cognitive assessment; may need to interview family members for information regarding changes in the patient's affect and social and cognitive behaviors; include a family history
      a. Affect: sad mood, apathy, agitation
      b. Cognitive: somatic concerns, thoughts of death, distorted perceptions, and negative outlook on life
      c. Motivational behavior: psychomotor retardation, restlessness, wandering, fatigue, social withdrawal
      d. Physical: sleep disturbances, changes in appetite, headaches and dizziness
   2. Assess for recent changes/losses (i.e., residence, lifestyle, financial resources, health, significant relationship losses)
   3. Assess for suicidal ideation
   4. Assess for hallucinations and/or delusional thinking
   5. Administer the Beck Depression Scale, Zung's Self-Rating Scale, Geriatric Depression Scale
   6. Administer the Folstein MiniMental State Assessment Tool
   7. Obtain medical evaluation to rule out physical basis for symptoms

★Most commonly used in older adults.

E. Nursing diagnoses
1. Self-esteem disturbance: related to multiple losses
2. Violence, risk for: self-directed, related to emotional pain of depression
3. Spiritual distress: related to negative feelings of being abandoned by Supreme Being
F. Interventions
1. Suggest psychotherapy
a. Individual or group, outpatient or partial hospital day program
b. Inpatient hospitalization if patient is unable to comply with treatment plan, is potentially harmful to self or others, and/or is incapable of life-sustaining self-care
c. Cognitive therapy
d. Reminiscence
e. Spiritual support
2. Meet self-care needs
3. Provide opportunities to express feelings
4. Assess suicidal risk
5. Monitor and reinforce positive coping behaviors
6. Assist in identification of support systems
7. Provide family/caregiver support and education
8. Offer medications
a. SSRIs (serotonin re-uptake inhibitors) are usually the first-choice drugs in the treatment of depression
b. TCAs (tricyclic antidepressants) are also frequently used
c. Anti-anxiety and anti-psychotic agents are given to treat accompanying anxiety and psychosis
d. Saint John's Wort is an herbal remedy that is sold across the counter in health food stores and pharmacies; there are no current conclusive studies to support its long-term effectiveness

VII. SUICIDE

A. Definition: self-destructive behavior with the intent to end one's life
B. General information
1. Suicide rates are highest in the older adult (23% of suicides occur in the older adult)
2. Suicide rate is six times higher in white males than in the general population
3. Non-married, widowed, or divorced have a greater incidence of suicide
4. 80% of older adults who threaten suicide follow through
5. Indirect life-threatening behavior, such as non-compliance or starving to death, may be more prominent in nursing homes and accounts for a higher percentage of deaths in nursing homes in contrast to community dwellers
C. Causes
1. Progressive inability to cope with feelings of loneliness, isolation, anger, and losses of health, home, and significant others
2. Depression, low self-worth, hopelessness
D. Assessment
1. Assess for risk factors
a. Over age 65
b. Presence of chronic illness/pain
c. Living alone
d. History of previous suicide attempt
e. Family history of suicide or mental illness
f. Depression, especially with agitation
g. Significant losses within the past year
h. History of substance abuse

         i. Preoccupied with suicide in conversation
         j. Disposing of personal belongings
     2. Suicide assessment
         a. Intent
         b. Method
         c. Plan
         d. Lethality of plan

E. Nursing diagnoses
     1. Coping, ineffective individual: related to multiple losses
     2. Self-mutilation, high risk for: related to the inability to express emotional pain
     3. Social isolation: related to feelings of insecurity, loneliness

F. Interventions
     1. Implement suicide precautions if suicide intent is assessed to be imminent
     2. Treat depression with psychotherapy and/or medication
     3. Realize that once a patient is serious about suicide, the patient remains at a high risk despite therapy
     4. Refer patient for immediate professional mental health care as indicated
     5. Remove potential method of self-injury
     6. Assist patient in establishing effective support systems

VIII. SELF-ESTEEM/SELF-CONCEPT

A. Definition
     1. Self-concept: encompasses all that the person values, feels, and holds to be true about his/her identity
     2. Self-esteem: the individual's judgment of his/her own worth; it is based on feelings of being valued, loved, useful, and competent

B. General information
     1. Self-concept/self-esteem are learned behaviors developed through the interactions with environment, family, and cultural reference groups
     2. These concepts are based on numerous theories and, therefore, are not easily measured
     3. A person who is reality-oriented is one whose inner reality is consistent with external reality
     4. Ability to maintain a healthy self-concept/self-esteem in the older adult is determined by successful life experiences, social interaction, and the frequency and duration of threats to self-esteem
     5. Ageism can directly effect self-esteem/self-concept in the older adult

C. Assessment
     1. Assess patient's developmental stage according to Erikson's Developmental Theory (ego integrity vs. despair)
     2. Assess the patient's perception of self (i.e., "What do other people think of you?")
     3. Assess role relationships with family and social groups
         a. "Describe yourself."
        b. "How does your family view you?"
        c. "Can you describe what type of family you grew up in?"
        d. "What social groups do you belong to?"
        e. "If you could change one thing in your life right now, what would that be?"
     4. Assess spirituality: "What role does a higher being play in your life?"

D. Nursing diagnoses (to be considered when alterations in self-concept/self-esteem occur in the older adult)
     1. Grieving, anticipatory: related to loss of self-esteem
     2. Hopelessness: related to perceived potential loss of relationships
     3. Coping, ineffective individual: related to low self-esteem

E. Interventions
1. Use reminiscence/life review therapy
2. Identify patient support systems
3. Assess in building social network
4. Administer Life Satisfaction Questionnaire
5. Administer the Luebben Social Network Scale
6. Provide community resources and support systems to meet identified needs
7. Teach effective coping skills

IX. LONELINESS/ISOLATION

A. Definition
1. Loneliness: a painful emotion; it accompanies self-rejection and is an inner sense of longing, emptiness, and sadness
2. Isolation: environmentally created aloneness though situations induced by self and others; separating self from other human contacts
B. Causes
1. Isolation from friends and family often results from institutionalization
2. Isolation may result in depression and loss of self worth and self-esteem
3. Loneliness occurs most frequently in older adults who are living alone, who have chronic illnesses, and who have a perception of debilitation
4. Loneliness increases the risk for physical and mental deterioration; the greatest risk factors for loneliness and isolation are childlessness, loss of social roles, and loss of financial support
C. Assessment
1. Complete nursing history to include Ludden Social Network Scale
2. Assess for a decline in or lack of physical abilities
3. Assess for interaction with others: eye contact, initiation of social interaction, response when visitors arrive and leave
4. Assess for attention-seeking behaviors
5. Administer a social skill checklist
D. Nursing diagnosis
1. Social isolation: related to variety of causes (such as decreased interaction, incontinence, sensory deprivation, financial restraints, lack of social/community resources)
E. Interventions
1. Establish time to spend with the patient either in silence or conversation
2. Suggest a pet, when appropriate, to decrease loneliness
3. Utilize a life review
4. Establish a family/community program to manage/prevent social isolation and loneliness in the older adult

X. SUBSTANCE-RELATED DISORDERS

A. Definition: according to the DSM-IV, substance use disorders are classified as dependency and abuse; there is a difference between dependency and abuse in that abuse does not include the processes of tolerance, compulsion, and withdrawal (APA, 1994)
B. General information
1. It is estimated that between 20% to 40% of nursing home residents are alcoholics
2. Alcoholism in the older adult often goes unrecognized because of chronic illnesses that can confuse the diagnosis of alcoholism
3. Decreased social demands allow older adults to easily hide their drinking
C. Causes
1. No single factor has been identified as the cause of alcohol abuse/dependency; however, common theories include
a. Behavioral: a response to stress in the environment

      b. Social/cultural theory: hopelessness of living conditions leads to the use of alcohol as a means for coping

      c. Biologic theory: genetic and biochemical factors increase the susceptibility to alcohol abuse/dependency in certain individuals

D. Assessment

    1. Complete nursing history to include

      a. Family relationships

      b. Environmental factors

      c. Social relationships

      d. Physical examination, to include all systems with special emphasis on psychomotor, cutaneous, and cognitive

      e. Laboratory and nutritional analysis

E. Nursing diagnoses

    1. Coping, ineffective individual: related to impaired or non-existent support systems

    2. Social isolation: related to mistrust and mistreatment by others

    3. High risk for injury: related to motor and cognitive impairment

F. Interventions

    1. Monitor for acute withdrawal symptoms (vital signs, hydration, and seizures) and treat appropriately

    2. Increase nutrition and fluids

    3. Maintain nonjudgmental and supportive approach

    4. Encourage and assist in attending self-help groups

    5. Assist with identification of effective coping mechanisms and support systems

REFERENCES

Algase D: Cognitive discriminants of wandering among nursing home residents, *Nurs Res* 41(2): 78-81, 1992.

American Association of Retired Persons: *Alcohol abuse among people,* Washington, DC, 1994, AARP.

American Psychiatric Association: *Diagnostic and statistical manual of mental disorders,* ed 4, Washington, DC, 1994, The Association.

Arnold E, Bogg M: *Interpersonal relationships,* ed 2, Philadelphia, 1995, WB Saunders.

Baker FM: A contrast: geriatric depression versus depression in younger age groups, *J National Med Associa* 83:340-344, 1991.

Beck A: *Depression: causes and treatment,* Philadelphia, 1967, University of Pennsylvania Press.

Boyd M, Nihart M: *Psychiatric nursing: contemporary practice,* Philadelphia, 1998, JB Lippincott.

Brant BA, Osgood NJ: The suicidal patient and long-term care institutions, *J Gerontol Nurs* 16(2):15-18, 1990.

Brautigan R, Reno B: Depression in the older adult. In Luggen A, Travis S, Meiner S, editors: *NGNA core curriculum for gerontological advanced practice nurses,* Thousand Oaks, CA, 1998, Sage.

Burke M: *Gerontological nursing: care of the frail elderly,* St Louis, 1992, Mosby.

Carson V, Arnold E: *Mental health nursing: the nurse-patient journey,* Philadelphia, 1996, WB Saunders.

Drew B: No suicide contracts to prevent suicidal behavior in the in-patient psychiatric settings, *J Am Psychiatr Nurs Assoc* 5(1):23-28, February, 1999.

Ebersole P, Hess P: *Toward healthy aging: human needs and nursing response,* ed 5, St Louis, 1998, Mosby.

Eliopoulos C: *Gerontological nursing,* ed 4, Philadelphia, 1997, JB Lippincott.

Flowers ME: Recognition and psychopharmacologic treatment of geriatric depression, *J Am Psychiatr Nurs Assoc* 3(2):32-39, 1997.

Frierson RL: Suicide attempts by the old and the very old, *Arch Inter Med* 151:141-144, 1991.

Haber J: *Comprehensive psychiatric nursing,* ed 5, St Louis, 1997, Mosby.

Harvard Medical School: Update on mood disorders, part 2, *Harvard Mental Health Lett,* January, 1998, pp 1-5.

Isaacs A: *Lippincott's review series: mental health and psychiatric nursing,* ed 2, Philadelphia, 1996, JB Lippincott.

Kane R, Kane R: *Assessing the elderly: a practical guide to measurement,* Santa Monica, CA, 1981, Rand.

Klebanoff N: Wandering. In Loftis PA, Glover T: *Decision-making in gerontological nursing,* St Louis, 1993, Mosby.

Lueckenotte A: *Gerontologic nursing,* St Louis, 1996, Mosby.

McCall PL: Adolescent and elderly white male suicide trends: evidence of changing well-being, *J Gerontol Nurs* 46:S43-51, 1991.

Moody HR: *Aging: concepts and controversies,* Thousand Oaks, CA, 1994, Pine Forge Press.

Moore S: Grief and loss. In Luggen A, Travis S, Meiner S, editors: *NGNA core curriculum for gerontological advanced practice nurses,* Thousand Oaks, CA, 1998, Sage.

Murray RB, et al: *Health assessment promotion strategies through the life span,* ed 6, Stamford, CT, 1997, Appleton & Lange.

Philipose V: Addressing cognitive issues. In Tyson SR, editor: *Gerontological nursing care,* Philadelphia, 1999, WB Saunders.

Samter J: Crisis intervention. In Luggen A: *Core curriculum for gerontological nurses,* St Louis, 1996, Mosby.

Townsend M: *Essentials of psychiatric mental health nursing,* Philadelphia, 1999, FA Davis.

Townsend M: *Nursing diagnosis in psychiatric nursing,* ed 2, Philadelphia, 1991, FA Davis.

US Department of Health and Human Services: *Depression in primary care: detection and diagnosis,* Washington, DC, 1993, Government Printing Office.

Yesavage JA, et al: Geriatric depression scale. In Corcoran K, Fischer J: *Measures for clinical practice, a sourcebook,* New York, 1987, The Free Press.

Zung W: Self-rating depression scale, *Arch Gen Psychiatr* 70:63-70, 1965.

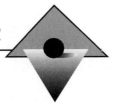

CHAPTER 22

INTEGUMENTARY PROBLEMS

Ann Schmidt Luggen

LEARNING OBJECTIVES

Upon completion of this chapter, the reader will be able to:

- Describe skin problems that occur with aging
- Discuss causes of pruritus and corresponding nursing interventions
- Differentiate between seborrheic and actinic keratoses
- Differentiate between three skin cancers prevalent in older adults
- Describe the clinical course of herpes zoster
- Discuss prevention and care of pressure ulcers

I. NORMAL AGING CHANGES OF SKIN

A. Epidermis: outer layer of skin becomes thin, fragile, shiny, flat
B. Dermis: layer below epidermis; supportive layer of connective tissue with hair follicles, sweat and sebaceous glands, nerve fibers, muscle cells, blood vessels; becomes less elastic, less supple, decreased blood flow, decreased proliferation of cells, diminished sensation, decreased sweating, decreased sebum production; loss of axillary and pubic hair in females, head hair thins and loses melanin—hence the gray color; chin hair grows because of decreased estrogen (Box 22-1)
C. Nails: become hard and thick, brittle, dull; vertical ridges develop because of decreased water content, calcium, blood supply

II. AGING SKIN PROBLEMS

A. Xerosis (dry skin)
  1. Cause: loss of sebum production, a protectant from dehydration
  2. Treatment: rehydrate epidermis with
    a. Vaseline, zinc oxide
    b. Mineral oil, ointments after bathing
    c. Limit soaps; use superfatted soaps without hexachloraphene (e.g., Dove, Caress)
    d. Lotions TID
    e. Increase room humidity to 60%
B. Pruritus (itching)
  1. Cause: eczema, seborrhea, psoriasis, hypothyroidism, hallucinations/dementias, impetigo, and scabies; pruritus is a symptom, not a disease; contributing factors are heat, temperature changes, sweating, fatigue, stress, illness (e.g., chronic renal failure, liver disease, iron-deficiency anemia).
  2. Treatment
    a. Cool compresses of saline solution
    b. Oatmeal compresses
    c. Epsom salts bath

BOX 22-1   **Cultural Aspects**

- Caucasians gray and wrinkle earlier than other races
- Mongolian spots (irregular-shaped gray areas) are very common in African Americans (90%) and Asians and Native Americans (80%); less so in Caucasians (9%)

Seen on lower back, buttocks, thigh

Occasionally arm, abdomen

      d. Lubriderm or Nutraderm lotions

      e. Avoidance of vigorous toweling

C. Keratoses

  1. Seborrheic keratoses

      a. Benign growths of face, scalp, trunk

      b. Occur commonly in older adults >65 years of age

      c. Superficial, raised, circumscribed lesions

      d. Thicken, darken over time

      e. Greasy appearance; "waxy blob"

      f. Can be picked off but return

  2. Actinic keratoses (solar keratoses)

      a. Precancerous lesions

      b. Cause: sun exposure

      c. Occur on sun-exposed areas: face, ears, nose, head, hands

      d. Skin thickens, crusts, has red-brown color, scaly patch

      e. Should be removed surgically

D. Skin cancers

  1. Basal cell (most common skin cancer)

      a. Appears in persons >50 years of age

      b. Cause: sun exposure, chronic irritation (eyeglasses), chronic ulceration

      c. Incidence highest in light-skinned individuals

      d. Slow-growing skin cancer

      e. First appears as pearly papule with blood vessels, or scar-like

      f. Ulcerates; disfiguring

      g. Rare metastasis

  2. Squamous cell (second most common skin cancer)

      a. Cancer of epidermic keratinocytes

      b. Common in fair-skinned older (>60) men with sun exposure

      c. Cause: radiation exposure, chronic stasis ulcers, scars (injury), chemical carcinogens (e.g., hydrocarbons)

      d. Presents as flesh-colored nodule

      e. Later, reddens, is scaly or hard wart-like, gray, or ulcerated, indurated with raised defined borders

      f. Metastasizes, requires excision

  3. Melanoma

      a. Cancer of melanocytes

      b. Increasing prevalence

      c. Metastatic; high mortality rate

      d. Cause: sun exposure, especially severe burn at a young age

      e. Presents on legs, backs of women; backs of men

      f. Develops from moles; pre-existent or new moles

      g. Diagnosis: asymmetrical, ragged border, multi-colored, mottled change in size or shape of mole

      h. Treatment: surgical excision, chemotherapy, radiation therapy

E. Pressure ulcers
   1. Definition: chronic disorder of bed-bound, debilitated elders; commonly found from the waist down
   2. Prevalence: 23% in long-term care settings; 30% in acute care
   3. Cause: ischemia and anoxia of skin tissue from persistent pressure
   4. Characteristics: series of events beginning with erythema (redness), edema, blister formation, ulceration
   5. Contributing factors: poor nutritional status, lack of subcutaneous fat, steroid therapy, immobilization, heat, moisture, age >70
   6. High risk: patients with femoral fractures (66%), quadriplegia (69%), critical care patients (33%), and residents in skilled nursing facilities (23%)
   7. Assessment: visual and tactile; prevention is key
      a. Establish baseline skin assessment, document
      b. Identify potential areas of breakdown
      c. Assess hyperemia (redness); recheck in 1 hour
      d. Note location, color, size, and use tools (see References, Pressure Ulcer Tools)
      e. Assess nutrition and serum albumin; <3.5 g/dl correlates with pressure sore severity
   8. Intervention
      a. Cost of healing pressure sore estimated to be $20,000
      b. Time to heal 60-year-old patient about 100 days
      c. Eliminate friction, moisture, encourage weight shifts q15 minutes; turn frequently q1h
      d. Good nutrition vital; need proteins, carbohydrates, vitamins
      e. Debridement of necrotic tissue
      f. Wound cleansing, appropriate dressings
      g. Mattress foam, air, gel, or water
      h. Sheepskin or pillows to keep ankles apart, heels off bed
      i. Change incontinent-soiled sheets promptly
F. Scabies
   1. Definition: parasitic mite *(Sarcoptes scabies)* that burrows under skin; communicable infection causing irritation and pruritus; incubation period 4 to 6 weeks
   2. Signs: intense itching; fine, wavy dark lines on finger webs, wrist, elbow, axilla, genitals; may present in different forms: blisters, eruptions
   3. Spread: direct contact
   4. Diagnosis: skin scrapings
   5. Assessment: on admission to any institution: acute care, long-term care
G. Herpes zoster (shingles)
   1. Definition: infectious, acute, vesicular painful inflammation of dorsal root ganglia by reactivated varicella zoster virus (cause of chickenpox)
   2. Occurs in >50 age groups, .5 to 1.0/100 people
   3. Increased incidence in patients with lymphoma, leukemia, AIDS because of diminished immune response
   4. Risk factors: increased age, physical or emotional traumas, debilitated state, systemic illness, immunosuppression
   5. Clinical: onset of fever and malaise with vesicular lesions occurring unilaterally along a dermatome; 1 to 4 days before there may be severe pain, itching, and burning in the same area; lesions progress to pustules, scab, heal 7 to 14 days later; post-herpetic neuralgia may occur and last months to years
   6. Diagnosis: characteristic lesions and Tzanck test of vesicular fluid
   7. Complications: infection of the ophthalmic branch of the trigeminal nerve or oculomotor nerve; may cause corneal and scleral damage and loss of vision

8. Management
   a. Pain: begin aspirin or acetaminophen (Tylenol) by mouth q4h for mild pain; codeine for moderate pain
   b. Acyclovir: antiviral q4h × 7–10 days; will decrease pain and healing time if begun early
   c. Steroids may be given to prevent post-herpetic neuralgia
   d. Post-herpetic neuralgia treatment
      (1) Topical capsaicin (Zostrix)
      (2) Amitryptyline (Elavil) + perphenazine (Trilafon) for months
      (3) TENS units may be helpful
      (4) Cool compresses to affected area
      (5) Pain may be so severe that clothes are painful

REFERENCES

Dennis C: Maintaining wellness of skin. In Tyson SR, editor: *Gerontological nursing care,* Philadelphia, 1999, WB Saunders.

Ebersole P, Hess P: *Toward healthy aging: human needs and nursing response,* ed 5, St Louis, 1998, Mosby.

Wold GH: *Basic geriatric nursing,* ed 2, St Louis, 1999, Mosby.

Pressure Ulcer Tools

Braden Scale

US Department of Health and Human Services: *Clinical practice guideline: pressure ulcers,* Rockville, MD, 1992, AHCPR

Norton Scale

Norton D, McLaren R, Exton-Smith AN: *An investigation of geriatric nursing problems in the hospital,* London, 1962, National Corporation for Care of Old People.

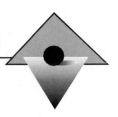

CHAPTER 23

SENSORY PROBLEMS

Ann Schmidt Luggen

LEARNING OBJECTIVES

Upon completion of this chapter, the reader will be able to:

- Describe the sensory changes and problems that occur with aging
- Conduct an assessment of the sensory system
- Discuss nursing management of sensorineural problems of older adults

I. HEARING LOSS

A. Incidence/prevalence
    1. Affects 28 million older adults
    2. Increases with aging
    3. Loss is gradual and insidious
    4. Prevalence
       • >30% of individuals aged 65-74
       • >45% of persons aged 75
       • >85% institutionalized older adults
B. Definition
    1. Conduction loss
       a. Defect or disease of external or middle ear that affects transmission of sound to inner ear; air conduction decreased; bone conduction normal; cerumen accumulates in external ear canal and contributes to the problem
       b. Otosclerosis: conductive loss affecting 1:100 elders, women > men; linked to childhood otitis media, measles; surgery may add improvement in hearing along with use of a hearing aid
    2. Sensorineural loss
       a. Cochlear problem with hair cells or cochlear nerve; irreversible although new cochlear implants may help; drugs with ototoxic effects include gentamycin, streptomycin, furosemide, salicylates, ibuprofen
       b. Presbycusis: progressive degeneration of inner ear over 5 to 10 years; decreasing acuity of hearing; difficulty discriminating high-pitched consonants (f, g, s, t sound); contributing factors are noise exposure, familial/genetic causes, arteriosclerosis, diabetes mellitus, ototoxic drugs, and Meniere's disease
       c. Tinnitus: high- or low-pitched tingling sound affecting L > R ear and men > women; may be accompanied by vertigo with nausea and vomiting, suggesting involvement of vestibular apparatus of ear, may occur with presbycusis
    3. Mixed loss
       a. Conductive and sensorineural
       b. Assessment reveals decreased air and bone conduction

C. Normal age-related changes in hearing
   1. Auditory system: external, middle, inner ear structures; VIII cranial nerve; auditory brainstem and auditory cortex in temporal lobe
   2. Primary dysfunctional changes caused by change in outer hair cells of the cochlea
   3. Tympanic membrane stiffens
   4. Inner ear cells degenerate
   5. Degeneration of ganglion cells and VIII cranial nerve fibers
   6. Inner ear membrane calcifies
   7. Cochlear blood supply diminishes
D. Consequences of hearing loss
   1. Affects communication with others
   2. Cannot hear music, laughter
   3. May lead to depression, social isolation
   4. Safety issues: unable to hear smoke alarm, telephone
   5. Loss of self-esteem
E. Clinical changes
   1. Loss of pure tones
   2. Cannot understand normal speech
   3. Cannot localize sound
   4. Difficulty listening with both ears
F. Assessment
   1. In patient's room or home, note loud TV, inability to hear telephone, patient talking loudly especially on telephone
   2. Assess acuity in normal quiet environment
   3. Observe for depression, isolation, hostility
   4. Assess motivation for assistive device intervention
   5. Examine for cerumen accumulation, otitis, membrane bulging, or perforation
   6. Use Weber and Rinne tests for air and bone conduction with 512 Hz tuning fork
   7. Refer to specialist in audiometry for further screening if deficiencies found
G. Management
   1. Touch patient to get attention
   2. Speak distinctly face to face, speaking to the "good" ear, unhurried, not shouting, in quiet setting, keeping voice tone low (cannot hear high-pitched sounds well)
   3. Involve family, friends, in strategizing
   4. Use Debrox (carbamide) for cerumen accumulation
   5. Use mineral oil at night to soften hardened wax
   6. Advise avoidance of inserting any object in ear
   7. Refer to ENT specialist (ear/nose/throat) for cerumen impaction
   8. Enhance telephone ringer, door bell, alarm clock
   9. Refer to audiometry specialist for hearing aid
   10. Hearing aid will facilitate communication, decrease loneliness and social isolation
   11. Hearing dogs are available for elderly hearing-impaired patients who live alone in the community
   12. Cochlear implants are available

II. VISION LOSS

A. Incidence and prevalence
   1. >90% of adults >65 need vision correction
   2. 65% have presbyopia, the most common change, difficulty with accommodation
   3. 60% have hyperopia, farsightedness
   4. 65% to 70% have astigmatism, increased curvature of cornea, distorting vision at all distances

5. 20% have myopia, nearsightedness
6. Cataracts, most common disorder of eye in older adults; two thirds of population >60 and 90% of the population >70 years of age
7. About 3 million people with low vision are unable to read
8. Adults 45 to 65 require a corrective lens change about every 2 to 3 years
9. Some individuals 60 to 70 get "second sight" and can see without glasses

B. Age changes of eyes
1. Loss of accommodation: presbyopia
2. Arcus senilis: calcium deposits and cholesterol salts deposits with a gray-white ring at the iris edge
3. Miosis: diminished pupil size because of sclerosis of the pupil sphincter and atrophy of the iris muscles; causes diminished visual fields and diminished peripheral vision; results in decreased light on retina and decreased vision in dim light situations
4. Color vision: lens yellows and filters out light; elders see blue and green as darker; also may be caused by drug toxicity (e.g., digoxin)
5. Lens opacity: increased light scatter causing glare; difficulty with night driving; decreased light to the retina
6. Entropion: lower lid flaccidity with inward-turned lashes that irritate cornea; requires surgical intervention
7. Ectropion: upper lid flaccidity causing inflammation and tearing; requires surgical intervention
8. Diminished tear secretion: caused by failure of the lacrimal pump; occurs particularly in postmenopausal women; causes dryness, irritation, discomfort; the eye cries less but waters more

C. Eye disorders common with aging
1. Cataracts: most common eye disorder in older adults
   a. Loss of transparency of lens
   b. Progressive, painless
   c. Heightened sensitivity to glare, blurring of vision, halos, clouded vision, decreased acuity of vision
   d. Corrective lens used until cataract "matures" enough for surgery (outpatient) with local or topical anesthesia; only one eye operated on at a time
   e. Eye patch after surgery for one day and at night for several weeks.
   f. Intraocular pressure (IOP) increases should be avoided for 2 to 3 weeks (e.g. bending, lifting, straining)
   g. Eyedrops after surgery
   h. Second eye can be done 1 to 2 months after completion of first surgery
2. Glaucoma: second leading cause of blindness in United States, major cause of blindness in African Americans; risk factors include race, family history, advanced age, myopia, retinal vascular disturbance, steroid use, diabetes mellitus
   a. Disease characterized by increased intraocular pressure (IOP) from fluids that may damage the retina
   b. Affects peripheral vision, resulting in tunnel vision
   c. Eventual blindness if untreated
   d. Symptoms are rare; irreversible damage can occur before recognition
   e. Tests for IOP easily done and should be done on all people >40 years of age
   f. Two primary types of glaucoma
      (1) Primary open-angle glaucoma accounts for 80% to 90% of cases in the United States (described previously)
      (2) Acute narrow-angle glaucoma accounts for 10% of U.S. glaucomas; more common in Asians, Native Alaskans, Chinese, and far-sighted people; this glaucoma has symptoms: redness and pain in eye, headache, nausea and vomiting, corneal edema, diminished vision immediately

g. There are secondary glaucomas caused by previous or concurrent eye disorders; characterized by anatomical or functional block of outflow of intraocular fluids, increasing the pressure; about 10% of glaucomas are these

h. Management

   (1) Screening conducted by eye specialists (ophthalmologist, optician)

   (2) Pilocarpine (mydriatic) eyedrops or an anticholinergic drug may precipitate severe eye pain with acute narrow-angle glaucoma; requires immediate ophthalmologic intervention

   (3) Drugs used to treat glaucoma include topical beta-blockers, such as timolol (Timoptic) or betaxolol (Betoptic); also acetazolamide (Diamox), methazolamide (Neptazane), dorzolamide (Trusopt), pilocarpine (IsoptoCarpine, Piloptic, Pilocar), and apraclonidine (Iopidine).

   (4) Any side effects of these drugs should be monitored and then reported to the ophthalmologist

   (5) Drugs must be taken indefinitely

   (6) Eye evaluation should occur every 6 months

   (7) Magnifying glasses, tinted lens

   (8) Large-faced clocks, watches, telephones

   (9) Large print books, talking books

3. Macular degeneration (senile macular degeneration):

a. Prevalence is about 30% of elders aged 75 to 81

b. Risk: Caucasians, smokers, patients with hypertension

c. The macula is a small area in the center of the retina where visual acuity is best

d. Macular degeneration (MD) occurs mostly in older adults

e. MD is the number one cause of legal blindness in the United States in adults >55

f. Cause is unknown; prognosis is poor

g. Two forms

   (1) Dry form: may be caused by inadequate vascularity to the eye; only central vision is lost; peripheral vision stable

   (2) Wet form: is caused by neovascularization (?), abnormal growth of blood vessels under the retina; vision damaged by leaking blood, which distorts the retina causing severe vision loss; laser surgery can seal blood vessels to prevent further loss

h. Assessment

   (1) Signs of central vision distortion; objects increase or decrease in size or straight lines appear bent

   (2) Determine motivation for low vision intervention

i. Management

- Refer to ophthalmologist
- Counsel use of magnifying lens, high-intensity lighting
- Advise telescopic lens may be needed for street signs
- Refer to counseling
- Refer to vision rehabilitation specialist
- Use bright colors, contrasting strong colors (not beige on white)
- Don't move furniture in room of patient with poor vision
- Become politically active; get sounds with traffic walk lights in every community

4. Diabetic retinopathy

a. Leading cause of blindness in adults

b. Occurs with long-standing DM, >15 years; causes blindness in 8000 in United States/year

     c. Symptoms include
- Decreased visual acuity
- Contrast sensitivity decreased
- Decreased color perception
- Decreased dark/light adaptation
- Scotomas (spots or lights)
- Glare disability

     d. Cause: hemorrhage in small blood vessels in vitreous humor similar to neovascularization in macular degeneration

     e. Management
- All diabetic patients should have yearly eye exams by an ophthalmologist
- Photocoagulation should be done by retinal specialist
- Maintain good control of diabetes mellitus

5. Detached retina
   a. Definition: forward displacement of the retina from normal position against the choroid
   b. Symptoms: spots moving across the eye, flashes of light, perception of a coating over the eyes
   c. Intervention
   - Must be prompt to prevent further damage, loss of vision
   - Bedrest, possible surgery
   - Can recur, occur in opposite eye

6. Floaters
   a. Definition: dots, lines, clouds in front of vision
   b. Occurs after age 50
   c. Clumps of debris in vitreous humor in front of retina
   d. Cause is degeneration of vitreous gel, hormonal (?)

7. Drug toxicity to eye
   a. Many drugs can cause toxicity to eyes
   b. Selected drugs
      (1) Cardiac
          - Digitalis, propanolol, quinidine, verapamil
      (2) Antihypertensives
          - Hydrochlorothiazide, chlorothiazide, hydralazine, alpha-methyldopa, spironolactone
      (3) NSAIDs (nonsteroidal antiinflammatory drugs)
          - Ibuprofen, salicylates, naproxen
      (4) Hypoglycemics
          - Tolbutamide, chlorpropamide
      (5) Antipsychotics
          - Haloperidol, chlorpromazine
      (6) Antidepressants
          - Tricyclics
      (7) Other
          - Dicumarol, heparin, morphine, vitamin D, vitamin A

III. TASTE (GUSTATION)

A. Taste facts
   1. Diminished taste and smell begins about age 60
   2. Taste depends about two thirds on smell ability
   3. It requires an intact nerve supply (facial nerve VII, glossopharyngeal IX)
B. Normal changes
   1. Decreased number of papillae
   2. 30% decrease in taste buds by age 70; begins at age 40

3. Decrease in salivary gland production, leads to dry mouth (xerostomia)

4. Major tastes: sweet, sour, salty, bitter—sweet, sour most affected by age

C. Taste problems

1. Unpleasant or strange taste; loss of taste, dysgeusia

2. Unpleasant smell, dysomnia

D. Causes of taste problems

1. Cigarette smoking

2. Poor oral hygiene

3. Infections in mouth

4. Vitamin deficiencies: niacin, riboflavin, vitamin C

5. Head injury

6. Medications

7. Nasal polyps

8. Sinusitis

E. Urgent taste problems

1. Hallucinations of taste or smell: CNS disorder or pharyngeal or esophageal cancers

IV. SMELL (OLFACTORY)

A. Smell facts

1. There is diminution of sense of smell with aging

2. 1:2 people >65 have lost sense of smell; fewer males than females

3. More sense of smell is lost than taste

4. Requires intact nerve supply, cranial nerve I

5. Olfactory nerves are only sensory nerves capable of regeneration

6. Unpleasant smell, dysosmia; no smell, anosmia

B. Causes of decreased or lost sense of smell

1. Nasal sinus disease

2. Repeated viral infections

3. Head trauma (minor cause)

C. Assessment: head/nose

1. Check fit of dental prostheses

2. Assess chewing ability

3. Note papillae

4. Note tongue size

5. Gingivitis, caries

6. Stomatitis

7. Hydration and color of mucous membranes in mouth and nose

8. Discuss gastroesophageal reflux, regurgitation

9. History of smoking

10. Swelling of mucous membranes of nose

11. Lesions of nose and mouth, gums, leukoplakia

D. Diseases affecting taste and smell

1. Allergy: 23% suffer loss of smell; in United States 20 to 30 million have allergic rhinitis

2. Alzheimer's disease

3. Asthma

4. Cancers

5. Epilepsy

6. Diabetes mellitus

7. Liver diseases

8. Parkinson's disease; may be very early sign of PD

9. Chronic renal failure

10. Viral infections

    11. Vitamin deficiencies

    12. Zinc deficiency

    13. Radiation therapy to the head

E. Drugs affecting taste and smell

    1. Anesthetics

    2. Antibiotics

    3. Anticonvulsants

    4. Antidepressants

    5. Antihistamines

    6. Antihypertensives

    7. Antiinflammatories

    8. Antineoplastics

    9. Beta-blockers

    10. Bronchodilators

    11. Calcium channel blockers

    12. Lipid-lowering agents

    13. Vasodilators

F. Management: focus on maintaining nutrition, safety, and social issues

    1. Serve very flavorful foods such as bacon and cheeses

    2. Increase the texture of foods; avoid bland liquid, soft diets

    3. Increase the smell of foods (breads)

    4. Perform meticulous oral hygiene

    5. Review medications

    6. Assess home environment

      • Gas cooking and heating (gas smells)

      • Faulty heaters

      • Contaminated foods

      • Smoke detectors

    7. Evaluate social areas

      • Body odor smells

      • Urine smells in living environment or on body

V. Touch

A. Touch facts

    1. Need for touch continues throughout life; increased in later years

    2. Tactile stimuli send nonverbal messages; caring touch communicates trust, care, sense of worthiness

    3. Patients will have individualized preferences about touch

      • Tweaking a cheek may cause anger

      • Pat on the back may be considered demeaning

    4. There are many kinds of touch from soft and light to deep and firm

    5. Usually touching the hand or upper arm is successful

    6. There are cultural differences in touch: Native Alaskans, Hispanics, French, and Jews are high-touch peoples in contrast with others; handshakes may be limit of touch for some

    7. Need for touch may increase as other sensory deficits increase

VI. Thermal Sensitivity

A. Thermal facts

    1. Palms of hands and soles of feet decrease in ability to sense heat and cold

    2. Assess these areas for bruises, burns, pressure

3. Older adults become increasingly sensitive to cold; institutions often are kept cold for the employees; residents need long-sleeved clothing and sweaters to maintain heat

4. See Chapter 17 on hypothermia/hyperthermia

VII. SENSORY OVERLOAD

A. Sensory overload facts
1. Increased neuro-excitability with aging
2. Increased secretion of neurotransmitters
3. Over-arousal occurs with sudden changes such as
    a. Hospitalization (institutionalization)
    b. Accidents
    c. Environmental demands
4. Those who marginally adapt are especially vulnerable

B. Signs of sensory overload
1. Racing thoughts
2. Attention scatter
3. Inability to sit still
4. Aberrant thoughts

C. Management
1. Sit with the person
2. Quiet room, decreased noise levels
3. Dim lights
4. Engage patient in non–demanding repetitive activity
5. Walking

REFERENCES

Brant BA: Sensory disorders. In Stone JT, Wyman JF, Salisbury SA, editors: *Clinical gerontological nursing,* ed 2, Philadelphia, 1999, WB Saunders.

Ebersole P, Hess P: *Toward healthy aging: human needs and nursing response,* St Louis, 1998, Mosby.

Tyson SR, Tyson SL: The five senses: sensation and perception. In Tyson SR, editor: *Gerontological nursing care,* Philadelphia, 1999, WB Saunders.

U.S. Department of Health and Human Services: *Cataracts in adults: management of functional impairment,* #93-0542, Rockville, MD, 1993, AHCPR, PHS.

Wicks MS: Older clients in the community. In Ayers M., Bruno A, Langford R, editors: *Community-based nursing care,* St Louis, 1999, Mosby.

Wold GH: *Basic geriatric nursing,* ed 2, St Louis, 1999, Mosby.

CHAPTER 24

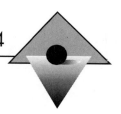

MEDICATIONS

Shirley S. Travis

LEARNING OBJECTIVES

Upon completion of this chapter, the reader will be able to:

- Define three aspects of drug misadventuring that affect nursing practice
- Recognize principles of pharmacokinetics/pharmacodynamics affecting mecication use among older adults
- Discuss the risks for adverse reactions to medications among older adults
- Recognize compliance issues that are most relevant for older adult clients

I. DRUG MISADVENTURING

A. Defined in the broadest sense to include all that can go wrong in the process of using a medication, including polypharmacy, adverse effects, and compliance issues

II. BACKGROUND INFORMATION

A. Nursing home (NH) residents receive an average of 6 drugs/day with 45% taking 7 or more and 20% taking more than 10

B. Greater than 60% of all visits to a physician for patients age >50 include renewal, continuation, or prescription of at least one medication

C. Prescription use (both likelihood of having a prescription and the number of medications) increases with age

D. One in 13 prescriptions received from office-based physicians involves a potentially inappropriate medication

III. POLYPHARMACY

A. Defined as the use of excessive or unnecessary medications with associated increased risk of drug interactions and other adverse effects

B. Causes of polypharmacy
1. Inadequate diagnosis
2. Illogical or inappropriate prescribing
3. Multiple prescribers without adequate lines of communication for effective monitoring
4. Failure to discontinue medications that are ineffective or no longer necessary as the patient's condition changes
5. Failure to agree on a therapeutic endpoint
6. Inadequate or ineffective family/patient education

BOX **24-1**   **Dosing Adjustments**

Aspirin can increase the effect of anticoagulants, penicillins
Antacids can decrease the effect of aspirin
Antidepressants can increase the effect of narcotics
Meperidine can decrease the effect of glaucoma medication

IV. PHARMACOKINETICS/PHARMACODYNAMICS

A. Pharmacokinetics: defined as the study of processes that affect drug concentration in the body, including drug absorption, distribution, and clearance by biotransformation or elimination
   1. Absorption: movement of a drug from the site of administration into the body
   2. Bioavailability: the amount of the drug administered that reaches the systemic circulation compared to the amount that reaches the circulation after intravenous administration
   3. Distribution: the amount of the drug distributed throughout the body in the extracellular and intracellular spaces with distribution to the well-perfused organs occurring most rapidly
   4. Volume of distribution: a hypothetical volume, an estimate of the fluid volume required to distribute a drug evenly throughout the body; is affected by a number of age-related changes in the body and drugs that decrease extracellular fluid
   5. Drug clearance: the kidneys and liver are the major sites of drug elimination from the body; both are affected by age-related changes in physiology
   6. Drug half-life: the time required to decrease the amount of a drug in the body by half; related to volume of distribution and clearance
B. Pharmacodynamics: defined as the quantifiable effects a drug has on its target receptor relative to the drug dose or concentration; physiological aging changes receptor systems and often necessitates suggested dose adjustments (Box 24-1)

V. ADVERSE DRUG REACTIONS

A. An adverse drug reaction (ADR) is any undesirable or unintended effect occurring with medication dosages at any dosage or drug concentration; 2 to 3 times more likely to occur in older than in younger adults (Box 24-2)
B. Causes of ADRs
   1. Interindividual variability
   2. Altered pharmacokinetics or pharmacodynamics or both
   3. Medications with a narrow toxic-therapeutic range (e.g., digoxin)
   4. Drug interactions and additives
   5. Number and severity of chronic illnesses
   6. Drug-disease interactions
   7. Number and types of medications prescribed
C. Drug-drug interactions: a result of the polypharmacy associated with advanced age; characterized as those that alter the pharmacokinetics of another drug or alter the pharmacodynamics of the drug
D. Drug-nutrient interactions: over-the-counter medications (OTCs), vitamins, and foodstuffs can affect absorption and interact with prescription medications
E. Drug-disease interactions: underlying pathology can alter the effects of medications
F. Elders in long-term care are at increased risk of ADRs

VI. NONCOMPLIANCE RISK FACTORS

A. Multiple medications
B. Recent prescription changes
C. Inability to name prescriptions
D. Multiple practitioners

BOX 24-2   Adverse Drug Reactions

Signs and symptoms of adverse reactions to a drug may differ in older adults
Adverse reactions may not be noted immediately after giving a drug
Adverse reactions to a drug may occur after the drug is discontinued
An adverse reaction to a drug may occur precipitously even though the older adult has taken the drug for
   some time

BOX 24-3   Drug Review

A substantial proportion of antimicrobial use (systemic and topical) in long-term care facilities is considered inappropriate
Eye drops for glaucoma are an important and often overlooked source of systemic adverse medication
   effects
Careful monitoring and titrating doses of drugs is essential

BOX 24-4   Self-Medication Errors

Giving an incorrect dose
Misunderstanding instructions
Discontinuing or inappropriately continuing medications without consulting the physician
Currently using prescriptions or OTCs recommended for a previous illness or problem

---

    E. Vision deficit
    F. Inability to perform a simple calculation
    G. Inability to judge an appropriate twice-daily dosing schedule

VII. ASSESSMENT

    A. Review all medications (prescription, OTC, herbal supplements, folk remedies, etc.) at least
       every 6 months (Box 24-3)
       1. What is the purpose of the drug?
       2. Has the aphorism "start low, go slow" been followed in dosing?
       3. Are there any patient allergies that have not been reported?
       4. Are there drug-drug interactions that need to be checked?
       5. Has the most effective route of administration been selected?
    B. Assess patient and/or family knowledge of medications and the ability to
       1. Follow instructions
       2. Monitor for adverse effects
       3. Make decisions about contacting the physician
    C. Assess the environment for proper storage, delivery systems, and memory prosthetics (Box
       24-4)

VIII. POSSIBLE NURSING DIAGNOSES FOR PATIENT'S MEDICATION USE

    A. Noncompliance with medication regimen: related to visual deficit
    B. Self-care deficit, medication: related to diminished cognitive functioning
    C. Injury, risk for: related to an adverse drug reaction (e.g., hypotension, dehydration, dizziness)

IX. NURSING INTERVENTIONS TO FACILITATE DESIRED EFFECTS OF PHARMACOLOGICAL AGENTS

    A. Identified in National Nursing Intervention Classification System
       1. Medication *administration:* helping patients locate or create memory prosthetics, such as
       pill dispensers, calendars, check-off systems

2. Medication *management:* understanding the therapeutic goal and the pathophysiology of the disease to be treated; using this goal for monitoring the efficacy of the drug
3. Medication *prescribing:* nonprescribing nurse should recognize principles of pharmacoeconomics that may affect the drug selection behaviors of the primary care provider
   a. Unit cost of the drug
   b. Cost of administering the drug (special skills and assistance needed)
   c. Impact of drug's pharmacokinetics (e.g., half-life and patient characteristics) on the cost of the drug
   d. Costs associated with managing side effects
   e. Costs associated with monitoring the patient (lab work, home/physician visits)
   f. Costs associated with augmentation of treatment failure (e.g. consultations)
B. Patient teaching content
   1. Drug names (generic and brand)
   2. Drug indications
   3. Dosage
   4. When and how to administer the medication
   5. Contraindications
   6. Adverse effects and drug interactions
   7. Storage
   8. Demonstration and return demonstration opportunities
   9. Anticipatory counseling about OTCs
   10. Creating a portable medication record to share with all providers

REFERENCES

American Medical Directors Association: *Pharmacotherapy companion to the depression clinical practice guideline,* Columbia, MD, 1998, American Medical Directors Association.

Aparasu RR, Fliginger SE: Inappropriate medication prescribing for the elderly by office-based physicians, *Ann Pharmacother* 31:823-829, 1997.

Bernabei R, Gambassi G, Lapane K, et al: Characteristics of the SAGE database: a new resource for research on outcomes in long-term care, *J Gerontol Med Sci* 54A:M25-M33, 1999.

Cargill JM: Medication compliance in elderly people: influencing variables and interventions, *J Advan Nurs* 17:422-426, 1992.

Eliopoulos C: *Gerontological nursing,* ed 4, Philadelphia, 1997, JB Lippincott.

Howanitz E, Pardo M, Smelson D, et al: The efficacy and safety of clozapine versus chlorpromazine in geriatric schizophrenia, *J Clin Psychiatr* 60:41-44, 1999.

McCloskey JC, Bulechek GM, editors: *Nursing interventions classification,* ed 2, St Louis, 1996, Mosby.

Miller CA: Frail elders: handle with care when using medications, *Geriatr Nurs* 19:239-240, 1998.

Nicolle LE, Bentley D, Garibaldi R, et al: Long-term Care Committee: antimicrobial use in long-term care facilities, *Infect Contr Hosp Epidemiol* 17:119-128, 1996.

Pepper GA: Drug use and misuse. In Stone JT, Wyman JF, Salisbury SA: *Clinical gerontological nursing: a guide to advanced practice,* ed 2, Philadelphia, 1999, WB Saunders.

Podrazik PM, Schwartz JB: Cardiovascular pharmacology of aging, *Cardiovas Dis Elderly* 17:17-34, 1999.

Rathore SS, Mehta SS, Boyko WL, et al: Prescription medication use in older Americans: a national report card on prescribing, *Fam Med* 30:733-739, 1998.

CHAPTER 25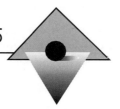

PAIN

Ann Schmidt Luggen

LEARNING OBJECTIVES

Upon completion of this chapter, the reader will be able to:

- Differentiate between acute and chronic pain
- Describe some of the fallacies of nurses' beliefs about pain
- List some of the pain treatment modalities that nurses can use to manage pain

I. PAIN DEFINITION

    A. Unpleasant sensory and emotional experience associated with actual or potential tissue damage

    B. Whatever the patient says it is

II. INCIDENCE/PREVALENCE

    A. 25% to 50% of community-based elders have pain

    B. Up to 85% of residents in long-term care report pain

    C. 73% of hospitalized medical patients say pain was excruciating

III. CLASSIFICATION OF PAIN

    A. Acute: usually of sudden onset, short-lived, or transient; easily treated with medications for short duration

    B. Chronic: constant pain or of long duration; usually accompanied by depression especially if pain is poorly managed

IV. CLINICAL SIGNS

    A. Acute: increased pulse, respiration, blood pressure, diaphoresis, visible facial expression of grimace or tension, crying, guarding, restlessness, immobility of body part, fetal position

    B. Chronic: no change in vital signs even with moderate to severe pain of long standing; chronic pain becomes an entity and illness state; patient may report sleeplessness, depression, anxiety, inactivity, appear stoic

    C. Pain in cognitively impaired older adult: person may exhibit behaviors different from usual behavior (e.g., demonstrative person becomes quiet, passive; quiet nonverbal person becomes talkative; happy person sad; sedentary person active, etc.)

V. CAUSES OF PAIN

    A. Acute: surgery, procedures, acute incidents such as fracture, myocardial infarction, appendicitis, etc.

        1. Clinical signs are not dependable for assessment of pain in older adults

        2. Anecdotal evidence that elders have silent MIs and painless acute appendicitis are well known

B. Chronic: arthritis is most common cause of pain in older adults; neuralgias from diabetes and peripheral vascular diseases; cancers, which are a common illness of older adults

VI. PAIN COMPONENTS

A. Physiological/sensory
B. Central
   1. Includes memory and past history of pain
   2. Significance of the pain to the patient (e.g., small cut vs. cancer diagnosis)
   3. Beliefs about pain (need to "be a man")
   4. Culture (God is making you suffer for your misdeeds)
   5. Coping abilities (amount of control over pain)
   6. Level of anxiety, presence of depression
   7. Gender
   8. Level of consciousness

VII. PAIN ASSESSMENT

A. Pain tools
   1. Tools that have been used in research and in clinical settings and have been found useful in assessment and evaluation of pain in older adults
   2. Each patient will have a preference for the one that is most easy to use; it should be used consistently to assess pain
B. Pain descriptions
   1. Following areas should be explored with every patient who has pain or suspected pain at a time when he/she is comfortable
      a. Determine location of pain, quality (use a word descriptor such as "aching" or "burning")

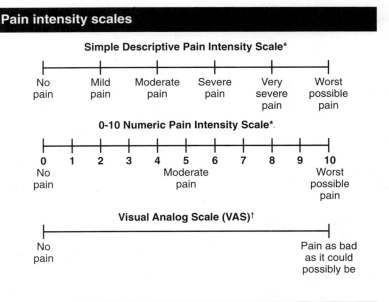

Figure 25-1   Pain intensity scales.
(From US Department of Health and Human Services, Public Health Service, Agency for Health Care Policy and Research, Rockville, MD, AHCPR Publication No. 94-0593, March, 1994.)

b. Intensity (rating scale) (Figure 25-1)
c. Duration, pattern, or variation (every morning)
d. How is pain expressed (stay in bed longer, don't cook any more)
e. What aggravates the pain (rainy weather)
f. What makes it better (hot baths)
g. Pain medications tried in the past; what pain medications make it better

C. Pain observation
1. Note patient's behaviors when in pain, when pain is relieved; note guarding, expressions; tension, etc.
2. Observations will be different for each patient

D. Pain impact
1. What can the patient no longer do because of pain (ADLs, social life)
2. Is the patient irritable, depressed, sleeping; marital relationship affected?

VIII. PHARMACOLOGICAL MANAGEMENT OF PAIN

A. Medications to be avoided in older adults
1. Demerol (meperidine): lowers seizure potential level, causes confusion
2. Talwin (pentazocine): confusion, disorientation
3. Methadone: long half life; accumulates over time
4. Darvon (propoxyphene): confusion

> **START LOW
> GO SLOW**

B. Rule of thumb with older adults: **start low, go slow**
C. Mild to moderate pain
1. Acetaminophen (non-antiinflammatory), aspirin (antiinflammatory)
a. Use aspirin with caution in older adults
b. <4000 mg acetaminophen/day for older adults
2. NSAIDs
a. GI upset, bleeding can be an issue with these drugs
b. Piroxacam (Feldene) has long half life—use with caution
c. Indomethacin (Indocin) can cause kidney problems—use with caution
d. Cox-2 inhibitors said to prevent GI problems—unclear (Celebrex, Vioxx)
3. Codeine added to acetaminophen
a. Oxycodone (Percodan, Tylox): useful
4. Levorphanol (Levodromoran) used less often because of long half-life and potential accumulation in older adults, causing over-sedation

D. Moderate to severe pain
1. Medications
a. Morphine: drug of choice for moderate to severe pain
b. Oxycodone (Oxycontin) and hydromorphone (Dilaudid): recommended oral medications for severe pain
c. Fentanyl (Duragesic) patch: useful for NPO patients
2. IM medications should be avoided because of uneven absorption and pain of injection
3. Nurses fear addicting patients; however, percentage of those addicted is <1%
4. Nursing management of opioids
a. Constipation: always start a bowel regimen with opioids
b. Nausea: offer antiemetics to start; nausea will disappear in time
c. Sedation: check other medications, remove those with sedating effect; observe for over-sedation; wake patients for next dose of pain medications when sleeping

d. Principle for pain management: give pain medications round-the-clock; stop pain before it becomes severe

e. Oral route: for pain medications is less expensive

f. Rectal route: underused; many opioids come in this form; this is a useful route especially when the patient is nauseated

g. Patient-controlled analgesia (PCA): most patients with pain feel little control over their pain; this is one way for them to manage their own pain

h. PCA lockouts: keep patients from accidentally taking too much pain medication

i. Breakthrough pain management: manage pain before it can "break through"

> ## Principle for Administration of Pain Medication: Give Around-the-Clock

IX. NURSES' KNOWLEDGE OF PAIN

A. Nurses fear addicting patients, fear giving narcotics, give less than prescribed doses or minimal dose; result: patients suffer

B. Nurses underestimate patients' pain; result: patients suffer

C. Nurses make incorrect assumptions about patients' pain because patients do not behave according to nurses' expectations of patients in pain; result: patients suffer

D. Nurses and patients believe that pain is a natural part of aging; result: patients suffer

X. NONPHARMACOLOGICAL MANAGEMENT OF PAIN

A. Touch: a natural method of comforting; promotes relaxation; said to promote healing

B. Relaxation: helps control pain by relieving tension that enhances pain; useful combined with other pain relief methods

C. Meditation: relaxes and focuses thinking; provides distraction from pain

D. Imagery: focusing on a thought, word, picture; works especially well if it is something meaningful to the patient; used with relaxation; can picture the pain leaving the body in an image such as a ball of fire

E. Massage: deep or superficial stimulation; interferes with pain sensation; very helpful in certain situations; each patient's therapy should be individualized to his/her preference

F. Heat/cold: useful for many pains; cold good for "hot" pain of inflammation, injury; heat useful for muscle strain, aching pain of arthritis

G. Acupuncture/acupressure: counter-stimulation of pain impulse; blocks pain sensation; may produce endorphins, a natural pain narcotic produced by the body

H. TENS, transcutaneous electric nerve stimulation: electrical stimulation delivered by electrodes over the painful area; patient can control increases or decreases of vibration, tingling sensation that blocks pain; many older adults find this treatment successful, especially after surgery or for lower back pain

I. Distraction: TV, radio, watching sports, movies, reading, puzzles, games; nurses who see patients appearing happily distracted by visitors should not assume that they are pain free; distraction is a successful therapy for mild pain

REFERENCES

Ebersole P, Hess P: *Toward healthy aging: human needs and nursing response,* St Louis, 1998, Mosby.

McCaffery M, Pasero C: *Pain clinical manual,* ed 2, St Louis, 1999, Mosby.

US Department of Health and Human Services: *Acute pain management: operative or medical procedures and trauma, Agency for Health Care Policy and Research clinical practice guideline,* Rockville, MD, 1992, USDHHS, Public Health Service.

ORGANIZATIONAL AND HEALTH POLICY ISSUES

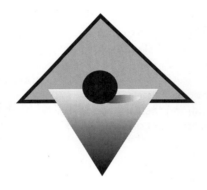

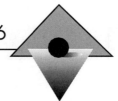

CHAPTER 26

HEALTH CARE DELIVERY SYSTEMS

Sue E. Meiner

LEARNING OBJECTIVES

Upon completion of this chapter, the reader will be able to:

- Discuss common elements of nursing case management
- Identify areas of a social support system assessment
- Discuss communication needs with inter- and intradisciplinary team members
- Discuss community resources available to the disabled older adult
- List five types of community-based health delivery systems
- Differentiate levels of care among the institutional-based health care systems
- State the various subacute care categories

I. COMPONENTS

   A. Case management: encompasses many different models of care delivery
      1. History
         a. Spans over 100 years: most prominent figure was Lillian Wald, founder of American Public Health Nursing in New York City in the 1890s
         b. Case management programs: developed after diagnostic related groups (DRGs) and HMOs in an effort to reduce the cost of health care delivery in 1980s and 1990s
      2. Case finding and affect on the patient
         a. Bonding: trust develops between patient and nurse case manager
         b. Working: patients, especially older adults, look at newer ways of achieving self-care and accepting care from others
         c. Changing: behavior modification through concern, support, and sharing of knowledge between older adult and nurse case manager
         d. Cost-effective: less emergency room visits, primary care visits, hospital admissions, and shortened length of stay through case management
      3. Screening/intake can be done to identify those who could benefit from nursing case management services
      4. Assessment of the acuity of older adults' need for services, using physical, cognitive, functional, social, and economic parameters
      5. Care planning strategies that will meet the mutually agreed upon needs of the older adult
      6. Service arrangements for continuity of care in the most cost-effective location (e.g., private home, relatives' home, extended care, etc.)

      7. Monitoring and follow-up using multidisciplinary and interdisciplinary team members, according to older adults' needs

      8. Evaluation using quality outcome measures

B. Social support system: provides, among other items, the subjective feeling of belonging, being accepted, loved, valued, and needed

      1. Relationship to health and well-being is established

      2. Assessment of social support systems

         a. Type of support provided

         b. Source of support

         c. Function that is served by the support

         d. Characteristics of that supportive relationship

      3. Examples of social support systems

         a. Familial support system: siblings, children, grandchildren, etc.

         b. Organized religious support systems

         c. Caregivers or helping professional support systems

C. Accessibility to health care delivery systems

      1. Patients with physical limitations to accessing health care services should be identified through community case-finding sources (e.g., church, senior center, etc.)

      2. Patients with transportation limitations to accessing health care services need referral to funded transportation services (e.g., Area Agency on Aging, disabled persons' transport services, and/or community-operated transportation for the elderly)

      3. Patients with financial limitations to accessing health care services need to be referred to social services in the catchement area where the person is currently living

      4. Patients' cultural/language barriers can lead to limitations in accessing health care services

         a. Interpreter in the specific language should be sought

         b. Investigating the cultural beliefs and health care practices of patients with cultural/language barriers to services should be undertaken by health care providers

         c. Contact should be ongoing with a family member or significant other who has an understanding of the patient's cultural needs

      5. Legislation related to community resources: Americans with Disabilities (ADA) Act of 1990 is an expansion of the Rehabilitation Act of 1973 and prohibits discrimination against qualified people by organizations that receive federal grants or other forms of financial assistance; the act addresses five areas (Titles I-V) that promote the rights of people with disabilities and allow individuals to use local, state, or federal regulations to fight discrimination; Titles II, III, and IV include

         a. Title II, Public Services and Transportation: prohibits discrimination in public transportation programs

            (1) Paratransit services must be provided for the disabled who cannot use public ground transportation systems

            (2) All bus and rail systems must be accessible

            (3) A 20-year period has been allowed for systems to comply with all regulations because of the complexity and costs of transportation services

         b. Title III, Public Accommodations: privately operated enterprises must provide public accommodations for the disabled; private clubs are exempted from coverage by the Civil Rights Act of 1964 as are religious organizations

         c. Title IV, Telecommunications: Federal Communications Commission (FCC) must provide interstate and intrastate telecommunications services to speech- and hearing-impaired people; these Telecommunications Devices for the Deaf (TDD) services would allow speech- and hearing-impaired people to communicate on a functional level equivalent to the non-impaired

    D. Information and referral networks
        1. Collaborative sharing of sources of information and multidisciplinary referrals for needs outside of a single discipline
            a. Provides a more complete continuum of services for patients
            b. Contacts government and private health care agencies to obtain names and contacts information for referral services
            c. Maintains names, addresses, and phone numbers for future referral needs
            d. Is important in assessing the patient/family receptivity to a referral
                (1) Explores values, cultural beliefs, and health care behaviors and practices to determine congruency
                (2) Identifies positive and/or negative experiences with referrals in the past
                (3) Informs the patient/family of their role in the referral and any conditions that may be present with a specific referral
                (4) Allows the patient/family to select options when available
            e. Recognizes barriers to accessing some referral sources
                (1) Communication issues: foreign language as the only language, sensory deficits that interfere with communication (e.g., hearing or visual deficits)
                (2) Transportation issues: ability to obtain public or private means
                (3) Hours of operation: congruency with patient/family schedule
    E. Interdisciplinary collaboration
        1. Essential in maintaining quality care for older adults
        2. Identifies interdisciplinary team members that will be involved in care
        3. Communicates goals to be accomplished by the team
        4. Delineates expectations and how each discipline will deliver services
        5. Determines the methods for documentation of each member of the team and the form and frequency of communication among intra- and interdisciplinary team members
        6. Determines evaluation methods to be used to measure outcomes of care
    F. Least restrictive placement
        1. Complete assessment must be made before determination of residential transfer from one place to another (e.g., hospital to home vs. hospital to extended care facility)
        2. Functional capacity should be used to guide placement choices presented to the patient needing additional care (inside the home or in another facility)
    G. Discharge planning
        1. Old definition: the process of planning for referral and intervention upon discharge from one facility to another
        2. New definition: planning for resource use, resource planning, needs planning, or case management
        3. Main function is to promote continuity of care regardless of place of care, using referral sources whenever possible

II. COMMUNITY-BASED CARE

    A. Home health care/visiting nurses: provide long-term assessment with service provisions (e.g., OT, PT, ST, and equipment), supportive home-based services, and counseling
    B. Senior centers/area agencies on aging: usually provide non–health care services, except for health promotion and education programs, nutritional support in centers or through home-delivered meals, and social support provided through group activities and day trips; supported by Title 20 funding from Administration on Aging (AOA), Title III Older Americans Act, and state and local governments
    C. Day care services: for older adults with needs that range from frequent observation within a structured program of activities to overseeing of non-acute nursing needs (rehabilitation and some personal care may be included) in centers that are open during the day hours with or without transportation components

D. Foster care homes for older adults: individuals agree for minimal compensation to take care of an older person in a private home where minimal assistance with ADLs is needed
   1. Standards and guidelines are set by states if licensing is required; may fall into the personal care home because the resident does not need intense medical or nursing care
   2. Payment is often made through subsidized programs, such as the Community-Based Alternatives Program or the Medicaid Nursing Facility Waiver Program
   3. Advantages include homelike atmosphere, lower costs of care, resident's ability to maintain independence and self-worth, similarity to an extended family setting
E. Group home care: for completely independent older adults where no hands-on personal care is given
   1. Services can include meals, housekeeping, laundry, finance management, and transportation needs
   2. Self-care is essential for this lower cost environment
F. Geriatric assessment centers: provide older adults and families with services that range from physical, functional, psychosocial to economic assessment for determining the ability for self-care with independent living capabilities; referral to other health care delivery modalities when appropriate
G. Homemaker, chore, and personal services: assessed by persons from local area agencies on aging or other health and welfare sources
   1. Government assistance can be provided to maintain independent living for older adults
   2. Funded by Social Security Act, Title 18; Medicare, Title 19; Medicaid, Title 20; and the Older Americans Act, Title III
H. Respite care: provides short-term relief for caregivers in home or institutional facilities when relief from 24-hour-a-day care is required
   1. Short-term respite care given on a regular basis can prevent institutionalization because of caregiver exhaustion
   2. Relief of caregiving responsibilities may include housekeeping, transportation, shopping, cooking, paying bills, and heavy physical care
   3. When heavy physical care and safety issues require the caregiver to become homebound with the ill person, respite care is periodically a necessity
   4. Sources of respite care
      a. Nursing homes (for a weekend or a few weekdays)
      b. Adult day-care centers, which can provide up to 8 hours of respite care during the day time
      c. Home health aides or hospice volunteers as a source of respite

III. INSTITUTION-BASED CARE

A. Nursing homes: provide regulated (state health departments and offices on aging, Federal Certification for Medicare, Medicaid, OBRA) long-term living and care along with a full range of services (most common type of long-term facility)
   1. Medical/nursing
   2. Rehabilitation/convalescence
   3. Psychological/social
   4. May provide religious, hospice, and/or respite care
B. Rehabilitation facilities: aim to prevent complications of physical disability resulting from either acute or chronic illnesses; restore and maintain a high level of functioning and/or adaptation to an altered lifestyle
   1. Use a multidisciplinary approach
   2. Provide continuity of care
   3. Focus on restorative care and prevention of secondary complications
      a. Disuse syndrome, risk for: related to immobility or weakness
      b. Mobility, impaired physical: related to intolerance to activity, decreased strength or endurance, pain, perceptual/cognitive impairment, neuromuscular or musculoskeletal impairment, depression or severe anxiety

   c. Injury, risk for: related to sensory/motor deficits or lack of awareness of environmental hazards
   d. Self-care deficit: related to intolerance for activity, fatigue, pain, or discomfort, perception/cognitive impairment, neuromuscular or musculoskeletal impairment, depression or severe anxiety
   4. Emphasize quality of life
C. Acute care facilities: provide services to a disproportionately high rate of older adults per capita, with nearly 13% of the population using 36% of health care services, 33% of all hospital stays, and 44% of all days of care in hospitals
   1. Older adults are at higher risk for complications and decline in function in acute care because of decrease in reserves and ability to cope with physical and psychosocial stressors
   2. There can be complications such as falls, infections, change in mental status, incontinence, decreased functional abilities, and decreased muscle mass and tone
   3. Specialized acute-care geriatric unit benefits include unit design to compensate for common physical and sensory challenges and to promote orientation to the surroundings
   4. Geropsychiatric units and mental health services in acute care address both mental and concomitant chronic medical problems while assessment, medication titration, and group therapy are initiated as appropriate
D. Subacute care facilities: result from cost controls and managed care
   1. Transitional subacute care: involves a short stay (5 to 30 days) with high nursing acuity (5 to 8 hours/day); requires medical care and monitoring; serves as a step-down facility to the acute care of the hospital
   2. General subacute care: requires weekly medical monitoring with moderate nursing acuity (3.5 to 5 hours/day) and rehabilitative activities (1 to 3 hours/day); short-term intravenous therapy (antibiotics)
   3. Chronic subacute care (60 to 90 days): requires biweekly medical monitoring with moderate nursing acuity (3.5 to 5 hours/day) for older adults with little hope of functional independence or recovery; patients may be transferred to long-term care (head injuries, stroke, oncology requiring chemotherapy)
   4. Long-term transitional subacute care: can be provided in an acute care setting (swing beds) with medically complex patients needing skilled nursing care (e.g., ventilator patients)

REFERENCES

Burke MM, Walsh MB: *Gerontologic nursing: wholistic care of the older adult,* St Louis, 1997, Mosby.
Clark L, Fraaza M, Schroeder S, et al: Alternative nursing environments: do they affect hospital outcomes? *J Gerontol Nurs* 21(11):32-38, 1995.
Ebersole P, Hess P: *Toward healthy aging: human needs and nursing responses,* ed 5, St Louis, 1998, Mosby.
Farrell K: Interdisciplinary/intradisciplinary team building and development. In Luggen AS, Travis SS, Meiner SE, editors: *NGNA core curriculum for gerontological advanced practice nurses,* Thousand Oaks, CA, 1998, Sage.
Farrell K: Referrals. In Luggen AS, Travis SS, Meiner SE, editors: *NGNA core curriculum for gerontological advanced practice nurses,* Thousand Oaks, CA, 1998, Sage.
Hogstel MO: *Community resources for older adults: a guide for case managers.* St Louis, 1998, Mosby.
Johnny R: Accessibility of community resources. In Luggen AS, editor: *NGNA core curriculum for gerontological nurses,* St Louis, 1996, Mosby.
Koroknay VJ: Rehabilitation principles. In Luggen AS, editor: *NGNA core curriculum for gerontological nurses,* St Louis, 1996, Mosby.
Luggen AS: Community networks. In Luggen AS, editor: *NGNA core curriculum for gerontological nurses,* St Louis, 1996, Mosby.
Luggen AS: Long term care. In Luggen AS, editor: *NGNA core curriculum for gerontological nurses,* St Louis, 1996, Mosby.
Satin D: *The clinical care of the aged person: an interdisciplinary perspective,* Oxford, UK, 1994, Oxford University Press.
Stanhope M, Lancaster J: *Community health nursing: promoting health of aggregates, families, and individuals,* ed 4, St Louis, 1996, Mosby.

CHAPTER 27

FEDERAL REGULATIONS

Ann Schmidt Luggen

LEARNING OBJECTIVES

Upon completion of this chapter, the reader will be able to:

- Discuss the components of the Older Americans Act of 1973
- Explain what OBRA is
- Describe the survey process
- List residents' rights and the role of the ombudsman

I. OLDER AMERICANS ACT (1973)

   A. Nutrition programs
      1. Congregating low-cost meals at senior centers and nutrition sites
      2. Home-delivered meals
   B. Transportation
      1. Programs with bus or van for grocery shopping or medical appointments
   C. Social service needs of older Americans
      1. Physical and mental health services
      2. Housing issues
      3. Training, research to disseminate knowledge of aging
      4. Long-term care ombudsman
      5. Information and referral services
   D. Training, research, and other projects
      1. Expand and disseminate knowledge about aging
      2. Expand and disseminate effective services and programs

II. NURSING FACILITY REGULATION

   A. History
      1. States were primary regulators of quality of care
      2. Some states provided poor quality of care
      3. In 1990, OBRA (Omnibus Budget Reconciliation Act of 1987) was enacted
      4. OBRA 1987 was written by HCFA (Health Care Financing Administration) to address quality of care issues in intermediate and skilled care facilities
      5. States continue their own separate regulations; many stricter than federal regulations
      6. Nursing homes must follow both federal and state regulations or
         a. Be fined
         b. Lose licensure
         c. Lose certification status

B. Survey
   1. State survey occurs every 12 to 18 months
   2. Team visit
   3. Unannounced visit
   4. Multi-day (3 to 4 day) inspection
C. Survey process
   1. Focus is on resident outcomes
   2. Paper and chart reviews
   3. Building inspection
   4. Federal surveyors may inspect state surveyor performance and come at the same time or directly following
   5. Regulations must be met "consistently" without significant deviation or a "deficiency" is received for each regulation that is not complied with
   6. Any "deficiency" requires a response from the nursing home administrator with a proposed plan of correction; this occurs within a designated time frame
   7. Deficiencies must be posted in a public place in the nursing home
D. Survey team
   1. Consists of nurses, dietitians, and/or sanitarians
   2. Rates facility on a 3-year survey history, report card
   3. Reviews representative sample of residents; some interviewable, some non-interviewable
   4. Surveyors examine quality of care, quality of life, resident rights', problems such as privacy, dignity, and staff response to residents' needs for attention
   5. Surveyors review the environment
      a. Activity areas
      b. Treatment areas
      c. Common areas (lounges, hallways)
      d. Emergency power supply, water availability
      e. Residents' rooms
   6. Surveyors also review
      a. Medications and rationale (e.g., Prilosec for reflux)
      b. Laboratory test followup (e.g., thyroid function tests with synthroid medication)
      c. Dining room quality of life and care, type of diets
      d. Closed records (residents discharged or died)
      e. Dietary services
         • Sanitation
         • Delivery
         • Food choices, palatability
         • Food temperatures
      f. Resident rights
         • Telephone availability
         • Mail service
         • Snacks
         • Roommates and room arrangements
         • Personal financial matters
         • Health professional contacts
         • Resident decisions about care and treatment
         • Safety
         • Complaints
E. Minimum Data Set (MDS)
   1. OBRA (1987) mandated a standardized interdisciplinary assessment tool, MDS, in all nursing homes
   2. In 1990, the first MDS and accompanying resident assessment protocols (RAPs) were used

3. MDS must be completed within 14 days after resident admission or when a significant change in the resident's condition occurs
4. Each discipline assesses its components (e.g., nutrition status—dietitian)
5. Nursing (LPN/RN) completes most of the MDS
6. RAPs identifies problem areas concerning each resident based on information from the MDS (e.g., problem must be addressed in the medical record/care plan)

III. OMBUDSMAN PROGRAMS
A. Office on Aging provides state or local ombudsman
B. Ombudsman's role is to ensure protection of residents' rights

IV. CAREGIVER REGULATIONS
A. Registered Nurse (RN)
1. Skilled nursing services provided through the direction of an RN
2. Graduate of an approved professional school of nursing
3. Licensed as an RN in the state of practice
4. Similar regulations for LPN
B. Certified Nurse Aides (CNAs)
1. OBRA regulations require certification of aides, implemented in 1990
2. CNAs are unlicensed staff members
3. OBRA sets standards for training and approves all certification training programs
4. States keep CNAs in a register
a. Maintain records of qualifications of CNAs
b. CNAs must be registered with the state
C. Administrator
1. Nursing home administrators must be licensed by the state
2. States set standards for education/experience required for licensure/maintenance of licensure
3. There is great inconsistency in states' requirements

V. PEW COMMISSION
A. Pew Health Professions Commission and University of California, San Francisco Center for Health Professions created a task force on health care workforces
B. Regulations supported by Pew Charitable Trusts reported 95 recommendations to improve the regulatory system
1. States to regulate health care workforces
a. Standardized
b. Accountable to the public
c. Effective and efficient
2. Regulatory systems
a. Protect the public from harm
b. Regulate bodies accountable to the public
c. Respect consumer rights to choose health care providers
d. Provide flexible, cost-effective health care systems

VI. JOINT COMMISSION ON ACCREDITATION OF HEALTHCARE ORGANIZATIONS (JCAHO)
A. Private voluntary accreditation
B. Provides "deemed" status for Medicare (in compliance with Medicare Conditions of Participation established by Health Care Financing Administration [HCFA] for acute care and home care)
C. JCAHO measures performance of organizations against standards set higher than most licensure requirements
1. Seeks high quality of care, not minimal level care
2. Is outcome focused

REFERENCES

Flanders SC The effects of OBRA 1987 on the financial performance of the nursing home industry. In Romeis JC, Col RM, Morley JE, editors: *Applying health services research to long-term care,* 1996, New York, Springer.

Ignatavicius DC: *Introduction to long-term care nursing,* Philadelphia, 1999, FA Davis.

Pratt JR: *Long-term care,* Gaithersville, MD, 1999, Aspen.

Rini AG: Health policy: financial resources and regulatory and legislative issues. In Luggen AS, Travis S, Meiner SE, editors: *NGNA core curriculum for gerontological advanced practice nurses,* Thousand Oaks, CA, 1998, Sage.

CHAPTER 28

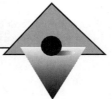

REIMBURSEMENT MECHANISMS

Patricia M. Kelly

LEARNING OBJECTIVES

Upon completion of this chapter, the reader will be able to:

- Describe historical development of health care reimbursement systems
- List components of major reimbursement plans for older Americans
- Delineate the different types of reimbursement
- Utilize the current terminology of health care financing

I. DEVELOPMENT OF HEALTH CARE REIMBURSEMENT IN AMERICA

A. Time line

1935   Social Security System established to provide for retirement

1945   Any American who becomes disabled to get benefits

1965   Medicare Part A became part of the Social Security System, National Health Insurance Policy; the Hill-Burton Act provided construction money that obligated hospitals to give reciprocating "free care of same cost" that could be provided over several years

1966   Medicare Part B added, with a monthly premium and an 80/20 reimbursement pattern (Medicare pays 80% of the bill and the patient pays 20%)

1967   Rising cost of co-insurance and deductible on Medicare Part A didn't decrease service volume; health care facilities increased prices to cover the patient's 20%, which was expected to be unrecoverable

1972   Medicaid legislation for medically indigent financed by state and federal governments

1984   Diagnosis-Related Groupings (DRGs) established to decrease Medicare payments (prospective payment initiated); set at the median health care charge from selected sites around the country per each diagnosis; health care facilities took the set amount of dollars and equated it to the number of hospitalized days covered per diagnosis; began the cycle of "quicker and sicker," increased home health use; hospitals started trimming costs to decrease costs; Part A now capped by DRGs; Part B capped by a reasonable value-based formula system ("MD takes assignment" means physician agrees to Medicare reimbursement value as the fee for service)

1985   Hospice added to Medicare Part A to transfer inpatient care to care given at home—pain/symptom control, specific for terminal noncurative (palliative care) patients; requirement is signed statement of "less than 6 months to live"; if misjudged and patient lives longer than 6 months, company still has to provide service

1988   Physician visits and x-rays added to Medicare Part B

1989   Omnibus Budget Reconciliation Act (OBRA) enacted; mandate for Health Care Financing Administration (HCFA) to address Medicare cost control; HCFA directed to develop an assessment tool to standardize the collection of patient data; this clinical data would drive the reimbursement of providers; this change in the structure of financing moved Medicare from a "fee for service" model to a capitated payment model with goal to actually cut Medicare spending; act also required standards for training and required certification of nursing assistants in long-term care facilities and home health agencies

1990   Re-evaluation of median cost of DRGs because of health care facility's decreased costs to provide care; insurance companies moved to adopt DRG type model and reduce lengths of stay

1994   Health care reform movement initiated to reduce federal expenditure on care (Medicare/Medicaid) and provide health care access to uninsured or underinsured Americans

1995   Health Care Financing Administration (HCFA) mandated use of a standardized assessment process for all long-term care facilities; in long-term care facilities, the federally generated forms were the Resident Assessment Instrument (RAI), which includes the Minimum Data Set (MDS), and the Resident Assessment Protocols (RAPs); facilities were given the mandate to computerize this assessment process so that clinical data could be used to change reimbursement systems for long-term care

1996   Balanced Budget Act enacted to restructure reimbursement methods for Medicare Part A; opened new options of Medicare plans to include managed care options; mandated reimbursement systems to change to a Prospective Payment System (PPS) for ambulatory care, long-term care (LTC) facilities, home health agencies, and rehabilitation hospitals; the LTC facilities were the first to experience the shift to the PPS system of reimbursement; Medicare was to pay the LTC facility a higher daily prospective rate and then place the LTC facility as the gatekeeper of services, putting them at risk for paying other health care providers out of the daily PPS rate; only the physician could continue to bill Part B, other providers delivering service to the Medicare Part A beneficiary would have to bill the nursing home for payment; coverage for advanced practice nurses was included so that APNs could make the physician visits to nursing home and be paid 85% of the Medicare allowable

1997   Medicare-certified skilled nursing facilities/nurse facilities (SNF/NF) were required to electronically transmit MDS data on all residents in the SNF/NF, regardless of the payment source, to state data banks; the state, in turn, would collate data and send information to the federal level to create a national database on all residents residing in long-term care facilities across the country; state departments of licensing and regulation allowed to utilize the database to guide surveyors in monitoring the care needs of residents and to quickly identify and intervene with facilities that have poor resident outcomes

1998   HCFA began implementation of PPS reimbursement system on a 4-year phase-in plan; the PPS system consolidates routine care, ancillary services, and capital costs into one payment; the payment methodology is based on assessing the resource needs of individual beneficiaries; all skilled nursing facilities (SNFs) will receive the same payment for services rendered to individuals with similar needs (except for geographic, urban/rural, and market value adjustments); payment is based on a clinical intensity category called Resource Utilization Groups (RUGs); using information collected by the MDS, patients are classified into one of 44 possible RUG categories, each with a corresponding per diem reimbursement rate as beneficiaries of the Medicare program who are eligible for Part A services in a long-term care facility; with regulations on November 5, 1999, coverage was expanded for advanced practice nurses in all practice settings, removing the restrictions on rural/urban practice differences and who employed the APN

   B. Final rule
      1. HCFA published final rule requiring home health agencies to electronically report data from the Outcome and Assessment Information Set (OASIS)
      2. OASIS will provide data that will allow for the identification of appropriate clinical outcomes and reimbursement rates tied to the clinical assessment; implementation of this prospective payment system has been delayed until after 2000 so the Y2K work can be completed at the state and federal levels

II. Sources of Reimbursement

   A. Medicare
      1. Medicare Part A: the hospital insurance part of Medicare; it helps pay for care in hospitals, skilled nursing facilities, and for home health and hospice care; the insured pays no premium but must enroll for Medicare benefits; eligibility: to be ELIGIBLE for Medicare, one must be a US citizen and any of the following be TRUE: the person is 65 years OR OLDER and receives benefits under Social Security (SS) or the Railroad Retirement (RR) system, OR client or spouse had Medicare covered through government employment, certain disabled persons are younger than 65, OR persons with permanent kidney failure
         a. Hospital services: semiprivate room, meals, general nursing and other hospital services, and supplies (but not private duty nursing, a television or telephone in the room, or a

private room unless medically necessary); for each benefit period, the insured pays $768 for a hospital stay 1 to 60 days, $192 per day for days 61 to 90 days, $384 per day for days 91 to 150 days, all costs for each day beyond 150 days; BENEFIT PERIOD: starts with hospital admission, includes day of discharge; ends when client no longer receives skilled nursing services for 60 days in a row; however, these 60 days do not include home health care services, only inpatient acute care, skilled nursing facility care, and rehabilitation

b. Skilled nursing facility (SNF) care: semiprivate room, meals, skilled nursing and rehabilitative services, and other services and supplies; for each benefit period, the insured pays nothing for the first 20 days, up to $96 per day for days 21 to 100, and all costs beyond the 100th day in the benefit period; to qualify for coverage, the beneficiary must have a qualifying 3-day hospital stay within the last 30 days, the bed must be classified as "certified" for Medicare, and the patient must require skilled care

c. Home health care: intermittent skilled nursing care, physical therapy, speech-language pathology services, home health aide services, durable medical equipment (such as wheelchairs, hospital beds, oxygen, and walkers), and supplies and other services; the insured pays nothing for home health and 20% of approved amount for durable medical equipment; to qualify for coverage, the beneficiary must have a qualifying 3-day hospital stay within the last 30 days, the agency must be "certified" for Medicare, and patient must require skilled care and must be "homebound"

d. Hospice care: pain and symptom relief and supportive services for the management of a terminal illness; home care is provided; also covers necessary inpatient care and a variety of services otherwise not covered by Medicare; insured pays limited costs for outpatient drugs and inpatient respite care

e. Blood transfusions: from a hospital or skilled nursing facility during a covered stay; insured must pay for the first 3 pints

f. Inpatient psychiatric care: covers mental health services in a Medicare-certified psychiatric facility

2. Medicare Part B: the medical insurance part of Medicare; it helps pay for doctor services that are medically necessary, outpatient hospital care, and some other medical services that Part A doesn't cover; the insured pays $45.50 per month (1999) for Part B coverage.

a. Doctors' services, inpatient and outpatient physician services, and supplies: pays for services of practitioners, such as clinical psychologists, clinical social workers, and nurse practitioners; the insured pays an $100 annual deductible, 20% of approved amount after the deductible, 50% for most outpatient mental health

b. Physical, occupational, and speech therapy: the insured pays an annual $100 deductible, 20% of the first $1500 of physical therapy, 20% of the first $1500 of occupational therapy, and all charges thereafter

c. Diagnostic tests: the insured pays nothing once the Part B deductible is met

d. Durable medical equipment: DME is equipment that meets the following requirements—can withstand repeated use, serves a medical purpose, is not useful to a person in the absence of an illness or injury, and is used in the home setting; DME requires a certificate of medical necessity and may require a prior authorization; Medicare will usually rent vs. buy because of "temporary need" expectation

e. Prosthetic and orthotic items: these replace all or part of the function of an internal body organ, such as artificial limbs, eyes, breast after cancer surgery, or correct a physical deformity, such as braces, diabetic shoes, corrective lenses after cataract surgery; prosthetics and orthotics require a written prescription, a certificate of medical necessity, and may require a prior authorization

f. Part B will also help pay for: x-rays, speech-language pathology services, kidney dialysis and kidney transplants, other organ transplants under limited circumstances (heart, lungs, or liver), limited ambulance services, emergency care, limited chiropractic services, medical supplies such as ostomy bags, surgical dressings, splints, or casts, and very limited outpatient drugs

g. Preventative medical services or health care services

(1) Screening mammogram: once a year; insured pays 20% of approved amount; insured does not have to meet the $100 deductible

(2) Pap smear and pelvic exam: once every 3 years, every year for high-risk persons or those who had an abnormal Pap smear in the preceding 3 years; insured pays 20% of approved amount for doctor services and no lab charges; insured does not have to meet the $100 deductible

(3) Colorectal cancer screening: fecal occult blood test once a year, flexible sigmoidoscopy every 4 years, colonoscopy every 2 years if at high risk for cancer of colon; barium enema can also substitute for these tests; insured pays 20% of approved amount after the annual Part B deductible

(4) Diabetes monitoring: includes glucose monitors, test strips, lancets, and self-management training; insured pays 20% of approved amount after the annual Part B deductible

(5) Bone mass measurements: covered for high risk only, insured pays 20% after annual Part B deductible

(6) Vaccinations: flu shot, once a year; pneumococcal vaccine, once (may be all that is ever needed); insured does not pay coinsurance or Part B deductible

(7) Hepatitis B: for those persons who are high risk for hepatitis; insured pays 20% of the Medicare-approved amount after Part B deductible

3. Medigap/Medicare supplemental insurance: plans offered by private insurance companies to fill the gaps in the original Medicare Plan coverage; federal law requires the Medigap policies be one of ten standard types and must be labeled with the letters A to J to make it easy for consumers to compare policies; generally A is least coverage and J is most; Medigap policies may cover some or all of the Medicare coinsurance amounts, some or all of the deductibles, and certain services not covered by the original Medicare plan at all, such as medications; the insured pays monthly premiums for this Medigap policy; Medicare SELECT refers to a type of Medigap policy that requires the person to use doctors and hospitals within a network in order to receive full benefits; medicare SELECT policies will generally have a lower premium than a standard Medigap policy

4. Medicare PLUS CHOICE: with the 1997 Balanced Budget Act, Medicare expanded the choices that people have related to benefits; recipients can now select original Medicare or choose Medicare Managed Care plans with options providing Medicare HMO, PSO, HMO with point of service, or PPO; the Medicare Managed Care plans maintain guidelines similar to any other managed care organization: select physicians, certain services, reduced use of specialists and testing procedures, and use of preferred providers (e.g., only certain hospitals/providers); plans may include extra benefits not usually covered by original Medicare Part A and B plans, such as prescription medications, dental care, dentures, eyeglasses, and hearing aids; insured may pay additional premiums, small co-pays, and pay more if they use a non-plan provider

B. Medicaid

1. Medicaid: joint Federal and State assistance program for poor Americans; federal government each year designates the income eligibility level; most health care costs are covered if one qualifies for both Medicare and Medicaid

2. For older adults and disabled, low-income people, Medicaid must pay the Medicare Part B premiums

3. Medicaid is a state-run program with matching federal monies

4. Mandatory services that states must offer

a. Inpatient and outpatient hospital care

b. Laboratory and radiological services

      c. Physician services

      d. Skilled nursing care at home or in a nursing home for people over age 21

      e. States must provide at least one of these optional services: prescriptions, dental services, eyeglasses, or intermediate facilities care

    5. Services vary from state to state

C. Supplemental Security Income (SSI)

    1. Additional monies provided monthly primarily for chronically ill, low-income recipients

    2. Money can be used as determined by recipient

    3. Certain disability qualifications are required

    4. Awarded 24 months after application filed

D. Out-of-pocket fee-for-service

    1. Older Americans are paying for a large portion of health care from their own savings

    2. Often have to "spend down" (divestment) to be eligible for some types of health care funding

    3. Original Medicare does not currently cover pharmaceuticals although Congress is discussing the option of offering a prescription coverage benefit

III. TYPES OF REIMBURSEMENT

A. Retrospective reimbursement: payment for services rendered based on cost of services received

B. Prospective payment system (PPS): reimbursement payment at a predetermined, fixed rate for a specific health care program or set of health care services available

C. Third party reimbursement for health care services: reimbursement from someone or some agency other than the individual receiving service, usually a form of public or private insurance

D. Fee for service: payment rendered on delivery of services; first party (client) pays the second party (health care provider)

E. Per diem payment: an agreed-upon cost per day for specific services or part of services (e.g., room and board charge in a hospital)

F. Diagnoses-related groups (DRGs): hospitalization payment based on determined amount of payment for a specific diagnosis

G. Capitation: payment for health services on the basis of a financial amount per person for a given period; payment does not vary by the volume or type of services provided; "covered life" is the person enrolled in this type of system

H. Managed care organization: an effort to provide preventive and curative health care to individuals or groups at the lowest health care delivery setting or long-term expense; primary example of this type of organization is an HMO; a monthly premium is paid for the membership and minimal fee for service charge when used

I. Resource utilization groups (RUGs): predetermined levels of reimbursement based on patient acuity and the staff needed to provide care to a particular mixture of patients/residents; both Medicare and Medicaid are moving toward reimbursement methods that account for the acuity and care needs of the patient/resident

IV. ADDITIONAL TERMS USED IN HEALTH CARE FINANCING

A. Carrier: handles claims for services by physicians and suppliers covered under Medicare Part B program

B. "Cherry picking": selective enlistment of individuals in better health or financial resources to participate in health care program (e.g., HMO)

C. Coinsurance: the 20% of Medicare Part B expenses not covered in the Medicare payment

D. Cost outliers: Medicare's definition—cost of client treatment greater than $36,000 or twice the DRG-specified cost for a diagnosis

E. Deductible: amount of health care expenditure before coverage paid by Medicare or other financial resource

F. Divestment: reducing assets by selling, giving away, or transferring to another person or business

G. Entitlements: federal programs produced through legislation with eligibility criteria for recipients, then funded by the federal government; examples: Social Security, Medicare, Aid to Families with Dependent Children

H. First party: in financial terms, the person incurring expenses

I. Fiscal intermediary: company that manages the financial aspects for another agency or organization; Medicare has a fiscal intermediary to pay and supervise health care institutions, then the Health Care Finance Administration pays them

J. Health care: comprehensive term used inclusively to describe any health-related type of medical, nursing, or facility services

K. Intermediaries: handle inpatient and outpatient claims submitted on one's behalf by hospitals, skilled nursing facilities, home health agencies, hospices, and certain other providers of Medicare Part A services

L. Managed competition: puts government and private health care providers in competition to reach the health care consumer by offering more cost-efficient services

M. Medically indigent: individuals or families unable to afford health care

N. "Merit want": providing health care to everyone, regardless of their ability to pay for it

O. Peer review organizations (PROs): groups of practicing physicians and other health care professionals who are paid by federal government to review the care given to Medicare clients

P. Preferred provider organization (PPO): second parties selected by third party to provide health care to an individual or group at reduced or pre-set rates

Q. Premiums: monthly charge for coverage (e.g., Part B of Medicare)

R. Primary payor: for older adults, it is usually Medicare; company primarily responsible for the majority of the health care expenses

S. Rationed health care: limiting certain health care services to individuals by refusing to fund or reimburse or offering limited funding/reimbursement by governments or health care plan (e.g., HMO or insurance company) for a particular service

T. Second party: the health care facility or person providing care and producing a bill

U. "Spending down": refers to older adults reducing or divesting themselves of assets to become eligible for Medicaid coverage, particularly for nursing home placement

V. Supplemental insurance: second insurance policy, which usually covers the deductible and the 20% not covered by the primary payor

W. Universal coverage: accessible health care for every American; funding and what health care services are being debated

X. Value added services: services provided to promote client care at the least costly health care delivery setting

REFERENCES

SNF Prospective Payment System: Available at *http://www.hcfa.gov/medicare/snfpps.htm.*

MDS 2.0 Technical Information Site: Available at *http://www.hcfa.gov/medicare/hsqb/mds20/default.htm.*

Keillor A, Nutten S: Systems across the continuum, *J AHIMA,* June 1999, pp 25-30.

Medicare health plan choices: Medicare news, HCFA special edition, National Medicare Education Program, October, 1998, Health Care Financing Administration.

US Department of Health and Human Resources: *Medicare supplemental insurance policies,* No HCFA-10115, Health Care Financing Administration, Baltimore, MA, 1998, USDHHR.

US Department of Health and Human Resources: *Your Medicare benefits, 1999 handbook,* No HCFA-10116, Health Care Financing Administration, Baltimore, MA, 1998, USDHHR.

PROFESSIONAL ISSUES

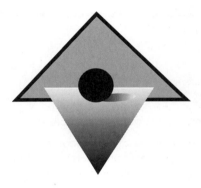

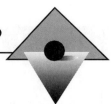

CHAPTER 29

SCOPE AND STANDARDS OF GERONTOLOGICAL CLINICAL NURSING PRACTICE

Sue E. Meiner

LEARNING OBJECTIVES

Upon completion of this chapter, the reader will be able to:

- Define the term *audit* as it pertains to patient outcomes
- Differentiate between structure, process, and outcome audits
- Identify the national voluntary accreditation organization actively involved in quality of health care delivery
- Name the standards and scope of gerontological nursing practice, as written by the American Nurses Association (1995)

I. THE AUDIT

A. Tool to systematically measure quality of care based on standards
B. Purposes are to improve patient care, educate, and enhance staff development
C. Standards for audits are agreed-on baseline conditions, demonstrating a level of excellence and forming a model to be followed
D. Types of audits include structure, process, and outcome

II. STRUCTURE AUDITS

A. Characteristics
   1. The most common type of audit in early efforts to measure quality of care
   2. Monitors the structure or setting in which patient care occurs
   3. Monitors resources in the patient care setting
   4. Ensures a safe and effective environment but does not measure the actual care that is given
B. Structural elements
   1. Physical setting of care
   2. Instruments used to deliver care
   3. Conditions through which nursing care is administered
      a. Organizational philosophy and objectives
      b. Organizational structure
      c. Financial resources

         d. Equipment

         e. Institutional licensure

         f. Expectations and attitudes of patients and employees

    C. Examples of structure audits

        1. Checking to see if patient call lights are working

        2. Examining the patient–nurse staffing ratio and/or patterns

        3. Evaluating the nurse's credentials

        4. Measuring staff turnover

        5. Reviewing accreditation reports

        6. Determining nurses' salary levels

        7. Evaluating sources of financial resources

        8. Evaluating the space, comfort, convenience of a facility's layout

        9. Evaluating the currency, type, safety of equipment and the staff's ability to use it

    D. Appropriate use of structure audits requires that process and outcome audits be considered in a total picture of the quality of care being delivered

III. PROCESS AUDITS

    A. Characteristics

        1. Task-oriented measure of how care is provided

        2. Focuses on adherence to practice standards

        3. Assumes that process of care indicates quality of care

    B. Process elements follow the nursing process with subsystems

        1. Taking a health history

        2. Conducting a physical examination

        3. Writing a nursing care plan

        4. Making a nursing diagnosis

        5. Charting

        6. Coordinating care

        7. Teaching and counseling

    C. Examples of process audits

        1. Reviewing charts to determine if nurses recorded patient teaching on fall prevention

        2. Assessing the use of teaching-learning principles during patient education

        3. Determining if patient problems were addressed by assessment data

        4. Evaluating if skin care was done according to written policies and procedures

        5. Determining if appropriate steps were taken before, during, and after the use of physical restraints

        6. Identifying multi-disciplinary participation in patient care conferences

        7. Evaluating the use of universal precautions in patient care

        8. Reviewing procedure manuals for adherence to ANA practice standards

    D. Examples of situations where the process audit is appropriate

        1. Where adverse outcomes occur frequently

           a. High-risk areas

           b. High-volume areas

           c. Problem-prone situations

        2. Where outcomes are attributed to factors outside of nursing control

        3. Where patient care continues for long-term periods (e.g., rehabilitation)

        4. When patients have complex and multi-factor problems

    E. Collection techniques for the process audit

        1. Observing caregiving activities

        2. Using caregiver's self-report

        3. Reviewing chart or records

        4. Interviewing the patient

IV. OUTCOME AUDITS

A. Characteristics
1. Determines the results of nursing interventions
2. Reflects changes in patient's health status
3. Assumes the outcome accurately demonstrates the quality of care that was given
4. May be based on goals for patient's psychological, emotional, and physical well-being

B. Outcome standards indicate what the patient will know, do, experience, or express verbally or physiologically (e.g., wound healing)

C. Outcome elements for the patient
1. Modification of signs and symptoms
2. Attitude and/or knowledge
3. Compliance with agreed-on health practices
4. Increase in skill level when self-care issues are present

D. Examples of outcome audits
1. Patient properly self-administering medications
2. Patient knowledgeable concerning fall prevention
3. Evaluation of patient's perceived nursing care
4. Identification of rates of infection on specific nursing units or areas
5. Documentation of length of stay (LOS) for specific disorders, injuries, or diseases on specific units

E. Interpretation of outcome audits
1. Many factors enter into the perception of outcomes
2. Often the outcome audit must be measured against the process audit

V. AUDIT METHODS

A. Retrospective
1. Obtained after the patient has received the services
2. Often conducted following the patient's discharge from the facility
3. Based solely on the patient's health record
4. Less time-consuming and usually less costly than the other audit forms
5. Accuracy depends on the completeness of recording by all caregivers

B. Concurrent: performed during care-giving, permitting corrective actions when deficits are identified

C. Prospective: future-oriented; directed toward current interventions, benefits later

D. Disciplinary: conducted by a single discipline (e.g., nursing or dietary)

E. Multi-disciplinary: conducted by an audit team consisting of more than one discipline (e.g., nursing and medicine)

VI. DECISION-MAKING AND METHODS

A. Audit responsibility
1. Individuals
2. Departments
3. Committees
4. External reviewers

B. Selection of audit topic(s)
1. Importance of the problem
2. Current problems at issue
3. High-risk areas
4. High-volume areas
5. Problem-prone issues

   C. Audit method selection
      1. Chart audit
      2. Observation audit
      3. Interview audit
      4. Combination
      5. Reports vary with reliability and validity of measurement tools
   D. Selection of audit subjects based on rationale for audit: who, how many subjects, over what time period, time involved for the audit, and cost factors
   E. Data collection
      1. Design of data collection by audit team/person
      2. Data collection by independent person/team
         a. Trained in data collection methods
         b. Validated for accuracy, reliability
   F. Data evaluation and analysis
      1. Who and how
      2. Data interpretation
      3. Establishment of baseline and/or trends
   G. Audit recommendations
      1. Communication: supervisors, audited people, interested or affected people
      2. Educational recommendations
      3. Change recommendations
      4. Reinforcement of positive practices
   H. Follow-up audits done to determine effectiveness of corrective action and for reinforcement of continual quality improvement (CQI)

VII. JOINT COMMISSION ON THE ACCREDITATION OF HEALTHCARE ORGANIZATIONS (JCAHO)

   A. Identification of factors as determinants of quality patient care
      1. Accessibility
      2. Timeliness
      3. Effectiveness
      4. Appropriateness
      5. Efficiency
      6. Continuity
      7. Privacy
      8. Confidentiality
      9. Participation of patient and family
     10. Environmental safety
   B. Essential requirements for patient care evaluation by the JCAHO
      1. Objectivity: measurable standards must be present before evaluation
      2. Clinical soundness: criteria must reflect achievable patient care, given the expertise and resources available
      3. Efficiency: professional nursing time must be used when necessary, and non–professional time should be used when no clinical judgment is needed
      4. Flexibility: variations are permitted when reported with good cause
      5. Documentation: written and reported decisions and evaluations must be present for review
      6. Action orientation: confirmed deficiencies must be analyzed, and appropriate corrective interventions must be implemented

VIII. STANDARDS OF CLINICAL GERONTOLOGICAL NURSING CARE (ANA, 1995)

A. ANA guidelines for quality assurance in nursing care are disseminated through established standards of nursing care, including specific standards for special practice areas such as gerontological nursing, among others
1. Standard I. Assessment: the gerontological nurse collects patient health data
2. Standard II. Diagnosis: the gerontological nurse analyzes the assessment data in determining diagnosis
3. Standard III. Outcome Identification: the gerontological nurse identifies expected outcomes individualized to the patient
4. Standard IV. Planning: the gerontological nurse develops a plan of care that prescribes interventions to attain expected outcomes
5. Standard V. Implementation: the gerontological nurse implements the interventions identified in the care plan
6. Standard VI. Evaluation: the gerontological nurse evaluates the aging person's progress toward attainment of expected outcomes

IX. STANDARDS OF PROFESSIONAL GERONTOLOGICAL NURSING PERFORMANCE (ANA, 1995)

A. Standard I. Quality of Care: the gerontological nurse systematically evaluates the quality of care and effectiveness of nursing practice
B. Standard II. Performance Appraisal: the gerontological nurse evaluates his/her own nursing practice in relation to professional practice standards and relevant statutes and regulations
C. Standard III. Education: the gerontological nurse acquires and maintains current knowledge in nursing practice
D. Standard IV. Collegiality: the gerontological nurse contributes to the professional development of peers, colleagues, and others
E. Standard V. Ethics: the gerontological nurse's decisions and actions on behalf of patients are determined in an ethical manner
F. Standard VI. Collaboration: the gerontological nurse collaborates with the aging person, significant others, and health care providers in providing patient care
G. Standard VII. Research: the gerontological nurse uses research findings in practice
H. Standard VIII. Resource Utilization: the gerontological nurse considers factors related to safety, effectiveness, and cost in planning and delivering patient care

REFERENCES

American Nurses Association: *Standards and scope of gerontological clinical nursing practice,* Washington, DC, 1995, The Association.

Joint Commission on Accreditation of Healthcare Organizations: *Accreditation manual for hospitals,* Chicago, 1989a, The Commission.

Joint Commission on Accreditation of Healthcare Organizations: *Accreditation manual for hospitals,* Chicago, 1992, The Commission.

Joint Commission on Accreditation of Healthcare Organizations: Characteristics of clinical indicators, *Qual Rev Bull* 15(11):330-339, 1989b.

Joint Commission on Accreditation of Hospitals: *Accreditation manual for hospitals,* Chicago, 1983, The Commission.

Kizilay, PE: Evaluation. In Leahy JM, Kizilay PE, editors: *Foundations of nursing practice: a nursing process approach,* Philadelphia, 1998, WB Saunders.

Lueckenotte AG: *Gerontologic nursing,* St Louis, 1996, Mosby.

Roberts KT: Audit procedures. In Luggen AS, editor: *NGNA core curriculum for gerontological nursing,* St Louis, 1996, Mosby.

CHAPTER 30

MANAGEMENT

Ann Schmidt Luggen

LEARNING OBJECTIVES

Upon completion of this chapter, the reader will be able to:

- Describe what policies and procedures are and their purpose in management
- Define common budgeting terms and describe the budget process
- Discuss different leadership styles
- Clarify different manager levels and describe manager tasks
- Define delegation, the delegation process, and barriers to effective delegation
- Discuss the communication process
- Describe causes of conflict and different methods of conflict management
- Explain the performance appraisal process
- Define QI and QA and differentiate between them
- List adult education principles and describe a good environment for adult learning
- Discuss change theory and how to manage change

I. POLICY AND PROCEDURE DEVELOPMENT

A. Policies and procedures are guides to accomplish goals and objectives
  1. Policy definition: general comprehensive statement used to guide decision-making
  2. Procedure definition: specific directive for implementing policy; a tool for standardization and evaluation
  3. Examples of policy and procedure (P & P)
    a. P & P on absenteeism
    b. P & P on handling grievances
B. Development
  1. Policy is usually developed at highest level of management; in participative management, there is input from knowledgeable managers and staff
  2. Procedures are developed by managers and staff who are knowledgeable about specific details of implementation
  3. Steps
    a. Determine that P & P is needed or a change is needed
    b. Assign development to appropriate person or committee
    c. Use appropriate sources of information
      • Current literature
      • Internet
      • Government documents, regulations
    d. Draft
    e. Review; send for review to departments, physician groups, those affected by policy

      f. Review by nurses who must interpret P & P in giving care
      g. Compile comments and redraft
      h. Send to legal department for review
      i. Send final draft to administration for signatures
      j. Distribute to all departments; include in all P & P manuals
  C. Unwritten policies
    1. Be aware of unwritten policies of the organization
    2. A consistent pattern of administrative behavior constitutes policy
  D. Origin of policies and procedures
    1. JCAHO (Joint Commission on Accreditation of Healthcare Organizations)
    2. Government regulations
    3. Labor contracts
    4. Professional standards

II. RESOURCE ALLOCATION/FISCAL PLANNING

  A. Definitions
    1. Resources: assets, supports such as dollars, time, people, materials
    2. Allocation: distribution and management of assets and supports
    3. Fiscal year: financially planned year
    4. Fiscal plan: systematic plan, informed best estimation of revenues and expenses
  B. Budgeting terminology
    1. Operating budget: the plan for the day-to-day activities of the unit, the organization; the expected revenues (income from sales of services and products) and expenses (cost of providing services and products); examples are salaries, food, utilities, and supplies; the personnel budget is the major expense in the operating budget
    2. Cost center: an area of accountability; a unit with its own identified costs and revenues; examples are a nursing unit, the laboratory, an x-ray department
    3. FTEs: full-time equivalents; 2080 paid hours of work per year; one full-time nurse working 40/hours/week equals 1 FTE; a nurse working one-half time, 20 hours, is 0.5 FTE
    4. Productive hours: paid time that is worked; examples are direct caregiving, education time, orientation
    5. Non-productive hours: paid time that is not worked; examples are vacation time, sick days, holidays
    6. Capital budget: major purchases, usually >$500, that have a useful life >1 year; examples are cardiac monitors and unit refrigerator
    7. Fixed and variable costs
      a. Fixed costs: salaries of management and some staff (e.g., minimal staffing in intensive care unit, OB unit), equipment depreciation, interest on loans, items that do not change when the patient census changes
      b. Variable costs: costs related to volume of patients (e.g., meals, linen, supplies, and some salaries); they may increase or decrease daily
  C. Budget/financial plan
    1. A financial forecast for 1 year, several years
    2. Guides use of human and material resources, products, services
    3. Based on objectives of organization, units
    4. Budget is simple, flexible
    5. Standard of performance for managers
    6. Motivates nurses with increased awareness of costs
  D. Budget process
    1. Determines productivity goal for the year
    2. Forecasts the workload, expected number of patient days

3. Budgeting patient care hours
4. Planning staffing schedule by shift, day of week
5. Determining productive and non-productive time
6. Estimating supplies, number and cost
7. Estimating services, number and cost
8. Determining capital expenses needed
9. Negotiating revision of budget
10. Evaluating variances from budget (difference between projected budget and actual budget); meeting objectives in terms of the budget

III. LEADERSHIP STYLES AND MANAGEMENT APPROACHES

A. Definition
1. Leadership: process of persuasion by which the leader or team induces the group to take action in accordance with the leader's purposes or the shared purposes of all
2. Leadership style: underlying motivation of the leader
B. Styles of leadership
1. Autocratic, democratic, laissez-faire leaders
a. Autocratic: decision-style in which the leader does not consider group input
b. Democratic: decision style in which the leader considers group input equally with the leader's and includes the group in the decision-making process
c. Laissez-faire: decision style used by a leader who allows the group to have autonomy (also called free rein)
2. Transactional leader
a. Focuses on day-to-day operations; managerial focus
3. Transformational leader
a. Visionary, empowering, motivating leader
b. Creates environment that allows productivity
c. Uses charisma, intellectual stimulation to allow followers to rise above personal needs to meet group goals
C. Manager
1. Definition: one with the authority to hire, transfer, direct, suspend, promote, discharge, reward, or discipline other employees
D. First-line manager
1. Definition: manager who is one level higher than employees supervised by the manager
2. Primary responsibility is providing the service or product—patient care
3. The service is provided via nursing staff, equipment, supplies, and the overall system
E. Middle manager
1. Definition: manager who has responsibility for lower-level manager; does not have direct responsibility for staff (e.g., department or division director)
2. Conveyor of information, a link from upper management and administration to the first-line manager and from lower managers to administration
3. Educator for first-line managers, a support
F. Executive/administrator
1. Definition: a position in the top level of an organization's hierarchy; a vice president, chief nursing officer
2. Roles
a. Leader: motivates subordinates to achieve the goals of the organization
b. Figurehead: ceremonial leader
c. Spokesman: speaks for the nursing division
d. Disseminator: distributes information to managers, staff
e. Entrepreneur: initiator of projects, development
f. Negotiator: formal and informal bargainer

G. Tasks of leaders and managers
1. Leader tasks
   a. Visionary
   b. Motivator
   c. Maintains unity
   d. Represents group, a symbol
   e. Develops trust
   f. Manages—plans, develops, uses decision-making, uses political judgment
2. Manager tasks
   a. Planning
   b. Organizing
   c. Directing (leading)
   d. Delegating (empowering)
   e. Controlling (evaluating)

IV. PLANNING AND DECISION-MAKING

A. Planning: definition
   1. Basic function of a manager
   2. Affects all management functions, such as organizing, staffing, directing, and evaluating
   3. Affected by human, financial, and material resources
   4. Influenced by organizational mission and purpose and the philosophy of nursing care
B. Purpose of planning
   1. Focus on objectives
   2. Facilitate control, avoid chance
C. Types of planning
   1. Daily plan: organization of activities (e.g., staffing)
   2. Strategic plan: market-oriented, future-oriented, life plan for organization
   3. Long-range plan: future-oriented, provides direction for organizational growth, more general than strategic plan (1 to 3 year plan)
D. Decision-making
   1. Intrinsic to manager functions of planning, organizing, controlling, and evaluating
   2. A complex conclusion relating to a specific situation
   3. Critical in problem solving
E. Decision-making process
   1. Identification of the problem or issue needing a decision
   2. Gathering of data related to the problem or issue
   3. Analyzing the situation, influences
   4. Determining potential solutions, alternatives
   5. Selecting one choice to implement
   6. Evaluating the outcome
F. Consensus building
   1. Japanese decision-making method
   2. Entails input from all concerned in decision (leaders, service-providers, and customers) over months or years
G. Intuition
   1. Right-brain activity wherein one perceives the possibilities inherent in a situation; one integrates information from different brain centers—facts and feelings; intuitive nurses have vision

V. DELEGATION

A. Delegation: definition
   1. A major element of the directing function of managers
   2. Transfer of work to a subordinate

3. Directing the work of others to accomplish a goal
4. Assignment of responsibility and authority for performing a task
B. Accountability/responsibility/authority
1. Accountability: explanation or justification of behavior of self or subordinates
2. Responsibility: obligation to do work at an acceptable level
3. Authority: right to give orders and expect obedience; also, entitlement to perform certain functions, such as in those given by state practice acts
C. Delegation process
1. Delegator sets broad goals; describes work clearly
2. Delegator tells subordinate what the goals are, objectives to be accomplished, rationale for assignment
3. Delegator sets limits, outcomes of work in terms of description and task assignment
4. Delegator allows subordinate to determine how to achieve goals
5. Delegator supports delegatee to determine if potential problems exist, helps with solving problems, and shows interest
6. Delegator gives rewards
D. Barriers to delegation in the delegator
1. Perfectionism or thinking that you can do it better yourself
2. Lack of ability to direct others; lack of experience
3. Lack of training the staff
4. Fear of risk-taking; not allowing mistakes
E. Barriers to delegation in the delegatee
1. Lack of competence, experience
2. Inability or refusal to take responsibility; shifts it back to 'boss' (upward delegation)
3. Work overload
4. Lack of organizational abilities
5. Lack of self-confidence

VI. COMMUNICATION PROCESS

A. Definition: interactive transfer of information, understanding to another person
B. Communication elements
1. Sender: one who wishes to give information
2. Receiver: one who needs or is to receive information
3. Message: idea or information to be conveyed
4. Process: involves the following
   a. Ideation: message or idea to send
   b. Encoding: manner in which the message is conveyed
      • Verbal
      • Written
      • Visual
      • Nonverbal
   c. Transmission and receipt: requires intact senses (visual, hearing)
   d. Decoding: mental ability to receive and interpret message
   e. Response: feedback of understanding message
C. Behavioral components of communication
1. Perception: one's own individual view of the world; varies among members of a group
2. Perceptual set: one perceives what one expects to perceive
3. Closure: filling in the "blanks" to complete an unfinished picture, sentence, information
4. Non-verbal communication: process of communication that is unspoken, unwritten; it is 93% of communication; includes
   a. Gestures
   b. Clothing
   c. Body types

        d. Personal artifacts

        e. Facial expression and eye behavior

        f. Spatial arrangement, environment, personal space

        g. Touching behavior

        h. Voice characteristics

        i. Culture and time

D. Communication flow: down, up, horizontal

    1. Downward communication flow: high-level administration to lowest level employee—typical hierarchical communication; examples are specific directives, organizational policy and procedures, employee handbooks, performance evaluation tools

    2. Upward communication flow: low-level employee to higher level employer; good for employee morale; methods are memos, suggestion boxes

    3. Horizontal or lateral communication flow: between peers and colleagues at the same level in the organization or in similar departments; provides social and emotional support and contributes to work groups

E. Grapevines

    1. Present in all organizations

    2. Informal flow of information

    3. Cannot eliminate

    4. More rapid than other communication methods

    5. 75% of grapevine information is correct

F. Communication barriers

    1. Poor listening habits, distractions

    2. Inconsistent signals

    3. Credibility issues

    4. Time and work demands

    5. Frame of reference differences

    6. Soft tone of voice

    7. Biases

G. Effective listening

    1. Be aware of one's own listening habits

    2. Tolerate silences

    3. Ask open-ended questions

    4. Encourage speaker with eye contact

    5. Encourage speaker with "yes" or "I see," or paraphrase speaker's words

    6. Avoid premature judgments

    7. Summarize to avoid misunderstanding

    8. Concentrate

VII. Conflict Management

A. Definition

    1. A natural occurrence that can be beneficial

    2. A problem of incompatible goals

    3. Perception of interference from another in one's achievement of goals

B. Causes of conflict

    1. Any situation or source

    2. Win-lose attitudes (I win; you lose)

    3. Perception of scarce rewards

    4. Task interdependence (e.g., group project and one member has not completed the respective part that is due)

    5. Threats: power variances between two people

    6. Group identification: cohesiveness in one group increases potential conflict between two groups (e.g., competition between committees)

7. Conflicting messages: perception misunderstanding or two different messages from two people to one person (e.g., subordinate with two bosses)

C. Managing conflict

1. Avoidance: hope it will go away (take two aspirin and call in the morning); may be effective; may be resolved without intervention
2. Compromise: negotiation or bargaining (when each is of equal status); usually a temporary solution; not a win–win solution
3. Forcing: one with influence mandates conflict resolution in a certain way; a power intervention; short-term solution without resolution
4. Collaboration: talking things over; integration of insights; a win–win solution; consensus
5. Confrontation: problem-solving method of discussion of conflict and attempt at solution or agreement
6. Smoothing: minimizes conflict and differences without solution; deescalates situation temporarily.

VIII. PERFORMANCE APPRAISAL

A. Definition: a control process to determine if employee performance is meeting employer objectives or standards

B. Purpose of appraisals
1. Maintenance of improvement of performance
2. Feedback to employee, insight
3. Comparison of performance with standards
4. Method to ensure quality of care
5. Motivation for employees to perform tasks to accompany organizational mission
6. Personnel decisions such as raises
7. Meeting accreditation, regulatory, and legal requirements

C. Process of performance appraisal
1. Standard of performance developed, derived from
   a. Job description
   b. Job analysis
   c. Job evaluation
   d. Qualitative and quantitative analysis of job activity
   e. Standard established by institution or professional organization or association
2. Performance standards based on appropriate knowledge, expected behaviors
3. Employee is informed of standards governing appraisal
4. ANA standards of practice may be used for performance standards
   a. Established and accepted performance standard ensures credibility of standard
   b. Established and accepted standard will hold up under legal action against appraiser
5. Formal performance reviews held at regular intervals
6. Actions for/against employee must be based on data from performance review (e.g., merit increases of salary, terminations)

D. Performance appraisal problems
1. Managers and employees dislike performance appraisals
2. Measurement is imprecise
3. Many U.S. companies do not use formal appraisals
4. Executives unlikely to be evaluated
5. Employees' opinions of appraisal rarely solicited
6. More research and theory development on performance appraisal is needed

E. Peer review
1. Definition: examination and evaluation of an employee's performance by an associate at the same level
2. Promoted as a component of professional practice
3. ANA Standards of Professional Performance supports peer review

    4. May be formal or informal
    5. May improve accuracy of performance appraisal
    6. May provide recognition
  F. Performance review process
    1. Identify comparable peers for reviewers
    2. Educate reviewers about process
    3. Clarify manager role in peer review process
       a. Manager "owns" process
       b. Support for peer appraisers
       c. Gathering of practice information
       d. Providing information to manager in making personnel decisions
    4. Review performance criteria
    5. Select aspects of performance to be appraised
       a. Use of nursing process
       b. Patient outcomes
       c. Use of policy and procedures
       d. Adherence to infection control principles
       e. Participation on unit committees
       f. Continuing education activities
       g. Professional organization activities
       h. Teaching skills
       i. Scientific knowledge base
       j. Documentation of patient information
       k. Ethical behavior
       l. Clinical competence, adherence to practice standards
    6. Select data-gathering method
       a. Observe
       b. Review charts
       c. Interview patients
    7. Have employee being evaluated
       a. Submit evidence of attainment of criteria or performance standard
       b. Identify areas of needed growth
    8. Develop or identify tool to collect data
    9. Select peers to gather the information
    10. Collect data
    11. Analyze data
    12. Share data with employee or supervisor and employee (if supervisor only, more distrust)
    13. Develop and communicate recommendations

IX. QUALITY IMPROVEMENT

  A. Definition
    1. A controlling management function involving setting standards, measuring performance against standards, reporting results, taking action (education, corrective action)
    2. Approach and commitment to continually improve organizational processes to meet and exceed customer expectations and outcomes
  B. Standard
    1. Baseline level of professional behavior or excellence that makes up a model to be followed and practiced
       a. Predetermined
       b. Established by an author
       c. Communicated to and accepted by employees affected by the standard
       d. Measurable, achievable
       e. ANA has *Standards for Nursing Practice*

C. Quality Assurance (QA)/Quality Improvement (QI)
   1. Adopted by JCAHO in the 1970s
   2. Every organization evaluated by JCAHO was to have a QA plan in place
   3. JCAHO had 10-step process used 1985 to 1991
   4. QI developed in 1990s by way of Medicare and Medicaid external peer review, using Peer Standard Review Organizations (PSROs); databases were upgraded, data elements standardized, practice guidelines adopted, and QI initiatives begun
D. Deming/Juran
   1. W. Edwards Deming introduced three key concepts:
      a. Organization-wide value of quality
      b. Worker empowerment for increased productivity
      c. Use of teams to implement change and problem-solving
   2. Joseph Juran developed Juran trilogy of quality planning, quality control, and quality improvement
      a. Directed by top management
      b. Organization-wide steering committee to develop initiatives for cost-effective improvements (Table 30-1)
E. Tools for quality data
   1. Flow charts
   2. Cause and effect diagrams
   3. Interviews, focus groups
   4. Audits
      a. Structure audit: monitors client care setting (environment, nursing service, finances) (e.g., patient call lights in place, staffing patterns)
      b. Process audit: measures care process; task-oriented, ensures that practice standards are fulfilled (e.g., assess care plans, policy and procedure manuals to establish that blood pressure checks occur as policy states)
      c. Outcome audit: determines results that occur from nursing interventions; the outcome should demonstrate the quality of care provided; considered most valid indicator of quality care (e.g., mortality, length of stay, patient stress level, satisfaction with care, cost of care); JCAHO uses outcome criteria in review of quality of care

X. EDUCATION AND TRAINING

A. Staff development
   1. Based on philosophy of adult education principles
      a. Learning is a continual process in life
      b. Learner is self-directed
      c. Learner is internally motivated
      d. Learner experiences are valued

TABLE 30-1

QA vs. QI

	QA	QI
Focus	Clinical problem-solving	Continuous improvement of performance
Structure	Organizations	Patient care
Involvement	Clinical departments	Hospital-wide
Other/Drive	Individual Ensures quality Externally driven	Process, systems Improves quality Internally driven
Responsibility	Of few	Of all

      e. Learner experiences are varied

      f. Task or problem centered

  2. Rapid changes in health care and changing roles in nursing require staff development and education

  3. Technology increases in complexity require staff development, education

  4. Physical processes and cultural, political, and spiritual learning are areas of study for nursing staff

B. Staff development process

  1. Management program to aid staff in development of skills and knowledge that enhance their value as employees and add to their own professional goals

  2. Includes

    a. Orientation

      (1) Content relevant to philosophy, goals, policy and procedures, personnel benefits, role expectations, physical facility

    b. In-service education

      (1) Refining and developing new skills related to job performance

    c. Continuing education (CE)

      (1) Learning experience focused on competence and knowledge to be used by employees in broad array of settings

    d. Job-related counseling

      (1) Promoting professional growth by helping staff give best job performance; aiding in promotion, assisting in formal training

C. Andragogical curriculum development

  1. Andragogy: adult learning science; purports that learners are facilitators of their own education and motivate their own achievement

D. Needs assessment

  1. Learners' perceived needs should be same as planners' perception of learner needs

  2. Needs survey planning

    a. Determines target population for needs survey

    b. Develops time line

    c. Determines cost of survey

    d. Calculates financial and human resources needed

    e. Performs analysis of time

    f. Provides anonymity

    g. Provides objectivity

  3. Survey addresses

    a. Content: specific topics of interest, need

    b. Design of learning activities: when staff can attend courses and what kind of learning options should be offered (e.g., workshop, self-learning modules)

    c. Learners' backgrounds: education, experiences

    d. Organizational needs: in terms of regulatory agencies, etc.

      (1) JCAHO

      (2) ANA standards for continuing education

      (3) State requirements for continuing education

      (4) Customer needs

      (5) Standards of practice

      (6) Institutional philosophy and objectives

  4. Other needs assessment models

    a. Observation

    b. Interviews

    c. Open group meetings

    d. Literature review

    e. Performance appraisals

E. Training vs. education
   1. Training: organizational method of ensuring knowledge and skill for a specific purpose, such as performing duties of a job; managers assume some responsibility for this
   2. Education: formal and broad in scope; develops individual broadly; managers not usually responsible for this type of learning
F. Andragogical learning environment
   1. Relaxed and informal, comfortable
   2. Collaborative with educators, expresses openness
   3. Teacher and class set goals
   4. Decisions made by teacher and student
   5. Teacher, self, and peers evaluate learning

XI. CHANGE THEORY

A. Definition
   1. Change: to alter, vary, transform
   2. Planned change: deliberate, collaborative effort of change agent and system plan to improve operations and functions of the system through knowledge
   3. Change agent: person or group that works to effect change
   4. Unplanned change: accidental change that occurs without planning, without input
B. Change theory
   1. Lewin Force Field Analysis: classic change theory (Kurt Lewin, 1951)
      a. Uses problem-solving and decision-making
      b. Views behavior as force that is dynamic, in delicate balance, working in opposite directions within a "field" or organization
   2. Forces must be assessed and analyzed and dealt with in a three-step process
      a. Unfreezing: changing the status quo (which is comfortable) by way of education, information, maintaining safety and security; need awareness of need to change
      b. Moving, changing; actual change: driving forces greater than restraining forces
      c. Refreezing: stabilization of change to a normal function; maintaining change; change process needs to end
   3. Driving and restraining forces help and hinder change
      a. Driving forces: assist or help change (e.g., motivation to change, improve)
      b. Restraining forces: prevent change (e.g., fear of failure, fear of losing present satisfaction, resistance to change)
C. Force field analysis
   1. Diagnose need for change
   2. Determine what actions are necessary to bring change
   3. First identify driving and restraining forces in the organization—list how strong, how weak each is
D. Resistance to change
   1. Attempt to maintain status quo
   2. Based on threat to security of established pattern
   3. Resistance stimulated by complacency, conservatism, perceived loss of power, ego, perceived loss of rewards
   4. Also supported by
      • No felt need for change
      • Disagreement with change
      • Feel cost of change outweighs benefit
      • Lack of information
      • Lack of trust
      • Fear of the unknown

E. Managing change
1. State precise objectives of the change
2. Analyze change and impact on people, environment, organization
3. Define intended outcomes
4. Develop clear strategies to achieve outcomes
5. Allow sufficient time to implement
6. Coordinate activities
7. Provide strong leadership for change; need political base of power
8. Lend strong support to change agent
9. Educate participants of change process
10. Involve all affected by change
11. Listen to all complaints about the change and deal with them

REFERENCES

Farley S: Leadership. In Swansburg RC, Swansburg RJ, editors: *Introduction to leadership and management for nurses,* ed 2, Boston, 1999, Jones & Bartlett.

Fisher M: Leadership skills. In Luggen A, Travis S, Meiner S, editors: *NGNA core curriculum for gerontological advanced practice nurses,* Thousand Oaks, CA, 1998, Sage.

Grohar-Murray ME, DiCroce HR: *Leadership and management in nursing,* ed 2, Stamford, CN, 1997, Appleton & Lange.

Jameson PA, Hornberger CA, Sullivan EJ: *Nursing leadership and management in action,* New York, 1997, Addison-Wesley.

Rocchiccioli JT, Tilbury MS: *Clinical leadership in nursing,* Philadelphia, WB Saunders.

Swansburg RC, Swansburg RJ: *Introduction to leadership and management for nurses,* ed 2, Boston, 1999, Jones & Bartlett.

Yoder-Wise PS: *Leading and managing in nursing,* ed 2, St Louis, 1999, Mosby.

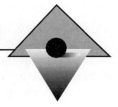

CHAPTER 31

RESEARCH

Joanne Kraenzle Schneider

LEARNING OBJECTIVES

Upon completion of this chapter, the reader will be able to:

- List three reasons why nursing research is important
- List four purposes of research
- Discuss the 17 steps of the research process
- Discuss the critique of a nursing research article
- Describe one process for research utilization in practice

I. IMPORTANCE OF THE ROLE OF RESEARCH IN NURSING (LoBiondo-Wood & Haber, 1998)

A. Improvement of nursing practice
B. Credibility of the nursing profession
C. Accountability of nursing practice
D. Changes in health policy

II. PURPOSES OF NURSING RESEARCH (Polit & Hungler, 1999)

A. Identification of phenomenon about which little is known
B. Description of phenomenon
C. Exploration of the characteristics of the phenomenon, how it is displayed, and factors with which it is related
D. Explanation or understanding of the components of the phenomenon and how it is theoretically related to other phenomena
E. Prediction and control of factors that are of interest to nursing

III. STEPS OF THE RESEARCH PROCESS (Polit & Hungler, 1999)

A. Conceptual phase involves reading, thinking, discussing, and conceptualizing
   1. *Identify the problem* to be solved or question to be answered; problems or questions may be identified from experience, social or political issues, collegial discussion, or a literature review
      a. Problem statement is a description of the dilemma or situation that needs investigation; the purpose of the problem statement is to provide understanding and direction
      b. Purpose statement is the goal of the study stated in declarative form; it is a broad statement that gives general direction
      c. Research question is the question to be answered by the study in interrogative form; research questions clarify and are more specific than purpose statements

        d. Research hypothesis translates the research question into expected outcomes; it is a prediction of the relationships between the variables being studied

   2. *Review the literature* to learn what is already known about the research problem and what studies have already been conducted; research journal articles are important aspects of the literature review; research journal articles are summaries of the highlights of investigations; they are critically reviewed and accepted for publication on a competitive basis

   3. *Define the theoretical framework* that identifies the relationships between variables; the purpose of theory is to describe or predict reality; theory makes the research findings meaningful

        a. Concepts are abstractions, or mental representations, formed by generalizing about human behavior and characteristics

        b. Constructs are abstractions inferred from situations, events, or behaviors; a slightly more complex abstraction than a concept

        c. Theory is a systematic, abstract explanation of an aspect of reality

        d. Variables represent the concepts within a research investigation

   4. *Formulate a hypothesis,* which is a statement of the expected relationships between the variables being studied; it is the predicted outcome of the study

        a. Independent variables are the presumed cause

        b. Dependent variables are the presumed effect

        c. Changes in the dependent variables are dependent on changes in the independent variable (Table 31-1)

B. Design and planning phase involves decision-making about the best way to address the research question

   1. Select a research design, or overall plan, for answering the research question

        a. Designs that address control over the independent variable

           (1) Experimental designs involve

- Manipulation of the independent variable by the investigator for at least some of the subjects
- One or more controls over the study situation, including a control group
- Random assignment to groups

           (2) Quasi-experimental designs involve manipulation of the independent variable but no control group or no randomization

           (3) Nonexperimental studies involve observation of the phenomenon under study as it naturally occurs

        b. Designs that address the type of group comparisons

           (1) Between-subjects designs compare groups of different subjects

           (2) Within-subjects designs allow comparisons of the same subjects more than one time

        c. Designs that address the number of data collection points

           (1) Cross-sectional designs involve data collection at one point in time

           (2) Longitudinal designs involve data collection at more than one point in time

        d. Designs that address the occurrence of independent and dependent variables

           (1) Retrospective designs focus on present dependent variables and independent variables that occurred in the past

           (2) Prospective designs focus on present independent variables and their effects on dependent variables in the future

        e. Designs that address the degree of structure

           (1) Structured designs specify the type of design before data collection (e.g., quantitative designs)

           (2) Flexible designs allow the design to evolve during data collection (e.g., qualitative designs)

   2. Identify the population or specify the group to which the results can be applied

        a. Population: the entire group of cases that meet the criteria for inclusion in the study

        b. Sample: the subset of cases that participate in the study

        c. Representativeness: how much the sample reflects the larger population

TABLE **31-1**

RESEARCH QUESTIONS/HYPOTHESES WITH THEIR CORRESPONDING INDEPENDENT
AND DEPENDENT VARIABLES

Research Hypothesis or Question	Independent Variable	Dependent Variable
Participants receiving a self-management program would increase compliance with inhaled medications (Berg, Dunbar-Jacob, & Sereika, 1997, p. 227).	Self-management program	Compliance with inhaled medications
Older adults who participate in a 14-week home-based resistance training program will significantly improve their postural control (Topp, Mikesky, Dayhoff, et al, 1996, p. 411).	14-week home-based resistance training program	Postural control
What is the effect of a behavioral medicine intervention on hardiness, social support, immune function, and perceived health status in persons with HIV (Nicholas & Webster, 1996, p. 395)?	Behavioral medicine intervention	Hardiness, social support, immune function, and perceived health status
Is there an increase in the risk of urinary incontinence after hip surgery (Palmer, Myers, & Fedenko, 1997, p. 9)?	Hip surgery	Risk of urinary incontinence
Bilirubin will be present in aspirates from nasointestinal tubes in a significantly greater amount than in aspirates from nasogastric tubes (Metheny, Stewart, Smith, et al, 1999, p. 191).	Aspirates from different types of tubes	Bilirubin
Fully nipple-fed preterm infants who receive a prescribed feeding regimen will have a higher caloric and protein intake and weight change than fully nipple-fed preterm infants who receive an ad lib feeding regimen (Pridham, Kosorok, Greer, et al, 1999, p. 86).	Feeding regimen (prescribed or ad lib)	Caloric and protein intake and weight change
Compared to pretreatment (baseline) measures, the cognitive-behavioral intervention will have a positive impact on patients' personal coping resources, pain-coping behaviors, and psychological well-being assessed after the treatment program (Sinclair, Wallston, Dwyer, et al, 1998, p. 317).	Cognitive-behavioral intervention	Coping resources, pain-coping behaviors, and psychological well-being
Women in the expanded treatment group (empowerment intervention plus group counseling) would report significantly less abuse (as measured by frequency and severity) in the 12 months following the pregnancy than women in the empowerment intervention only group or the comparison group (Parker, McFarlane, Soeken, et al, 1999, p. 60).	Group counseling	Abuse (frequency and severity)

3. Specify the method of measurement of each variable
   a. Biophysiologic measurement: assesses the physiologic status of the participant through the use of technical instruments and equipment
   b. Self-report: method of measurement where information is gathered by questioning participants directly
      (1) Unstructured interviews follow no preestablished format

(2) Structured interviews follow preestablished formats

(3) Self-report instruments may be questionnaires for self-administration and may be either open-ended or close-ended

c. Observation: method where the researcher directly observes the behavior of interest

4. Determine how the population will be sampled or the subjects will be chosen

a. Probability sampling: involves some form of random selection

b. Nonprobability sampling: involves selection by nonrandom methods

5. Finalize the research plan and have colleagues provide critique; before conducting the study, institutional review board approval must be obtained

6. Conduct the pilot study to make revisions and correct weaknesses; this allows testing of the sampling plan, the intervention, the methods of measurement and analysis and allows general testing of the adequacy of the entire research plan

C. Empirical phase involves the collection of data and the preparation of these data for analysis

1. Collect the data according to the research plan

2. Qualitative data preparation may involve transcribing all tape recordings, field notes, handwritten memos, etc.

3. Quantitative data preparation may involve reviewing data forms and coding the responses into numbers, according to specific coding rules, prior to data entry

D. Analytic phase involves analysis and interpretation to make the data meaningful; within this phase, the research question is answered

1. Analyze the data

a. Level of measurement used for each variable will partially determine the analyses performed

(1) Nominal measurement: classifies objects into categories (e.g., male and female)

(2) Ordinal measurement: ranks objects into an order relative to the order of the other objects, (e.g., severity level); the order must be meaningful

(3) Interval measurement: ranks objects, with the distances between these ranks as equal; interval level of measurement does not have a meaningful zero (e.g., the Fahrenheit scale); a zero is not the absence of temperature

(4) Ratio measurement: ranks objects, has equal distances between ranks, and has a meaningful zero (e.g., length)

b. Descriptive statistics: describe the variables

(1) Frequency distribution: an arrangement of the numeric values in order with a count of the number of times each value occurred

(2) Mean: the average of the scores computed by summing all the scores and dividing by the number of scores in the sum; used with interval and ratio level data

(3) Median: the point on a scale above which and below which 50% of the cases occur; used with ordinal level data or higher

(4) Mode: the value that occurs most frequently; used with nominal level data or higher

(5) Standard deviation: summarizes the average amount each value deviates from the mean and is used for interval and ratio level data

c. Inferential statistics

(1) Definition: those statistical tests that are used for hypothesis testing; two types are parametric and nonparametric

(2) Statistical significance: refers to a result that is so extreme that it is unlikely to have occurred by chance (Munro, 1997); a nonsignificant result means that the differences observed are likely due to chance fluctuations

(3) Common statistical tests to examine differences between group means

- t-test: involves the evaluation of the means and distributions of two groups (independent t-test); paired t-test involves the evaluation of the means and distributions of two measurements for the same group (correlated t-test) (Munro, 1997)

- Analysis of variance: involves comparing several groups on a particular measure (Munro, 1997)
- Multivariate analysis of variance: involves comparing several groups on multiple measures

    (4) Common statistical tests to examine relationships between variables
- Correlations: describe relationships between variables; correlation ranges from -1.00 to $+1.00$; positive correlations range from .00 to $+1.00$, which indicates how much two variables go up and go up down together; negative correlations range from .00 to -1.00, which indicates how much one variable goes up as the other variable goes down or vice versa; the higher the absolute value of the correlation, the stronger the relationship (e.g., $+.70$ is stronger than $+.30$ and $-.70$ is stronger than $-.30$)
- Multiple regression: predicts or explains a dependent variable by examining its relationship with multiple independent variables

2. Interpret the results or make sense of the results and examine the implications of these results; consideration should be given to the theory, the research questions/hypotheses, the accuracy of the data, and the representativeness of the sample

E. Dissemination phase involves communicating and using the findings
1. Communicate the findings by publishing the study as a journal article or presenting the findings at conferences as a paper or poster
2. Use the findings by recommending how the findings can be incorporated into practice and disseminating the findings to practicing nurses

IV. RESEARCH CRITIQUE OF RESEARCH ARTICLE

A. Introduction: includes the research problem/question and purpose, review of the literature and theoretical framework, and hypotheses
1. Are the problem statement and the purpose clearly stated?
2. Do the research questions match the problem statement and the purpose?
3. What is the research problem/question?
4. Is it significant to nursing?
5. Does the literature review thoroughly cover the previous research?
6. Does the content of the review relate to the research problem/question?
7. Does the review have a logical flow?
8. Does the review simply summarize earlier work or critique the pertinent research?
9. Does the review present the gaps in the literature and relate those gaps to the current study?
10. Are the major features of the theory or the conceptual framework described?
11. Is the theory appropriate for the research problem/question?
12. Are the deductions from the theory or conceptual framework logical?
13. Is the research problem/question stated in the form of hypothesis?

B. Methods: includes the research and sampling design, methods for data collection, description of the intervention, and description of the instruments
1. What type of design is used and is the research design appropriate for the research problem/question?
2. Does the design involve an intervention and is it described clearly?
3. What type of procedures did the researcher use to control external or situational influences?
4. What are the limitations of the design used?
5. What was the target population?
6. Was the sample selected to appropriately represent the target population?
7. How were the participants recruited?

      8. Did any other factor affect the representativeness of the sample?
      9. Are the sample size and the basic characteristics of the sample described?
     10. Is the sample size large enough?
     11. To whom can the results be applied?
     12. How were the data collected?
     13. Who collected the data and were these collectors appropriate?
     14. Were the data collectors trained appropriately?
     15. Did data collection place a burden on the participants that may have affected the quality of the data?
     16. What type of data collection instruments were used and were they described thoroughly?
     17. Was the type of data collection (self-report, observation, biophysiological) appropriate for the research problem/question?

C. Results: involves examining the statistical analyses of a quantitative study and the categories/themes of a qualitative study
    1. Quantitative research
      a. Did the researcher present the descriptive statistics?
      b. Were there inferential statistics used and were they appropriate for the research problem/question?
      c. Did the researcher provide rationale for the type of statistical analyses conducted?
    2. Qualitative research
      a. Was the categorization scheme described?
      b. Is the analysis parsimonious?
      c. Are the categories and theme described clearly?
      d. Does the study result in a meaningful description of the phenomenon being studied?

D. Discussion: involves the review of the findings, explanations for the results, implications, and recommendations
    1. Are the important results discussed?
    2. Does the researcher give explanations for the results? Are these explanations logical?
    3. Are alternative explanations offered?
    4. Does the researcher tie the findings to the theory or conceptual framework?
    5. Does the researcher offer implications for nursing practice, theory, or future research?
    6. Are the implications appropriate?
    7. Does the researcher provide recommendations for future research?
    8. Does the researcher provide recommendations for nursing practice?
    9. Are the recommendations appropriate?

V. Research Utilization or the Process of Transforming Research Findings Into Nursing Interventions (Estabrooks, 1999); Research Utilization Involves a Review and Critique of the Current Studies

A. Select a topic generally driven by a practice problem
B. Retrieve the relevant literature, particularly the related studies
C. Read the theoretical articles before the studies
D. Read and critique the studies
E. Make a decision regarding the use of each study in the synthesis of the research findings; the decision should involve
    1. Overall scientific merit
    2. Type of participants used in the study and similarity to the population to which the findings will be applied
    3. Relevance to the research problem/question
    4. Summary tables as a help during synthesis

F. Decide if the findings are appropriate for use in practice

G. Develop a research-based practice protocol

H. Implement the practice change

I. Evaluate the change by collecting and analyzing data with regard to the change; modify practice as necessary

REFERENCES

Berg J, Dunbar-Jacob J, Sereika SM: An evaluation of a self-management program for adults with asthma, *Clin Nurs Res* 6(3):225-238, 1997.

Estabrooks CA: The conceptual structure of research utilization, *Res Nurs Health* 22:203-216, 1999.

LoBiondo-Wood G, Haber J: *Nursing research: methods, critical appraisal, and utilization,* ed 4, St Louis, 1998, Mosby.

Metheny NA, Stewart BJ, Smith L, et al: pH and concentration of bilirubin in feeding tube aspirates as predictors of tube placement, *Nurs Res* 48(4):189-197, 1999.

Munro BH: *Statistical methods for health care research,* ed 3, Philadelphia, 1997, JB Lippincott.

Nicholas PK, Webster A: A behavioral medicine intervention in persons with HIV, *Clin Nurs Res* 5(4):391-406, 1996.

Palmer MH, Myers AH, Fedenko KM: Urinary continence changes after hip-fracture repair, *Clin Nurs Res* 6(1):8-24, 1997.

Parker B, McFarlane J, Soeken K, et al: Testing an intervention to prevent further abuse to pregnant women, *Res Nurs Health* 22:59-66, 1999.

Polit DF, Hungler BP: *Nursing research: principles and methods,* ed 6, Philadelphia, 1999, JB Lippincott.

Pridham K, Kosorok MR, Greer F, et al: The effects of prescribed versus ad libitum feedings and formula caloric density on premature infant dietary intake and weight gain, *Nurs Res* 48(2):86-93, 1999.

Sinclair VG, Wallston KA, Dwyer KA, et al: Effects of a cognitive-behavioral intervention for women with rheumatoid arthritis, *Res Nurs Health* 21:315-326, 1998.

Topp R, Mikesky A, Dayhoff NE, et al: Effect of resistance training on strength, postural control, and gait velocity among older adults, *Clin Nurs Res* 5(4):407-427, 1996.

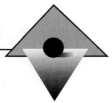

CHAPTER 32

ELDER ABUSE

Alice G. Rini

LEARNING OBJECTIVES

Upon completion of this chapter, the reader will be able to:

- Define and describe the several types of elder abuse
- Discuss the responsibilities of the nurse who encounters a patient experiencing an abusive situation
- Explain the importance of legal and ethical issues in dealing with elderly persons at risk of abuse or who are experiencing abuse

I. DEFINITIONS

A. Abuse: act of physical or mental maltreatment that threatens or causes harm to an elderly person whether by action or inaction

1. Assault: putting an elderly person in fear of impending abuse or violence; does not include actual touching; usually consists of physical or verbal threats
2. Battery: in law this is unwanted or offensive touching, can often include violent acts of beating, hitting, pushing, or throwing objects that hit the elderly person; may also be non-injurious touching
3. Passive abuse: commonly called neglect (see following discussion)

B. Neglect: a type of passive abuse that may include withholding of medication, medical treatment, food, and personal care necessary for the well-being of the elderly person; also includes behavior that ignores the person's obvious need even though the neglectful person is present

C. Financial abuse: theft or conversion of money or anything of value belonging to the elderly person; persons most commonly involved are relatives and care givers; the theft may be accomplished by force, stealth through deceit, misrepresentation, fraud, or undue influence on financial decisions made by the elderly person

D. Psychological abuse: also known as mental or emotional abuse; may include name-calling, verbal assault, threats of violence, neglect, or institutionalization; may include a deliberate effort to dehumanize the elderly person often with an intent to drive the person to mental illness or suicide

E. Self-neglect: generally a function of diminished physical or mental ability; includes not taking medication, avoiding medical treatment, being unable or unwilling to provide for food and personal hygiene; in this situation there may be an ethical question of how much to intervene with self-neglect behavior if the elderly person is competent and simply chooses not to perform this care

F. Sexual abuse: forced or exploitative sexual conduct or activity; demand for sexual favors by use or threat of force; anyone can be a sexual abuse perpetrator, including family members, caretakers, health care providers, criminal sexual predators, or other persons with access to the elderly person

II. Nursing Responsibilities

A. Detecting abuse in patients
   1. Elderly persons are often reluctant to report any kind of abuse because they often fear that they will be abandoned
   2. The incidence of abuse of all kinds is likely under-reported, underestimated, and not well documented
   3. Injuries, weight loss, and other problems may be signs of abuse but are often thought to be consequences of the aging process rather than abuse or neglect
   4. Reporting is sometimes difficult because patients, families, and other caretakers are uncooperative or doubtful that abuse or neglect is occurring
   5. Psychological and sexual abuse are difficult to identify because there may not be demonstrable evidence; these types of abuse are often found along with other types of abuse or exploitation
   6. Change in appetite or depression are common with all kinds of abuse and neglect
   7. Detection of a sexually transmitted disease in a person otherwise unlikely to be so infected may be a sign of sexual abuse
   8. Finding of genital/perineal trauma in an elderly person who is not sexually active is additional evidence of sexual abuse
   9. May be difficult to obtain evidence or a complaint because persons who are victims of any kind of abuse or exploitation are often reluctant to report

B. Reporting abuse and neglect
   1. Many states have mandatory reporting requirements regarding the abuse, neglect, exploitation, or conversion of financial assets of elderly persons; some only apply to elderly persons in long-term care facilities, leaving those residing in the community unprotected by such laws; more recently, many state legislators have realized that elderly persons outside long-term care facilities are vulnerable and have extended reporting laws and other detection and deterrence strategies to such persons
   2. Nurses, nursing home administrators, physicians, podiatrists are required to report actual or suspected abuse or neglect; in states with mandatory reporting requirements, it is a violation of the practice law to have knowledge of abuse of any kind and to *not* report; anyone, not only health care professionals, can report abuse to an appropriate state agency
   3. In some states, incidents of abuse of any kind are mandated to be reported regardless of where the elderly person is living—whether in long-term care, one's own home, the home of a relative or friend, or some other arrangement; some states have permissive reporting of such abuse, meaning that to report, the nurse must have permission of the abused person or his/her guardian unless there is an emergency; emergency situations are usually covered by domestic violence laws; some states have determined that abuse and neglect occurring in long-term care facilities are criminal offenses
   4. State and federal laws relating to physical and chemical restraints often include reporting requirements with regard to their misuse

C. Confidentiality
   1. Many states have enacted laws to protect persons who have been sexually abused from unnecessary publicity because most persons find such abuse embarrassing and shameful
   2. Persons in counseling related to sexual abuse are protected in some states from the disclosure of communication that has occurred between the counselor and the patient; information related to that communication may be disclosed only with the consent of the patient; such laws include protection from release of information about the sexual abuse at a trial; information may be re-leased *in camera* (in the judge's presence only) should such information be needed in a case against the accused perpetrator, and the judge can order it released

D. Nursing intervention and accountability
  1. Nurses should have a working knowledge of the law in the state(s) of practice regarding all kinds of abuse and violence in terms of reporting, safety of patients, and the nurse's role in complying with the law
  2. For one's own protection and also for the patient, nurses should ensure that institutions and agencies that provide care for the elderly and for which nurses work have policies and procedures concerning the nurse's and other provider's roles in dealing with elder abuse, neglect, and exploitation; such information should be available at orientation and in policy books for later reference
  3. Do not assume that "normal" or "nice" appearing families, caretakers, and others with access to the elderly are unaware of or uninvolved in acts of general or sexual abuse should diagnostic signs indicate such abuse; alternatively, don't expect that everyone is an abuser because of the excessive media hyperbole regarding general and sexual abuse issues
  4. In mandatory reporting states, the nurse is always required to report observed or suspected incidence of abuse; otherwise nurses should follow state law and agency policy; nurses must use judgment as to whether injuries to elderly persons are the result of abuse, neglect, or exploitation and then report appropriately in *good faith;* good faith means that any report must be in the best interests of the patient and based on a true belief that abuse or neglect has occurred, not for retribution or revenge against others for real or imagined bad acts
  5. Nurses should maintain close working relationships with patients and their families so that subtle nuances of behavioral change are evident, and there is a greater willingness to communicate and confide should problems occur
  6. Should photographs be necessary, nurses should know who has the authority to take them; if the nurse cannot do so, he/she could assist in ensuring that the appropriate photographs are taken and to witness that such photographs actually depict the problems in question
  7. Nurses concerned about patients in the community who may be experiencing abuse, neglect, or exploitation may encourage and support patients in seeking help, reporting problems, and achieving a safe environment
  8. Nurses should participate in the education of other nurses, nursing students, health care and other professionals, unlicensed personnel, and the public about abuse and the sources of assistance in avoiding or stopping it
  9. Nurses should involve themselves and other nurses and nursing associations in legislative efforts to prevent and prosecute violence, abuse, and neglect

III. PROFESSIONAL AND LEGAL ISSUES

A. Knowledge of the law of the state(s) in which one practices will help to avoid improper or incorrect responses in detecting abuse or neglect
B. If a nurse is required to testify about findings or patients concerning abuse, neglect, or exploitation, he/she should first be sure to seek legal counsel before responding to subpoenas or court orders; nurses need to know their own rights as witnesses, as professionals, and in relation to patients regarding information and when they must disclose such information and when such information may or must be withheld or discussed only *in camera;* nurses should also make sure that agency rules are observed; however, if one is a witness, one cannot refuse a court order to testify
C. Nurses have certain responsibilities with regard to confidentiality of patient information, and they must avoid breaching that confidentiality even when called to do so by a court; some states' practice laws prohibit breaching patient confidentiality except in very limited circumstances
D. Nurses may be involved in collecting evidence to document abuse, neglect, or exploitation, most commonly in emergency departments, home care, and some other community settings; nurses must understand the importance of careful collection, adequate testing, and proper

documentation; the *chain of custody* of evidence is also of importance because the adequacy of evidence and its admissibility in court depends on the evidence being in the proper hands and not tampered with before it is analyzed by appropriate laboratories and other authorities

REFERENCES

Black HC: *Black's law dictionary,* ed 6, St Paul, MN, 1991, West Publishing Company.

Brent NJ: *Nurses and the law,* Philadelphia, 1997, WB Saunders.

Frolick LA, Barnes AP: *Elderlaw,* Charlottesville, VA, 1992, The Michie Company.

Rini AG: Abuse. In Luggen AS, Travis SS, Meiner S: *NGNA core curriculum for advanced practice gerontological nurses,* Thousand Oaks, CA, 1998, Sage.

CHAPTER 33

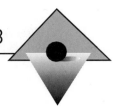

ADVOCACY

Alice G. Rini

LEARNING OBJECTIVES

Upon completion of this chapter, the reader will be able to:

- Discuss the role of the nurse as a patient advocate in health care settings
- Describe the advocacy roles played by others in the health care system
- Describe the effect of advanced directives on patients in health care

I. DEFINITIONS

 A. Advocate: one who pleads for, supports, or recommends on behalf of another

 B. Surrogate: acting as an agent or proxy for another such as a patient; one who represents and acts for a patient in making health care decisions

 C. Nurse advocate: nurse who acts in an advocacy role in the professional health care situation; support of patient as a free agent with the right of self-determination; the American Nurses Association in its Code of Ethics promotes nurse advocacy for all patients

II. NURSE IN AN ADVOCATE ROLE

 A. Nurses must understand that health and illness represent different concepts and different experiences for each person and that a caregiver's approach must be based on a particular patient's experiences and expectations

 B. Patients today are more informed and more educated about their health problems; public sources of health care information have made health care consumers aware of new drugs and treatments; this has been an empowering experience for many persons

 C. Legal tools have also provided power and self-direction for patients; however, many of them, particularly elderly, disabled, or functionally impaired patients, may still need the important advocacy activities of a caring nurse to navigate the health care system

 D. Advocacy should not be confused with paternalism; paternalism means treating others as if they were unable to make decisions on their own; the advocate supports and represents the patient's wishes

III. OTHER ADVOCATES IN THE HEALTH CARE SYSTEM

 A. Patients' rights representatives: employees in hospitals and other health care agencies who are hired to protect the patient's rights

 B. Ombudsmen: employees in health care agencies or with private and/or government agencies who investigate complaints, report findings, and negotiate resolution

 C. Institutional review boards and ethics committees: protect patients if they are research subjects or are taking part in certain treatment protocols

 D. Educational and advocacy groups or organizations: may not be within or exclusive to the health care system but work to empower patients of health care and other services; a good example is the United Seniors Association, who recently went to federal district court to restore the ability of Medicare beneficiaries to privately contract with their health care providers

IV. HEALTH CARE SURROGATES

A. Surrogates advocate for patients by virtue of a legal appointment by a declarant; they are provided for by state laws that address such matters through advance directives

B. Such state laws were mandated by the federal act known as the Patient Self-Determination Act of 1991

C. State laws provide specific opportunities for competent persons to make advance directives that provide for care at a time when a person becomes terminally ill and cannot contemporaneously make decisions about care; such laws also provide for the appointment of a health care surrogate or a durable power of attorney for health care who will make decisions for the patient should he/she become unable to do so

D. Relationships between health care providers and surrogates

1. A surrogate appropriately appointed should be respected as the decision-maker for the patient at the time the patient can no longer make decisions; information that would normally be provided to patients and/or families should also include the surrogate; nurses should know their agency policy regarding relationships with legally appointed health care surrogates

2. If there is a question whether the appointed health care surrogate is acting as the principal (for the patient who appointed surrogate) indicated by the document appointing the surrogate or if the surrogate is not acting as the principal would have acted were the principal able to do so, then nurses should question these issues in accord with institutional/agency or state policy

E. Surrogates and guardians

1. A surrogate or proxy decision-maker is a one who acts as an agent for a principal or declarant; surrogates are appointed by the principal or declarant usually in a written document typically in the form of a durable power of attorney or a health care surrogate designation; appointment may also be done by state action

2. A guardian is appointed by a court pursuant to state law that allows the state to use its *parens patriae* (power to act as a parent) to protect those who cannot make decisions for themselves; guardians are vested with the power and charged with the duty of taking care of the person, his/her property, and safeguarding the rights of another person who, because of some limitation, cannot manage his/her own affairs

3. Guardianship laws evolved early in legal history to protect persons who were incapable of managing their own affairs; such laws address the office, duty, and authority of a guardian; guardianship is less common now because of the availability of advance directives, declarants' abilities to appoint surrogates themselves, and other common law decisions that have developed other ways of dealing with problems of decision-making

REFERENCES

Black HC: *Black's law dictionary,* ed 6, St Paul, MN, 1991, West Publishing Company.

Frolick LA, Barnes AP: *Elderlaw,* Charlottesville, VA, 1992, The Michie Company.

Kenney JW: *Philosophical and theoretical perspectives for advanced practice nursing,* Boston, 1996, Jones & Bartlett.

Rini AG: Surrogate advocacy. In Luggen AS, Travis SS, Meiner S, editors: *NGNA core curriculum for gerontological advanced practice nurses,* Thousand Oaks, CA, 1998, Sage.

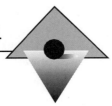

CHAPTER 34

RIGHTS

Alice G. Rini

LEARNING OBJECTIVES

Upon completion of this chapter, the reader will be able to:

• Define the concept of rights
• Discuss how patient rights affect nursing practice
• Analyze how patient rights may be exercised in health care settings

I. DEFINITIONS

    A. Right: something to which one has a just claim or title, whether legal, moral, or by custom; something to which one is justly entitled

    B. Right: power, privilege, or demand that one person can assert and another person must recognize; a capacity residing in one person of controlling, with the assent and assistance of the state, the actions of others

        1. Client/patient rights: generally considered civil rights in that they (1) belong to every citizen of the state or country and (2) are capable of being enforced and, if violated, provide compensation to a person through a civil action in a court of law

        2. Personal rights: generally mean those rights of personal security, life, limb, body, and health

II. PATIENT BILL OF RIGHTS

    A. Bills of Rights are guides for institutions in dealing with clients/patients who enter such institutions; these Bills of Rights do not have enforcement mechanisms through courts and statutes but are generally required to be in place as part of the accreditation requirements

    B. Bills of Rights for hospitalized or institutionalized patients are not guaranteed by constitutions or other laws and, therefore, differ from those constitutional rights well understood by most people

    C. Hospitals and nursing homes that, as a matter of policy, adopt a Patient Bill of Rights are held to the standards stated in the list of rights by those who rely on the Bill of Rights as a legitimate expectation; this includes patients, families, and courts who have held hospitals and other institutions liable for injury for improperly implementing policies meant to protect patients

    D. Rights in long-term care

        1. Omnibus Reconciliation Act 1987 (OBRA 1987) provides for long-term care reform affecting facilities that participate in Medicare and Medicaid

        2. Reforms under this act relate to quality of care and residents' individual rights

        3. Residents have a right to due process before being transferred to other levels of care, but courts have determined that not all transfers are violations of rights but may be made on the basis of the patient's condition

4. Due process is a course of formal proceedings carried out in accord with established and known rules and principles; for hearings or other proceedings to be considered due process, patients need to have prior knowledge of the rules under which the hearing will take place and the opportunity to have legal representation

5. OBRA 1987 also addresses the need for Pre-Admission Screening and Annual Resident Review (PASARR) to prevent inappropriate institutionalization so federal funds are not used to care for people who do not belong in long-term care facilities; this idea is related to the public policy of favoring deinstitutionalization of people with mental disabilities who may be in nursing homes because of an improper placement

III. WHAT IS INCLUDED IN PATIENT RIGHTS?

A. Privacy and confidentiality: these two concepts are separate and distinct although they may be used interchangeably; they are two rights identified by the Joint Commission on Accreditation of Healthcare Organizations (JCAHO) and are, therefore, incumbent on health care providers to observe
  1. The American Nurses Association Code for Nurses addresses the right to privacy and confidentiality of patient information in its second item; it calls for the nurse to safeguard the right to privacy and protect confidential information
  2. The right of privacy is considered a constitutional protection; although it is not explicit in the constitution, it is interpreted by the Supreme Court to arise from the Fourteenth Amendment's concept of personal liberty, which relates to personal autonomy and freedom from intrusion
  3. Confidentiality has a statutory foundation that gives a certain legal status to relationships between and among certain individuals so that trust can be promoted in professional relationships; confidentiality is controlled by the person to whom an individual's private information is relinquished; this means the nurse to whom information is revealed has a legal (and moral) obligation to treat the information appropriately

B. Disclosure of confidential information
  1. Certain health-related information is required to be disclosed for the public's protection; this is governed by federal and state law (examples include infectious diseases and violent injuries)
  2. Reporting done in good faith, pursuant to law or at the direction of a court to the appropriate government agency, is permitted; the reporter of information will be given immunity from any action against himself/herself for breach of confidentiality, but the health care provider may have to prove the good faith and that the reporting was done in the correct manner
  3. Disclosure laws vary among states but generally apply to communicable diseases, abuse of others, gunshot wounds, crime-related injury, and cancer diagnoses (Box 34-1)

C. Right of access to information
  1. A health care facility that creates a medical record, considered to be a business record, owns and controls it but cannot refuse to release the information in it when an appropriate request is received
  2. Creation, use, and disposition of medical records are subject to many laws and regulations, both state and federal
  3. Patients and others have a right to obtain information contained in the medical record, including films, pathology slides, and other materials
  4. Patient has the right to access his/her medical records or authorize their disclosure to others, but the health care institution controls how the record is released; the institution may require
    a. Written consent
    b. Lead time for copying
    c. That the request comes through an attorney or physician, but unreasonable restriction to

---

BOX 34-1   Laws Requiring the Disclosure of Confidential Information

- 21 Code of Federal Regulations, Section 606.170 requires the reporting of adverse reactions to blood collections or transfusions
- 10 Code of Federal Regulations, Section 35.33 requires a report to the Nuclear Regulatory Commission of any misadministration of radioactive materials within 24 hours of discovery of the misadministration
- There is a common law duty to disclose information to appropriate people or authorities if such information could prevent injury or harm to others or innocent third parties
  Example: A patient is diagnosed with active tuberculosis and inconsistently complies with treatment; she lives with an elderly relative, who is told of the patient's diagnosis and the risk of infection
  Example: A child sex offender is released from jail; the residents in the local neighborhood are notified of the impending release and soon-to-occur presence of the offender even though it could be said that the offender has paid his price to society for his crimes
- The duty to disclose has been extended to psychiatric patients who threaten specific persons, information about infectious diseases such as herpes or AIDS although some states have legislated specifically against disclosure of AIDS information (if one has such information, it should only be disclosed to people who have a need to know for purposes of treatment and in some cases for the protection of personnel; however, personnel protection is extremely limited since the mandating of Universal Precautions)

---

    access may be construed as refusal to release, which does violate the patient's right to his/her information

   5. The American Hospital Association recommends that the patient's physician be notified if the record is requested, but the physician may not block the release unless there is some important contraindication; this may be considered a violation of privacy if the physician is no longer caring for the patient

   6. Any request for release of records should be in writing and the health care institution must comply within a reasonable amount of time

  D. Right of self-determination

   1. The right of self-determination is possessed by competent adults and is not lost when a person becomes incompetent; this right may be maintained by the use of advance directives and the designation of surrogate decision-makers

   2. The right of self-determination for an incompetent person is usually managed by the use of surrogate decision-makers; the legal standards for this are *substituted judgment* and *best interests*

     a. Substituted judgment: attempts to reach the same decision the patient would make if he/she had the capacity to do so; it is preferred by courts because it preserves self-determination

     b. Best interests standard: requires a decision that benefits the patient by promoting his/her current welfare without consideration of previously stated preferences; does not require that useless or nonbeneficial treatment be started or continued

   3. In protecting self-determination, it is important to understand the identity of the true patient; it must be determined if the patient is the older adult himself/herself, the family, or some other person or entity such as a guardian or supporting institution

   4. The right of self-determination includes the right to refuse treatment, to demand disclosure of information about treatment, and to choose to avoid life-sustaining or prolonging actions by health care providers

   5. When a patient refuses care by some means, such as verbally, in clearly stated words, or physically such as turning away, moving, or resisting, staff should report the action to a supervisory nurse; the supervisory nurse should consult agency policy, inform the physician or other appropriate agency personnel, determine the existence of advance directives, and discuss the matter with the family of the patient

E. Right to protection from harm
   1. Older patients, because of the fact of aging and possibly increasing frailty, have some greater risks than younger patients
   2. Conditions that increase one's risk of harm include nervous system impairment, loss of bone density, susceptibility to infection, differing responses to medication
   3. Nurses must take into account age-related differences in caring for older patients so that harm does not result from substandard care
   4. Preventive practices that aid in avoiding injury and illness are minimal expectations; measures that increase self-care ability are also important in preserving the older patient's right to protection
   5. Although no law provides for patient advocates or ombudsmen in health care institutions, the ANA Code for Nurses requires safeguarding the patient from incompetent, unethical, or illegal practice; additionally, the presence of an advocate or ombudsman provides an objective person to assist in resolving disagreements or disputes and provides for an atmosphere of patient support
   6. Nurses who have questions or problems with safety or protection issues may consult with supervisors, ombudsmen, or other agency-specified people to obtain guidance or answers to such practice questions

REFERENCES

Brent NJ: *Nurses and the law,* Philadelphia, 1997, WB Saunders.
Rosenblatt RE, Law SA, Rosenbaum S: *Law and the American health care system,* Westbury, NY, 1997, The Foundation Press.

CHAPTER 35

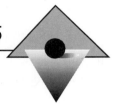

INFORMED CONSENT

Alice G. Rini

LEARNING OBJECTIVES

Upon completion of this chapter, the reader will be able to:

- Define consent and informed consent
- Discuss the role of the nurse in providing for informed consent from older adults
- Identify the barriers to informed consent

I. DEFINITIONS

A. Informed consent: a legal doctrine requiring the disclosure of information about a proposed treatment before obtaining consent for its performance

B. Capacity: the patient's functional ability to understand the nature of his/her medical condition, the risks of treatment or non-treatment, the risks and benefits of the proposed treatment, and the available alternatives

C. Competency: a legal judgment, rendered by a court and based on evidence, that determines whether a person is able to transact business or sign legally binding documents

D. Health care surrogate: one who has legal authority granted by the patient in a properly executed and witnessed document, usually prepared by an attorney, to make health care decisions for the patient; this is a narrow form of power of attorney in that it only grants consent power to another for health care decisions that the patient is unable to make at the time they are needed; being so appointed does not mean that additional powers may be vested in the same person

E. Power of attorney: a legal instrument authorizing one to act as the attorney or agent of another; this agent's power is terminated on the incompetence or death of the patient unless the power is *durable,* that is, it survives incompetence or death; a durable power of attorney can also be used to appoint a health care decision-maker

II. STANDARDS FOR INFORMED CONSENT

A. The professional standard limits the duty to disclose information to that which a reasonable medical practitioner would disclose under the same or similar circumstances
   1. This standard requires an expert witness in deposition or court to establish what the standard of informing is in the situation presented
   2. Physicians prefer this standard because the required information can be predicted in advance

B. The reasonable patient standard demands that the health care provider disclose such information as the patient would deem material to his/her decision whether or not to undergo a treatment or procedure
   1. Physicians have contested the patient-based standard, arguing that adopting such a rule would require the provider to guess what was important to each patient each time information was provided about a treatment

2. No expert witness is required in court because the standard to be established is that of the patient; this eliminates the need for expensive consultants in court
3. Establishing failure to provide informed consent under the reasonable patient standard includes
   a. The existence of a material risk that was unknown to the patient
   b. Provider's failure to disclose that risk
   c. An injury to the patient that was a direct result of the undisclosed risk

III. WHEN CONSENT IS REQUIRED

A. Consent is always required before any touching, including bathing, administering medications, measuring vital signs, performing medical and surgical procedures
   1. Nurses should use good judgment and common sense when providing care to patients who may or may not be well oriented to the health care setting
   2. Nurses should never assume that older patients cannot make their own decisions
   3. If there is a question of whether to proceed with care and risk charges of battery or some other intentional tort but avoid charges of neglecting the patient, nurses should seek guidance from supervisors or institutional policy
B. Consent may be implicit or understood in some situations
   1. On voluntary admission to a health care agency, there is implicit consent for routine procedures to be performed without specific consent for those procedures; however, nurses should be concerned about what is actually routine
   2. If a nurse begins to provide care or approaches the start of care and the patient cooperates or does not object, consent is implicit or can be understood as given from the patient's behavior
   3. A patient may revoke consent at any time by indicating refusal to be touched or treated; such refusal need not be written or spoken but may be by gesture or attitude; this does not mean that the patient should be left alone or ignored, but good judgment on timing, approach adjustment, or encouragement should be the nurse's strategy; the nurse should also find out what the patient is thinking or feeling
   4. Touching or continuing to treat subsequent to refusal by the patient is battery, a civil wrong (as distinct from criminal) related to unwanted touching
   5. Patients should be given specific information regarding what activity is proposed before its implementation, including information about medications; misleading the patient about the medications or ignoring questions may also be battery; even if the nurse believes the patient does not understand the explanation, the consent requirement is not waived; simple language can be used with the patient to provide a general explanation of the reasons for the activity or the need for the medication; family members or others who may be consenting on behalf of the patient should be fully informed about the treatment and its effect
   6. Specific consent is required when a procedure or treatment is invasive or has the possibility of side effects or complications
   7. Courts have generally ruled in favor of patients where treatments or procedures have been performed without specific consent
   8. If there is any doubt whether consent is needed, it is best to obtain specific consent; consent may be obtained from the patient who is competent, from responsible family members involved in the patient's care, or from a person holding power of attorney for the patient
C. Exceptions to the consent rule
   1. In an emergency
   2. When the patient waives the right to information
   3. When medical judgment is that information would be harmful to the patient and invokes the therapeutic privilege not to provide it; this action is taken very carefully
   4. Whenever information is not provided and consent is not obtained, it is important to document the decision-making process and outcome thoroughly

IV. WHO CAN CONSENT

A. Capacity must be present for consent to be valid; a patient cannot give consent if he/she does not have the capacity to understand the information provided on which the decision will be made; in such cases, surrogates or other family members are called on to provide consent where necessary

B. Competency is a questionable situation in consenting to health and medical care; merely because a patient cannot conduct business affairs may not mean he/she cannot understand the information needed to make medical decisions; health care providers need to make the decision whether or not the patient understands enough to consent

C. When consenting, if a patient's decision is consistent with his/her known values, incapacity cannot be determined merely because the preference is different from those of the caregivers

D. Physicians may determine capacity after consulting with other health care professionals as to their understanding of the patient's capacity

E. Because capacity is determined by a medical approach, not a legal one, the standard of "a reasonable degree of medical certainty" is used; if contested, a court would require that incapacity be manifested by clear and convincing evidence

F. Documentation should include how capacity was evaluated, the evidence for determining the level of capacity, and how often capacity should be re-evaluated

G. Only patients who are competent or have the capacity to consent may legally do so; consent from incompetent or incapacitated patients is ineffective

V. HOW TO OBTAIN CONSENT

A. Responsibility for obtaining consent belongs to the person performing the procedure or treatment requiring consent
   1. For medical or surgical procedures, physicians are responsible for providing appropriate information and obtaining consent
   2. If a nursing procedure is contemplated, the nurse should provide the information and obtain the consent; typically such consent is verbal for the common kinds of care received by most patients on a regular basis
   3. A health care institution has no responsibility for obtaining consent unless the physician is an employee of the institution or has delegated the responsibility to the nurse
   4. If the responsibility is delegated to the nurse, the nurse is then legally accountable for the information provided
   5. Health care facilities require nurses to verify that informed consent has been obtained; failure to make such verification may lead to liability for negligence on the part of the institution and the nurse
   6. Merely witnessing a signature does not create a duty on the part of the nurse to provide information related to informed consent

B. Nurses may provide information for the purpose of obtaining informed consent from a patient
   1. Such an activity does not exceed the scope of nursing practice
   2. Most institutions, however, prefer that nurses do not take on this responsibility because it exposes the institution to liability for the adequacy of that information
   3. Normally such liability is part of doing business as a health care institution, but it is difficult to provide information always consistent with what the physician had in mind and that exposure may be unreasonable to accept

REFERENCES

Brent NJ: *Nurses and the law,* Philadelphia, 1997, WB Saunders.
Furrow BR, Johnson SH, Jost TS, et al: *Liability and quality issues in health care,* St Paul, MN, 1991, West Publishing.

CHAPTER 36

LIMITATIONS ON TREATMENT

Alice G. Rini

LEARNING OBJECTIVES

Upon completion of this chapter, the reader will be able to:

- Discuss the right to refuse treatment
- Describe exceptions to the right to refuse treatment
- Explain the use and limitations of *Do Not Resuscitate* orders

I. DEFINITIONS

A. Terminal illness: a condition caused by an illness or injury that is incurable and irreversible and is likely to result in death within a short period of time; in such a situation, application of most treatments will only serve to prolong the dying process

B. Assisted suicide: making a means of suicide, such as medication or a weapon, available to a person with knowledge of the person's intent to end his/her life

C. Withholding and withdrawing treatment: honoring the refusal of treatments that a person does not want and that are more burdensome than beneficial; such recognition and compliance with the refusal is ethically and legally permitted even if such action hastens the time of death

D. Patient Self-Determination Act, 1991: federal law that requires hospitals, nursing homes, HMOs, and other health care agencies who receive Medicare or Medicaid funding to have written policies

1. Providing adult patients with the opportunity to consent to or refuse treatment

2. Informing patients concerning their rights under the state's law, including the opportunity to make advance directives and other decisions regarding treatment or non-treatment

3. Assessing for the existence of any advance directives and the same document in the medical record

4. Not conditioning the provision of care on the basis of the presence or absence of an advance directive

5. Complying with state law concerning advance directives

6. Providing educational programs to agency staff and the community on the law and advance directives

E. Advance directives: a written declaration or directive such as a living will or a durable power of attorney for health care that is recognized under state law and relates to the provision of care in case of incapacitation of the declarant; these documents are mechanisms for individuals to specify wishes concerning the withdrawing or forgoing of life-sustaining treatment in certain circumstances and/or the designation of a surrogate to make such decisions should the declarant be unable to make such decisions himself/herself

F. Brain death: a condition where all vital functions of the brain, brainstem, and spinal reflexes are irreversibly non-existent, as determined by accepted medical standards

G. Substituted judgment: acting according to what an incompetent person, if competent, would choose to do

H. Best interests decision: acting in such a manner as to support the maximum good or well-being of an individual who is incompetent; there is some question whether anyone can know what is best for another person and in law the best interests theory differs in process and outcome from substituted judgment (above)

II. LIMITATIONS ON TREATMENT

A. Despite the many available treatments for many diseases and the expanding technology that the health care establishment can claim, there are times when there are no more treatments that will benefit the patient, or the treatments will prolong life but at a great cost in terms of suffering; it is at such times that patients and their caregivers may determine that no further treatment is the only acceptable course of action

B. There is much controversy about limiting treatment; the medical establishment has always done "everything possible for the patient" whether or not such treatments had any effect on the course of the illness; there are those who believe that the cost of caring for persons with a doubtful future should be a consideration in what care is provided

III. DO NOT RESUSCITATE ORDERS (DNR)

A. DNR orders are legal and binding but must be justified as a patient request or be medically indicated; they often need more than one physician concurring on the order; medical futility—that is, treatment will have no beneficial effect—is a legitimate reason for a DNR order

B. Health care institutions should have formal, written policies on which to base DNR decisions, and they should be known to all employees and those with practice privileges in the institution

C. Standards of accrediting agencies require written policies made in consultation with medical and nursing staffs and other appropriate institutional personnel
   1. DNR policies must provide for decision-making, resolving conflicts, and prescribing roles for professional caregivers, family members, and others in the decision process
   2. The DNR decision belongs to the patient unless the patient lacks capacity
   3. When the DNR order is made, the supporting documentation must include the patient's current condition, prognosis, summary of decision-making, and who was involved
   4. DNR order should include a future time for review

IV. WITHHOLDING AND WITHDRAWING TREATMENT

A. Such actions are related to a patient's right to refuse treatment or withdraw consent for it

B. The right to refuse treatment extends to life-prolonging care

C. Refusal of treatment may be made regardless of the patient's health problem

D. The patient must have the capacity to refuse

E. Failure to respect and comply with a valid refusal of treatment or a request for withdrawal may result in a lawsuit against the providers of care

---

EXAMPLE: A patient had advised caregivers that she did not want to be "kept alive by machines." After experiencing respiratory and cardiac arrest, she was placed on a respirator. The family sued for invasion of privacy, pain and suffering, mental anguish, and unnecessary costs. The court said that treating against the patient's wishes is battery even if treatment is harmless or beneficial. *Estate of Leach v. Shapiro,* 489 NE2d 1047 (OH 1984)

V. ISSUES CONCERNING THE RIGHT TO REFUSE TREATMENT

A. Courts have not imposed life-sustaining or life-prolonging treatment on a patient where refusal is clearly expressed by the patient or a legitimate surrogate

B. Courts may make restrictions on the way withhold- or withdraw-treatment decisions are made

C. The patient's right to refuse treatment may be overridden when the state's interest is determined to be superior to the patient's; state interests include
   1. Preserving life
   2. Preventing suicide
   3. Protecting innocent third parties
   4. Maintaining ethical standards of the medical profession

D. There are questions about the withdrawal of nutrition and hydration; these issues are troublesome to ethicists and others
   1. The American Nurses Association issued a Position Statement entitled *Foregoing Nutrition and Hydration* in which it stated its belief that a decision to withhold or withdraw nutrition and hydration should be made by the patient or his/her surrogate in consultation with the health care team; the statement is very strong in its assertion that no matter what decision is made about nutrition and hydration, nurses must continue to provide high quality care, minimize discomfort, and promote the dignity of the patient; the statement expresses concern about the ethical and social issues surrounding food and water and attempts to distinguish between a patient who can take sips of water or small amounts of food and one who is unable to manage intake except by technological means; the issue of whether food and fluid are more burdensome than beneficial is also discussed, and the statement supports the premise that the benefits must outweigh the burdens for intervention to be justified; nurses whose moral values conflict with a decision to withhold or withdraw nutrition and hydration should be permitted to transfer care of the patient to another nurse
   2. Patients who are near the end of their lives often have a decline in appetite; it is important for nurses to realize that forcing food on such patients is inappropriate
   3. Hospice settings can do an excellent job of palliative care and minimizing pain and suffering; some patients are not aware of this service and sometimes believe their only choice is death to obtain relief; nurses must be aware of all alternatives for patients for whom there is not a treatment that will change the course of disease; hospice provides pain relief, multi-disciplinary interventions, and a peaceful, humane environment for a person's last days
   4. The American Dietetic Association takes the position that dietitians should be involved in the development of ethical guidelines for feeding permanently unconscious patients; clearly all the professions involved in patient care in a variety of ways should take part in patient care whatever decision is made regarding nutrition and hydration
   5. Nurses have the ethical obligation to act in the patient's best interests as evidenced by the patient's expressed values or through his/her family

E. Many states have addressed the withholding and withdrawal of artificially provided nutrition and hydration
   1. Competent persons may make such a decision in an advance directive or at the time the question arises in a health care agency
   2. Surrogates may make the same decisions as the advance directive declarant

---

EXAMPLE: A woman was severely injured and was in a persistent vegetative state (PVS). She received nutrition and hydration from a gastrostomy tube. Numerous friends and family testified to specific instances in which the woman had stated her desire not to be kept alive by artificial means. It was undisputed that she had irreversibly lost all cognitive functions although her brainstem continued to function. The state supreme court ruled that a person has a right to decline life-prolonging medical treatment, including artificially provided nutrition and hydration, but that the right is lost to incompetence. However, they further indicated that the right may be exercised by someone acting on the patient's behalf if the patient made her wishes known before becoming incompetent. This case supports substitute judgment as an effective means to preserve the rights of an incompetent patient to accept or refuse treatment. *DeGrella v. Elston,* 858 S.W.2d 698 (KY 1993)

REFERENCES

American Nurses Association: Position statement, "Foregoing nutrition and hydration," *http://www.ana.org/readroom/position/ethics/etnutr.htm,* 1999.

American Dietetic Association: Position statement, "Legal and ethical issues in feeding permanently unconscious patients," *http://www.eatright.org/alegal.html,* 1996.

Byock IR, Forman WB, Appleton M: Academy of Hospice Physicians position statement, "Access to hospice and palliative care," *J Pain Symptom Manage* 11(2):69-70, 1996.

Daly BJ: Withholding nutrition and hydration revisited, *Nurs Manage* 26(5):30-38, 1995.

CHAPTER 37

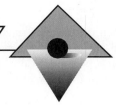

ADVANCE DIRECTIVES

Alice G. Rini

LEARNING OBJECTIVES

Upon completion of this chapter, the reader will be able to:

- Explain the purpose of advance directives
- Describe living wills, health care surrogates, advance directives, and other legal instrumentalities that may protect the interests of elderly persons should they be unable to do so independently
- Discuss the responsibilities and duties of nurses and other health care providers with regard to advance directives

I. DEFINITIONS

A. Advance directives: created by state statute, an advance directive is a written document that is made by a competent declarant in advance of need, directing health care providers in terms of the declarant's preferences regarding the acceptance or refusal of treatment under certain circumstances in the future, when the declarant can no longer make health care decisions; an advance directive may contain elements of a *living will* in that it directs what kind of life-sustaining treatment is acceptable or which should be withdrawn or foregone; an advance directive may also provide for and appoint a *surrogate decision-maker* who may make health care decisions on behalf of the declarant when said declarant can no longer make his/her own

B. Living will: written document prepared and executed by a competent declarant, which directs health care providers as to what kind of care should be provided, withdrawn, or foregone when the declarant is no longer able to make health care decisions for himself/herself contemporaneously with the need; form and process are created by state statute; a living will becomes effective when the declarant is terminally ill, in a persistent vegetative state, or is permanently unconscious according to state law definition; it is very important to understand that the presence of a living will does NOT mean that no care is desired, only that the patient may not want life-prolonging care (see also Chapter 36)

C. Durable power of attorney: includes appointment of a health care surrogate; a written document that designates and appoints another person to act as the agent of the competent person (principal or maker) executing the document in making health care decisions when the principal/maker of the document can no longer do so; form and process are dictated by state statute; depending on powers conferred, health care decision-making power only becomes effective when the principal lacks decision-making power; differs from a general power of attorney (see following)

D. Power of attorney: a written instrument that confers general and/or specific powers to another to act as an agent or attorney of the principal; is effective when made and is not based on the incompetence of the principal; is effective only for those duties and actions specified; is effective

233

only when the principal is competent and usually is revoked by operation of law when the principal becomes incompetent or dies

   E. Guardian: a person lawfully (and usually appointed by a court) invested with the power, and charged with the duty, of taking care of another person and managing the property and rights of that person, who, because of age, understanding, or self-control, is considered incapable of managing his/her own affairs; often a guardian is appointed for another person when that person is declared to be incompetent by a court of law

II. ELEMENTS OF ADVANCE DIRECTIVES

   A. The form of the document is critical

      1. A directive must be in writing

      2. The form is generally dictated by state law

         a. Alternative and variant forms may be acceptable as long as the document includes those elements required by law even if they do not use the exact same language

         b. To avoid rejection by health care providers or courts, it is the best practice to use the state-mandated form in the state of practice

         c. Health care providers should take care to ensure that advance directives presented as the intent of a patient are valid

      3. Documents should be executed and witnessed according to legal requirements

         a. The patient's signature must be witnessed by the legally mandated number of disinterested witnesses; such witnesses have no interest in the outcome of the care and are not beneficiaries of the declarant's will or trust

         b. An advance directive does not need to be prepared by an attorney, but there is a greater chance of validity if it is so prepared

         c. Employees or agents of health care institutions where the patient is receiving care may not be witnesses to advance directives; this includes nurses, physicians, admitting officers, or any other person associated with the agency

         d. Some states do not permit beneficiaries under the will of the declarant or other family members or close associates to be a witness for an advance directive

   B. Who can make an advance directive?

      1. Anyone who is competent/has decision-making capacity and wishes to provide direction for his/her care at a future time at which he/she might not be able to make health care decisions may make an advance directive

      2. Adults and emancipated minors are generally able to make advance directives

   C. Surrogates and agents

      1. The declarant may select any person he/she chooses for a health care surrogate decision-maker

      2. Agents/surrogates are often family members, but this is not a requirement

      3. Individuals appointing a surrogate may select a person whom they believe will make the most appropriate decisions, in the best interests of the declarant, and according to the declarant's specified wishes

      4. Employees and other persons associated with the health care institution in which the declarant is receiving care may not be agents or surrogates

   D. Revocation of advance directives

      1. A declarant may revoke a written advance directive by

         a. Verbally indicating it is no longer to be followed; issues of competence and decision-making capacity are important to consider in terms of how to deal with such revocation

         b. Physical destruction of the document by tearing, burning, or some other method

         c. Amending the original document so that provisions are changed that revoke the original provisions; this may not be in the original formal writing but may be in the writing of the declarant who may cross out or revoke passages and add new provisions

2. Once a declarant is no longer competent or has lost decision-making capacity, revocation or amendment is no longer possible

III. DUTIES OF HEALTH CARE PROVIDERS

A. Determine the presence of an advance directive during the initial assessment of the patient
B. Know the requirements of the state in which one practices as they relate to advance directives
C. Be aware of problems of validity of advance directives and question according to agency policy if there are suspicions of invalidity
D. Honor the provisions of valid advance directives and advocate for the patient with regard to those directives

REFERENCES

Areen J, King PA, Goldberg S, et al: *Law, science, and medicine,* Westbury, NY, 1996, The Foundation Press.
Black HC: *Black's law dictionary,* ed 6, St Paul, MN, 1991, West Publishing.
Brent NJ: *Nurses and the law,* Philadelphia, 1997, WB Saunders.
Eliopoulos C: *Gerontological nursing,* Philadelphia, 1997, JB Lippincott.
Rini AG: Advance directives. In Luggen AS, Travis SS, Meiner S, editors: *NGNA core curriculum for gerontological advanced practice nurses,* Thousand Oaks, CA, 1998, Sage.

CHAPTER 38

ALLOCATION OF RESOURCES

Alice G. Rini

LEARNING OBJECTIVES

Upon completion of this chapter, the reader will be able to:

- Describe what is meant by allocation of resources
- Discuss the manner in which scarce resources are allocated
- Evaluate the allocation or distribution of health care resources

I. DEFINITIONS

A. Scarce resources: in terms of health and medical care, these include access to providers, use of technology, availability of drugs, and other measures that contribute to the improvement of health of a health care consumer

B. Health insurance: complex assortment and system of insuring entities, including commercial, not-for-profit, health maintenance organizations, preferred provider organizations, and some governmental agencies, which assume some of the risk of health care cost in exchange for a premium paid by the beneficiary (except in the case of some governmental programs)

1. Health maintenance organizations: historically evolved from a variety of arrangements under which health care providers, including physicians, hospitals, and others are contracted to provide all agreed-upon care to employee groups or other groups of individuals for a pre-arranged fee; health maintenance organizations provide what is known as managed care

2. Managed care: any health coverage arrangement in which, for a pre-determined fee, a company sells a defined package of benefits to a purchaser, with services furnished to enrolled members through a network of participating providers who operate under written contractual or employment agreements, and whose selection and authority to furnish covered benefits is controlled by the managed care company

II. MANAGING SCARCE RESOURCES

A. Every society has to determine how best to use the resources available to it; scarcity is generally a pervasive issue

1. Production of goods and services requires an optimum mix of human, technological, and natural resources

2. An appropriate mix of goods and services to provide to the population needs to be manufactured or arranged; such goods and services offered are based on the needs, wants, and interests of the target population

3. Distribution of goods and services should be efficient; that is, costs should be appropriate and goods/services should effectively get to those who need them

B. Patterns of production and distribution

1. In socialistic societies, central planners determine patterns of production and distribution;

these are often ineffective in a near time frame because central planners do not predict or analyze the needs and wants of the population well; in the long term, also, central planning usually fails and produces extreme shortages, high prices, and consumer dissatisfaction

2. In kibbutzim and other tribal-type societies, production and distribution are cooperative and community based; these tend to be satisfactory because the community as a whole makes the decisions about production and distribution and the small size and homogeneity of the group served minimizes the chance of dissatisfaction with the process and products

3. The dominant mechanism in modern societies is the market system; markets can lead to a technologically cost effective and efficient allocation of resources; market efficiency requires a well-functioning legal system that can define and adjudicate claims over property rights and enforce contracts; markets also depend on certain norms of behavior and attitudes toward exchange and transactions; consumers must be aware of the quality of the product and the prices charged by each producer; there must be free entry and exit of producers in the market; there must not be significant barriers to entry or exit, either artificially created by government regulation or naturally occurring because of the nature of the goods

III. HEALTH CARE INSURANCE

A. Uncertainty is an inherent characteristic of many types of illnesses and accidents
   1. They and their associated costs are unpredictable
   2. Health care insurance cannot eradicate or even influence the uncertainty of illness, but it can reduce an individual's financial risks associated with illness

B. Uncertainty exists regarding the effects of treatment
   1. Although research can establish whether a procedure or treatment is effective, on average, its effectiveness for any single individual remains uncertain
   2. This uncertainty is an inherent aspect of health care services

C. Unpredictability or uncertainty regarding cost and outcome of an illness/accident means that health and health care decisions must be made in a context of risk

IV. HEALTH CARE INFORMATION

A. Information is one of the most important things consumers/patients want from health care providers to help deal with the element of risk
   1. Unable to diagnose themselves, consumers want information on what treatment will resolve their problems
   2. However, the patient/consumer very often has neither the information nor the knowledge to know what is wrong and what, if anything, is required to restore health
   3. The health care professional has this expertise and directs patients as to what treatments and procedures can be expected to restore their health; hence, there is an imbalance in the level of information, or an informational asymmetry, between the patient and the provider
      a. Informational asymmetries are a significant source of market failure in the health care sector because they give the providers considerably more power than the consumer
      b. Insurance doesn't necessarily mitigate the informational asymmetry
      c. In fact, with the advent of managed care, information may be less available to the consumer in that he/she may be unable to determine what treatment is covered for a particular health problem if he/she has been given information about all the alternatives and their effectiveness and the managed care organization limits the services available to the consumer based on the contract with the employer or through a Medicare-managed care plan

V. GOVERNMENT-SPONSORED HEALTH PLANS FOR OLDER ADULTS

A. Medicare: health plan available for older adults and certain disabled persons; every person over the age of 65 years who is eligible for Social Security retirement income is also eligible for Medicare

1. Medicare consists of two parts
    a. Part A, hospital insurance (HI): financed by a payroll tax paid by employers and employees; it is understood that the claim of an employer-paid part doesn't actually mean that working people are not bearing all the cost of the tax because employer-financed funds would likely be paid in salaries to workers if they were not first allocated to Medicare tax
    b. Part B, supplemental medical insurance (SMI): financed by a combination of premiums paid by beneficiaries and government general revenues; originally planned for a 50%-50% share for each, the cost of this program has escalated significantly because of reluctance to charge significantly higher premiums to Medicare beneficiaries; the share mix has changed to 25% paid by beneficiaries, 75% from general tax revenues
2. Medicare covers only about half of the health care expenditures of most elderly persons
    a. It has relatively high deductibles (it pays 80% of approved amounts after an annual deductible of $100)
    b. No cap on out-of-pocket expenditures
    c. No out-patient prescription drug benefit
3. Medicare is more expensive than most employer-based plans from which many retirees came
    a. To assist with the expenses not covered by Medicare, many beneficiaries also carry a supplemental insurance policy that will cover the 20% of Medicare-covered services that Medicare doesn't pay
    b. However, the supplemental policy also has a deductible and pays only 80% of the 20% not paid by Medicare
4. It is important to understand that Medicare-approved amounts paid for health care provided are significantly less than the actual charges for those services; this has been a source of animosity on the part of health care providers and continues to be so; these inadequate reimbursements for care have prompted some providers to opt out of the Medicare program

B. Medicaid: mandatory joint federal and state program in which federal and state support is shared based on the state's per capita income
1. The program provides basic medical care services to an economically indigent population who qualify for the program because of low income or who receive public assistance
2. Medicaid is funded by personal income, corporate, and excise taxes and is, therefore, considered a transfer payment from the more economically stable citizens to poor citizens
3. Medicare spending has grown at a rapid pace primarily because of the growth in the size of the covered population—growth in the elderly and disabled population requiring intensive care or long-term care services and use of medical technology to prolong the lives of extremely low birthweight infants and other severely compromised individuals who require extensive, often long-term, and expensive services

VI. MANAGED CARE

A. Managed care: population-based care system in which an organized care-providing group contracting with the managed care organization agrees to provide health maintenance and medical care to a defined population group
B. The population basis helps the insurer to determine, from actuarial data, the projected use of services by the population; such projections are used to establish premiums and other charges for benefits
C. In managed care, the insurer exerts considerable influence over the delivery, use, and cost of services
D. The financial incentives of providers in a managed care system are quite different from the incentives in the fee-for-service system prevalent in the past (fee-for-service providers are paid based on services rendered, thereby financially rewarding higher use [but not necessarily improper or medically unnecessary use])

1. Managed care uses a prospective or pre-payment concept in which a provider is paid a pre-determined, agreed amount to provide all the care persons in that provider's service need
2. It is called a capitation system in that payments are made by the insurer to the provider on a per-member basis
3. The provider receives the payment from the insurer whether or not any services are used by any of the members
4. If the provider's services provided exceed the pre-determined payment, the provider suffers financial loss, so the incentive is to control rather than promote use of services
5. If the provider uses fewer resources than payments received, the excess is retained as profit

E. The Health Maintenance Organization Act of 1973 (citation) provided loans and grants for the planning, development, and implementation of combined insurance and health care delivery entities; the Act also mandated a certain array of services
1. The legislation mandated that HMO options be offered by employers with 25 or more employees where such entities were available
2. Also mandated was that employers contribute a similar amount for employees in HMOs as they did for employees who remained in fee-for-service care
3. The federal funding and mandates stimulated the growth of HMOs

F. Medicare and Medicaid now offer managed care plans to their beneficiaries; in 1997, almost 5 million Medicare beneficiaries belonged to managed care organizations
1. Most older adults in managed care joined because they believed that the options offered, which were not available in traditional Medicare, would be worth the restrictions in choice
2. Recently, many managed care organizations and HMOs have withdrawn from Medicare because of low reimbursement from the government leaving many senior citizens without insurance; these persons will be able to select a managed care organization that is still in Medicare or return to traditional Medicare in January, 2000

REFERENCES

Rosenblatt RE, Law SA, Rosenbaum S: *Law and the American health care system,* Westbury, NY, 1997, The Foundation Press.

Shi L, Singh DA: *Delivering health care in America,* Gaithersburg, MD, 1998, Aspen Publications.

Sultz HA, Young KM: *Health care USA,* ed 2, Gaithersburg, MD, 1999, Aspen Publications.

CHAPTER 39

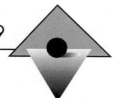

MENTAL COMPETENCY ISSUES

Alice G. Rini

LEARNING OBJECTIVES

Upon completion of this chapter, the reader will be able to:

- Identify the measures and instrumentalities to determine mental competency
- Discuss the legal rights of persons who have diminished mental competence or capacity
- Describe the duties of the nurse in caring for persons with mental incompetence

I. DEFINITIONS

A. Incompetence: a mental disability (as opposed to a legal one, such as being a minor) that renders a person unable to transact business affairs, to execute legal documents, or to provide testimony in legal proceedings; generally determined by a court

B. Incapacity: inability to understand the nature and effects of one's acts; one who lacks capacity may not give informed consent (see Chapter 35)

C. Decision-making capacity: defined by the President's Commission for the Study of Ethical Problems in Medicine and Biomedical and Behavioral Research as possessing a set of values and goals, being able to communicate and understand information, and having the ability to reason and deliberate about one's choices

II. PROTECTING INCOMPETENT PATIENTS FROM HARM

A. A patient with questionable mental competence is in greater peril than one who is competent so a nurse has a heightened duty of care

B. Patients who have diminished mental capacity do not lose their legal rights by virtue of the incapacity, so nurses providing care for such persons should not ignore issues of consent or intentional torts (see Chapters 35 and 43 for a detailed discussion of these issues)

C. Should a patient be admitted to a health care facility against his/her will, certain constitutional issues of due process arise and nurses must take care not to violate such rights; due process means that the patient and/or his/her family must be informed about the care proposed and have the opportunity to respond to it

D. If a patient with diminished mental capacity is at risk of harm from others in the health care facility, nurses must ensure the safety of the patient through more effective monitoring/observation and other strategies appropriate to the setting

E. If the patient is receiving mental health services, the nurse must take care to follow the law and institutional policy regarding seclusion and restraints; such methods should be used only to manage aggressive or self-destructive behavior and must be used very judiciously; should such methods be used, thorough documentation of the order and the reasons for use, monitoring, and the patient's responses must be documented

F. Using seclusion or restraints improperly, negligently, or failing to use them when needed leaves the nurse open to liability for any injury to the patient; even in the absence of injury, the nurse who secludes or restrains can be at risk of liability for false imprisonment (see Chapter 43)

III. CONFIDENTIALITY

A. There is always an ethical and legal responsibility to protect patient confidentiality and privacy; however, there are often greater protections needed when mental health issues are addressed; this is related to the notion that persons with mental health problems are viewed problematically by much of society; to avoid discrimination or poor treatment, there are stronger guidelines for the release of information about such patients

B. Some states have recommended or mandated by statute that health care institutions may not even reveal that a person is in the health care institution if that person was admitted to a mental health–related unit

C. In some cases, release of information is permitted; such cases include when the patient has given consent to release, if a court has demanded the records when abuse and neglect of children or other protected persons is suspected, or if the patient is to be involuntarily admitted for psychiatric care

D. There are also circumstances when confidentiality must be breached; they are very narrow and are meant to protect a foreseeable victim from harm intended by the mentally impaired patient; nurses who are aware of a patient's intent to injure a reasonably identifiable person are bound to make an effort to warn the potential victim using the appropriate channels of communication or to prevent the patient from accessing the potential victim

---

EXAMPLE   A graduate student was seeing a psychiatrist on campus and during one of the sessions indicated that he intended to kill another student, a woman. The psychiatrist was concerned about the matter and about his duty of confidentiality and discussed the matter with his colleagues who recommended that the campus police be notified. The campus police interrogated the student but did not find him "irrational" and so did not detain him. He killed the woman. The court, in a lawsuit against the University and the mental health professionals by the family of the woman student who was killed, found that there was a duty to warn third parties even if it meant that the usual standard of confidentiality was violated. *Tarasoff v. Regents of the University of California,* 529 P.2d 553 (Cal. 1974), *reheard en bank and affirmed,* 551 P.2d 334 (1976)

E. The requirement of confidentiality exists in order to encourage patients to be truthful with their therapists and be able to get help without fear that their mental health problems will be revealed to persons who have no need to know or where their reputation at work, school, or in the community would be impaired

IV. MAKING HEALTH CARE DECISIONS

A. Problems of health care decision-making exist when providers care for patients who lack mental competence or capacity; questions arise as to how to provide care or to withdraw certain life-prolonging care when it will not have a beneficial effect but when there is not a clear decision-maker

B. With an aging population and the known health problems that some of the old-old experience, it is expected that diminution of mental capacity sometimes associated with older age will become more of a problem; dementia in all its forms will impact the long-term care population

C. Nurses are well-advised to use the laws and methods accepted in other health care settings in terms of health care decision-making with patients who have mental health problems, diminished competence, or dementia; appointment of a surrogate or guardian by a court is one way to deal with this issue; other health care providers are comfortable working with close family members who are and have been caring for the patient in the past

D. When dealing with an impaired patient, health care decision-making is an important issue; most of the time working with families is acceptable; problems occur when individual family members disagree as to how care should be managed

E. When there is disagreement among family members, health care institutions and providers need to agree on whom they will consult; legal counsel may need to intervene; a legal guardian may need to be appointed

REFERENCES

Black HC: *Black's law dictionary,* ed 6, St Paul, MN, 1991, West Publishing Company.

Brent NJ: *Nurses and the law,* Philadelphia, 1997, WB Saunders.

Furrow BR, Johnson SH, Jost TS, et al: *Liability and quality issues in health care,* St Paul, MN, 1991, West Publishing Company.

Rosenblatt RE, Law SA, Rosenbaum S: *Law and the American health care system,* Westbury, NY, 1997, The Foundation Press.

CHAPTER 40

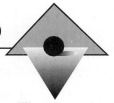

ORGAN TRANSPLANT ISSUES

Alice G. Rini

LEARNING OBJECTIVES

Upon completion of this chapter, the reader will be able to:

- Define anatomical gift and rationing
- Analyze the laws governing organ donation and transplantation
- Describe the nursing responsibilities in organ donation and transplantation

I. DEFINITIONS

A. Organ transplant: the replacement of diseased or damaged body organs, such as kidney, heart, liver, and lungs, with an organ from a human donor who died with his/her organ(s) intact and not diseased

B. Rationing: the distribution of a scarce resource based on certain decision-making processes or some societal agreement; rationing is necessary because of the scarcity of donated organs

C. Anatomical gift: a donation of all or any part(s) of the human body for the purpose of scientific investigation or transplant to a recipient

II. UNIFORM ANATOMICAL GIFT ACT OF 1987

A. Federal act enacted to alleviate the shortage of donated organs and to provide a model for states to enact their own laws for organ procurement, donation, and transplantation; since 1987, states have enacted their own laws modeled on the Uniform Act

B. Anatomical gifts of all or any part of the human body may be made by any individual over the age of 18; the gift takes place at or after death of the donor

C. The donation of an organ or body does not need to wait until after a testamentary will is probated

D. An anatomical gift that is not revoked by the donor before death is irrevocable after death and does not require the consent or concurrence of any other person after the donor's death

E. Certain close family members, legal guardians, and health care surrogates may make an anatomical gift of all or any part of a decedent's body

F. A donor of an anatomical gift may designate a recipient

G. If one donates all or any part of his/her body as an anatomical gift, he/she authorizes any reasonable medical examination to ensure acceptability of the organ for transplant or other purposes

H. Mandatory notification of all deaths to organ procurement agencies by hospitals and health care agencies became law in 1998 in order to increase the number of potentially available organs; because of this change from past practice, there has been a more than 5% increase in organ donations that may be at least partially attributed to the notification of such agencies of every death; this allows the procurement agency to determine the acceptability of the donation rather than the hospital or health care agency, which may not have adequate experience in such evaluation

III. Availability of Organs for Transplant

A. Fewer medical reasons exist for organ rejection at this time
   1. Organs donated by hepatitis-positive donors may be harvested and transplanted to hepatitis-positive recipients; the belief is that a relatively healthy organ is better than a failing organ and no disease that the recipient didn't have before is introduced
   2. However, persons who are HIV positive are not able to be organ donors
B. Research on why individuals or families consent to or refuse donation of organs was funded by the U.S. Department of Health and Human Services; the initiative that addresses the importance of potential donors to share their intent with their families is one outcome of that study
C. In 1999, approximately 62,000 persons were waiting for organ donations; however, only approximately 20,000 transplants occur each year; there are 5800 cadaver donations each year with an average of three organs per donation
D. A study by the Agency for Health Care Policy Research (AHCPR) found that few families discuss the issue of organ donation and fewer yet know whether or not other family members carried donor cards
   1. Although less than half of all families consent to donation of the organs of a decedent, 95% percent indicated that the intent of the dying family member who might be a potential donor would influence their decision
   2. Efforts to involve civic, business, and religious organizations to encourage organ donation by their members is effective and ongoing
   3. Sensitive and professional approaches by health care personnel from organ procurement agencies is also effective in obtaining donations
E. The Health Care Financing Administration (HCFA) holds organ procurement organizations (OPO) responsible for meeting a certain standard for the number of organs procured; such organizations are evaluated against their peer organizations on performance; critics of this type of incentive are concerned that the emphasis on numbers might precipitate the acceptance of organs of lesser quality or from patients or families who may be reluctant but coerced by assertive agency personnel; however, there is no evidence of such practices at this time
F. No health care is ever changed in terms of quality or quantity based on consent or refusal to donate organs

IV. Distribution of Donated Organs to Recipients

A. A recent proposal indicated that organs should be allocated based on patient need and what it refers to as sound medical judgment, rather than having the organs kept in the geographical area where they were procured; the premise is that patients should not have to be in a certain area of the country with a high transplant rate in order to have a good chance of getting an organ; however, some agencies believe that some people will be less likely to donate if they think the organs will not help local persons, especially hard-to-obtain organs such as hearts and livers
B. Criteria for organ allocation include objective and measurable medical criteria for placement on a transplant waiting list, standardized criteria for determining medical status, and the requirement that persons whose needs are most urgent have priority in organ receipt
C. Organs may not be sold or purchased; violation of this regulation is a felony

V. Public Access to Data About Transplant Activity

A. The Organ Procurement and Transplant Network (OPTN), a non-profit private sector network, operates by a contract with the Department of Health and Human Services (DHHS); the Omnibus Budget Reconciliation Act of 1986 requires that all hospitals performing transplants and organ procurement organizations follow the rules and regulations of the OPTN in order to receive Medicare and Medicaid reimbursement; this is a powerful inducement by the federal government because of its ability to withhold funds from health care institutions that have become dependent on such funds for patient care

B. Regulations provide for patients, physicians, and the public to have timely, accurate, and understandable information about the performance of local transplant programs so that all are able to measure quality and make decisions about transplants, should the need arise

C. OPTN Board of Directors includes both health care professionals and members of the public, including persons from nonmedical scholarly fields such as behavioral scientists, ethicists, the clergy, and policy analysts; Board composition also includes transplant recipients, those waiting for transplants, and family members of recipients; no more than 50% of OPTN Boards may be physicians

D. Secretary of DHHS may determine when transplant data and other information will serve the public interest and may release such information; this leaves the power to determine what information, if any, to disclose to citizens to the discretion of the Secretary

E. Public information is expected to include transplant outcome data within 6 months of the period to which the data apply; data include characteristics of organ transplant programs, waiting times for organs, non-acceptance of organs, and other information that would help persons make transplant decisions

VI. NURSING RESPONSIBILITIES

A. Nurses should be familiar with the rules and regulations about organ transplants as described previously and with notification of impending deaths and actual deaths required and to whom notification is made

B. Organ procurement agencies are generally available 24 hours a day so there is rarely any reason for notification of the appropriate agency not to be timely and accurately directed

C. Nurses must be aware of how and by whom patients and families are approached regarding organ donation; this is generally done by nurses and other professionals from the local organ procurement agency

D. Nurses should be familiar with organ donation processes so that they can answer questions that might be asked by patients and family members; they should also remain objective about organ donation and avoid either coercion or disapproval

REFERENCES

Fox CE: *Psychiatric, psychosocial, and ethical issues in organ transplantation,* presentation at Cleveland Clinic Foundation Fifth Biennial Conference, Cleveland, OH, October, 1998.

Furrow BR, Johnson SH, Jost TS, et al: *Bioethics: health care law and ethics,* St Paul, MN, 1991, West Publishing Company.

Improving fairness and effectiveness in allocating organs for transplantation, Rockville, MD, July, 1998, Office of Communications, HRSA.

National organ and tissue donation initiative, HHS fact sheet, Rockville, MD, April, 1999 (available www.organdonor.gov; www.hhs.gov).

CHAPTER 41

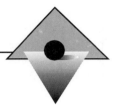

CODE FOR NURSES WITH INTERPRETIVE STATEMENTS (ANA)

Alice G. Rini

LEARNING OBJECTIVES

Upon completion of this chapter, the reader will be able to:

- Discuss the value of a code of ethics for nurses
- Evaluate how a code of ethics assists nurses in clinical decision-making
- Use the American Nurses Association (ANA) Code of Ethics in practice

I. CODE OF ETHICS FOR NURSES (AMERICAN NURSES ASSOCIATION, 1985)

   A. Code statements are based on beliefs about individuals, nursing, health, and society
      1. Statements deal with nursing behaviors and attitudes toward patients
      2. Nurses are expected to be responsible and accountable for their actions
      3. Similar concerns are found in the Standards for Gerontological Nursing Practice (ANA, 1995); the Standards call for the nurse to address mutual goals for the therapeutic, preventive, restorative, and rehabilitative needs of the older person
   B. Interpretive statements with the Code expand on it and provide examples and guidance so nurses will be assisted in adherence to the Code
   C. The Code does not carry the force of law through any constitution or statute but is evidence of practice standards and expectations of nursing actions and is therefore evidence of a standard of practice and can be introduced as such in a court of law; the Standards of Gerontological Nursing Practice (ANA, 1995) operate in a similar manner
      1. The Standards and Code are developed and accepted by professional nursing organizations and are generally regarded as evidence that the professional group expects adherence to them
      2. The Code and Standards are applicable to a variety of health care settings in which nurses care for gerontological patients
      3. Even though the Code and Standards are not law, it is worth noting that many of their statements have been adopted into statutes, regulations, and other legal documents; examples include laws regarding privacy, boards of nursing that describe competent practice, and judicial opinions that make up common law

II. INTERPRETING THE CODE OF ETHICS

    A. Statements in the Code are related to the nurse's behavior toward patients

    B. Responsibility for self is demanded

    C. In addition to the courts, the Code (as well as the Standards) can be used by other bodies and agencies to evaluate nursing practice

III. PROFESSIONAL CODES OF ETHICS

    A. The Code of Ethics for Nurses is unique to nursing and differs from such Codes adopted by medicine, law, and other professions

    B. Although the Code was adopted in 1985, it did not always get the attention it deserved; newer theories of nursing give more recognition and credibility to ethical theory, practice, and the need for such a Code

    C. Some nursing theorists incorporate ethics into their nursing theories; these theories include the concept of relating to patients as persons and moral beings rather than as objects

IV. MANAGING ETHICAL DILEMMAS

    A. Often Codes of Ethics are only addressed when there is an ethical problem

    B. Dilemmas actually often occur when the needs and obligations of some pledge, duty, or agreement conflict with similar needs of others or with one's own beliefs

    C. Health care institutions use ethics committees, members of the clergy, and other resources to assist in the management of ethical dilemmas

    D. It is important for nurses to understand and accept that there are often no right or wrong answers to ethical issues

REFERENCES

American Nurses Association: *Code of ethics for nurses,* Kansas City, MO, 1985, The Association.

American Nurses Association: *Standards for gerontological nursing practice,* Kansas City, MO, 1995, The Association.

Rini AG: Code of ethics for nurses with interpretive statements, In Luggen AS, Travis SS, Meiner S: *NGNA core curriculum for gerontological advanced practice nurses,* Thousand Oaks, CA, 1998, Sage.

Watson J: *Nursing: human science and human care—a theory of nursing,* Publication No. 15-2236, New York, 1988, National League for Nursing.

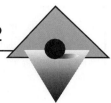

CHAPTER 42

PROFESSIONAL ACCOUNTABILITY AND COMPETENCY

Alice G. Rini

LEARNING OBJECTIVES

Upon completion of this chapter, the reader will be able to:

- Discuss nursing accountability in practice
- Describe appropriate delegation practices
- Explain the purposes and components of patient care documentation
- Analyze the relationship between nursing competence and accountability

I. DEFINITIONS

A. Accountability: state of being responsible or answerable to another or to some authority; nurses are accountable to their patients, employers, other professionals with whom they practice, and to the profession and the public

B. Competence: a state of possessing the requisite knowledge, ability, skill, and intent to perform certain activities; nurses who are competent to practice will have the appropriate education, experience, specific knowledge of the area of practice and kinds of patients, and a purposeful approach to performance of their professional activities

II. NURSING ACCOUNTABILITY FOR PATIENT CARE, DOCUMENTATION, DELEGATION, AND LEVEL OF KNOWLEDGE

A. Nurses are accountable for safe and appropriate patient care, documentation of care provided, appropriate and timely communication with other professional practitioners, maintaining an adequate level and currency of knowledge and skill to practice in the setting

B. Safe and appropriate patient care includes
   1. Making appropriate and timely assessments
   2. Providing for care based on the assessments and the plan of care developed by the professional nurse
   3. Ensuring that the care planned is carried out in a timely manner
   4. Delegating those aspects of care that can be delegated by law or by institutional policy; such delegation is predicated on the nurse's direct knowledge of the ability of the delegatee to perform the task delegated and the following criteria
      a. Delegation is understood to be the transfer of responsibility for performing a selected

task from a licensed nurse authorized to perform the task to another person who does not have the authority to perform the task absent the delegation

b. The task must be something that can competently be performed by the person to whom it is delegated and the nurse must be assured of that competence

c. No independent judgment should be needed to perform the task

d. The nurse must have completed an assessment of the patient for whom the task will be performed

e. The nurse retains accountability for the competent completion of the task

f. Whether or not a task can be delegated depends on the patient's condition, the competency of the person to whom the task is delegated, and the ability of the nurse to adequately supervise the person (see case study below)

5. Evaluating care in terms of a clinical pathway, projected outcomes, or other appropriate standard

C. Documentation of care provided is the timely recording, written legibly, of pertinent information about the patient in the official patient record using factual information and using only approved abbreviations

1. *Official patient record* is that record developed and maintained by a health care agency that provides legal proof of the nature and quality of care received by a patient during his/her relationship with that agency

2. Purposes of documentation

a. Accurately reflects care given

b. Demonstrates treatment results

c. Provides for coordination of care

d. Communicates clinical findings to all interdisciplinary team members

e. Provides a legal record of practice and decision-making with the patient

f. Furnishes data for a variety of uses

g. Is used in quality management reviews

h. Provides a record of services provided as a means of justifying reimbursement from insurers or private payers

---

CASE STUDY

A home health nurse was supervising the care of an elderly woman who had experienced several small strokes. She had some weakness of the lower extremities and occasional bladder incontinence with possible retention. The nurse included in the care plan, which was delegated to the various home health aides assigned to the patient by the home health agency, measurement of intake and output and careful observation of urinary continence and frequency and amount of voiding. The nurse generally visited every 2 weeks unless there was a problem that justified an earlier visit for which Medicare would pay. The home health aide recorded fluid intake and output on the agency-supplied forms. Twice the patient called the nurse and complained about lower abdominal discomfort. The nurse checked with the home health aide concerning the balance of intake and output and determined that it was normal. One evening, about 1 week after the nurse's home visit, the patient called 911 and was taken to the local emergency department where she was catheterized for 2200 ml of cloudy, yellow urine. Although it is unlikely that there would be a lawsuit for this, in terms of appropriate delegation, this nurse was negligent.

First, the nurse may have delegated assessments about the urinary continence that required more judgment about retention and incontinence than the home health aides were able to do. Second, the nurse knew that there were several home health aides caring for the patient but could not be assured that they all had the training and experience to manage the tasks. Third, the nurse knew that there were bladder problems but did not follow up on the calls from the patient about discomfort but only checked on intake and output. Many of the rules of delegation that have been promulgated by boards of nursing for the edification of licensed nurses in their states were violated in this situation.

3. Every entry in the patient record must have a time and date
   a. Supports that observations and assessments were done in a timely manner
   b. Supports that actions were taken in response to patient needs within an appropriate time frame
   c. Exact times, not ranges of time, should be used when documenting patient care
4. What should be documented
   a. Any action by a care provider taken in response to a patient problem or because of institutional routine or requirement
   b. Patient's response to any activity or treatment whether subjectively noted or objectively observed
   c. Actions taken to ensure patient comfort or safety
   d. Any unusual incident whether subjectively described by the patient or objectively observed
   e. Every observation about the patient by a care provider
   f. All treatments and procedures noted after they have been done
   g. Any information provided to the patient's primary care provider
   h. Ongoing assessments, including deviations from prior assessments
   i. Health teaching completed and the patient's response; cost of care is a significant issue and the act of teaching must be shown to have a beneficial outcome (e.g., learning) so as to justify its continuance
   j. Procedures done by others, diagnostic tests, and patient's response
   k. Statements by the patient in the patient's own words with quotation marks to ensure clarity
   l. Care provider's signature and credentials at the end of the note
5. Other documentation issues
   a. Never add documentation for another person or for something you do not know or have not seen personally
   b. Use every line in the record
   c. Always follow the standards of the institution, state of practice, accrediting bodies, and professional organizations
   d. Other providers need current information about what has gone before
   e. Appropriate documentation is an important expectation of licensing and accrediting bodies
   f. In case of a lawsuit, reviewers and courts look for regular, appropriate, legible, and timely assessments as well as timely and appropriate actions on them
   g. Regular, well-organized documentation is generally an indication of high quality care and is important to care continuity
   h. If there is irregular, inconsistent, or inadequate documentation, there is often an assumption of poor quality care by accreditors and courts
   i. Language used should be that which everyone generally understands, nonjudgmental in nature, and free of colloquialisms
   j. If some data were omitted, add the information as a new entry as soon as the omission is noticed; do not backdate or add to a previously written entry
   k. Never erase; cross out an error with one line so that it is not obliterated, note that the entry was an "error," and initial it (see case study opposite)
6. Electronic patient records
   a. In use in many health care systems
   b. Extent of use varies across the country and among health care settings
   c. Protection of confidentiality of records may be more difficult because health care providers are not accustomed to this kind of record-keeping; nurses must protect their record entry password and avoid permitting temporary use of it by others
   d. Nurses must not use the electronic system in an unauthorized manner but should always follow the guidelines the institution has developed for its use

CASE STUDY

A nurse, busily managing 15 long-term care patients with three nursing assistants, has carefully made assessments, administered medications, and provided appropriate treatments during her time on duty. She keeps the patient information with her, noted on a piece of paper she carries in her pocket. At the end of the shift, she speaks with the nursing assistants and obtains updated information from them about the patients/residents. She also documents her care in summary form on the patient's records, including noting vital signs on a flow sheet. About an hour after her shift ends, one of her patients experiences an ischemic attack. At the time of the attack, 4:30 PM, the patient's blood pressure is 200/110. The only blood pressure recordings by the day shift nurse are at 8:00 AM and noon, none higher than 140/90. The patient is a known hypertensive who has recently been experiencing instability in his blood pressure, and it was ordered to be measured every 2 hours. The patient is admitted to the hospital where he is diagnosed with a stroke. He does not recover. His family sues the long-term care facility and the nurse who cared for him. If the patient's chart is admitted to evidence, and it most likely will be, it is possible that the nurse will be held negligent. Even if the nurse claims she did blood pressure measurements on time, she did not record the information. Courts generally hold that if data are not documented, it is as if they were not done, and the nurse is deemed negligent.

    e. Nurses must know how to use and understand the power of electronic systems (e.g., nurses should be aware that built-in reminders and "expert commentary" are there to prevent errors and omissions and should not be ignored or overridden)

  7. Maintaining an adequate level and currency of knowledge and skill to practice in the setting

    a. Nurses should have appropriate continuing education; in some states such education is mandatory in terms of numbers of credits or hours but not content; nurses are well-advised to use continuing education opportunities to improve and update knowledge in their areas of practice

    b. Failure to maintain adequate and current knowledge may be grounds for malpractice liability if the lack of knowledge leads to inadequate or unsafe patient care

    c. Nurses are held to standards that may be promulgated by state licensing agencies, professional or specialty nursing organizations, institutional accrediting bodies, and the institutions themselves; such standards may be presented as the accepted level of practice by an expert witness in any legal action against a nurse or the institution for which the nurse works

III. ACCOUNTABILITY FOR NURSING ACTIONS

  A. Nurses can be held liable for their own actions even when following a physician's order

  B. Level of conduct for which a nurse is held accountable is referred to as the "standard of care"

  C. Standard of care is flexible and constantly changing, based on growing knowledge and expanding technology

  D. Nurses are held accountable for the standard of care in existence at the time they are providing care to a patient

  E. A majority of states recognize a national minimum standard of care and no longer consider local standards to control practice; what this means is that nurses working in small, rural settings are expected to have the same knowledge and act no differently than those in urban medical centers; it is understood, however, that available technology and other resources may not be equal in all settings

  F. Standard of care is that which a reasonably prudent nurse would do in the same or similar circumstances; such a standard is measured by what would be the accepted practice by a similarly educated and experienced nurse of average intelligence, judgment, foresight, and skill; it is important to note, however, that a nurse or an institution may not escape liability for improper practice if a lesser educated nurse is hired and continues to work in a specialty area for which that nurse is not adequately prepared (see H following)

G. The American Nurses Association has developed Standards of Care for nurses generally; nurses in specialty practice are responsible for developing and publishing guidelines specific to that practice; most have done so, including gerontological nurses

H. A nurse working in a specialty area is held to the standard of care in the specialty even if it is not his/her usual workplace

I. An individual institution may also develop standards of care to which it expects its employees to adhere; the standards are described in the institution's policies and procedures; an institution's standards may be higher than those of a professional organization, and, if they are, the nurse in the institution will be held to the higher standard; individual institutional standards *may not be lower* than those of the professional organization

IV. COMPETENCE OF PRACTICING NURSES

A. Requisite knowledge, ability, skill, and intent to perform certain activities are those factors that describe competence

B. Appropriate education
   1. There are many different routes to nursing practice; it is important to define the level of education required for gerontological nursing practice in all its functional parameters
   2. Required education must be based on bonafide job expectations so that such standards do not violate employment laws by being so high as to discriminate against certain federally protected groups; this is true even though one may think that quality of care may be compromised with lesser educated persons
   3. It is expected that differing levels of education may be required for different levels of job responsibility, the need to supervise others, or by the demands of job function

C. Experience
   1. Experience contributes to competence by virtue of the opportunities the nurse has had to make critical clinical decisions, take action on them, and see the consequences of the decisions and actions
   2. Care must be taken not to equate only experience with competence; merely having done something many times does not contribute to a nurse's broad-based competence; experience with a variety of patients and clinical situations in which the nurse's decisions and actions were appropriate and had positive outcomes is a much more meaningful criterion of experience

D. Specific knowledge of the area of practice and kinds of clients
   1. Gerontological nursing takes place in a variety of settings, including the home of the patient, long-term care facilities, hospitals, hospices, and others; each requires a different kind of practice with which a nurse must be familiar in order to be effective
   2. Different settings have differing levels of supervision, resources, and colleague support; the nurse must be able to manage his/her practice accordingly
   3. Gerontological patients must be understood to have great variety in terms of response to the aging process, level of health, ability to cope, and other life activities; they are not monolithic and must be approached with great respect for individuality; making decisions based on stereotypic beliefs is inappropriate for aged persons as well as any other definable group

E. Purposeful approach to performance of professional activities
   1. This means that nurses approach their patient care with consciousness and a problem-solving approach rather than an attitude of routine
   2. A purposeful approach fosters critical thinking about patient assessment and a depth of consideration about the interaction of all the patient's issues and problems; such an approach encourages the cross-referencing of ideas and information (much as a detective might do) to

integrate the sensory inputs from the patient and the environment with the intuitive skills the nurse has developed to best make effective clinical decisions about patient care

REFERENCES

American Nurses Association: *Standards of gerontological nursing practice,* Washington, DC, 1995, The Association.

Black HC: *Black's law dictionary,* ed 6, St Paul, MN, 1991, West Publishing Company.

Brent NJ: *Nurses and the law,* Philadelphia, 1997, WB Saunders.

Meiner SE: *Nursing documentation: legal focus across practice settings,* Thousand Oaks, CA, 1999, SAGE.

CHAPTER 43

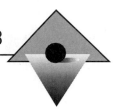

NEGLIGENCE AND MALPRACTICE

Alice G. Rini

LEARNING OBJECTIVES

Upon completion of this chapter, the reader will be able to:

- Discuss standards of care issues as applied to negligent actions
- Differentiate nursing negligence from medical malpractice
- Define specific terminology associated with a legal "tort"
- List the four elements of negligence

I. DEFINITIONS

A. Negligence: the failure to use such care and judgment as a reasonably prudent and careful nurse would use in the same or similar circumstances; doing something that a nurse of reasonable prudence would not do or not doing something that the nurse of reasonable prudence would do; conduct that falls below an established standard (see the *Standards of Gerontological Nursing Practice* and the *ANA Code of Ethics for Nurses,* which are accepted standards for practice)

B. Malpractice: professional misconduct or unreasonable lack of skill; usually applied to members of learned professions who fail to exercise that degree of skill, knowledge, and judgment commonly applied in the professional community; illegal or immoral conduct in the practice of one's profession

C. Tort: derived from the Latin *torquere,* meaning a civil wrong; an action, not in contract, resulting in an injury or damage for which the law provides a remedy in the form of money damages; goal of the law of torts is to protect persons from unreasonable and foreseeable risk of harm from others by enforcing duties that individuals have to each other

D. *Res ipsa loquitur:* a Latin term meaning "the thing speaks for itself;" it provides for an inference that a defendant is negligent because there is proof that the instrumentality causing the injury or the situation in which the injury occurred was in the defendant's exclusive control and that there was proof that the injury could not have occurred in the absence of negligence (Black, 1991)

E. *Respondeat superior:* a Latin term meaning "let the master answer;" a situation in which a supervisor may be responsible for the acts of a subordinate or a principal for the acts of an agent; if the care provided by the subordinate or agent is inadequate, and the supervisor or principal owes a duty of care, it will raise the concept of respondeat superior (Black, 1991)

II. THE LAW OF NEGLIGENCE

A. Elements of negligence
 1. Duty: legal or moral obligation; obligation to perform a certain service; something that one

person owes to another, typically one who has a responsibility to another; duty is an obligation that is recognizable in law

2. Breach: a failure to carry out the legal or moral duty; violation of an established standard required by a duty
3. Causation: fact of being the cause of something happening; act by which a certain effect is produced; connects the breach of duty with the injury that follows
4. Injury: any wrong or damage done to another, including physical, mental, interference with rights or property, damage to reputation, or invasion of a legally protected interest

B. Negligent conduct
  1. Acts of omission or commission
     a. Omission: failing to do something when a duty requires that the act be done; examples are failure to measure vital signs as needed based on patient assessment, neglecting to monitor patient's status, failure to document patient assessments and nursing actions
     b. Commission: doing something in a negligent manner or doing something that a reasonably prudent nurse would not do; examples are giving a medication incorrectly, coercing a patient to act in a certain manner by using misleading information, delegating a task to a nursing assistant without first determining the assistant's competence
  2. Negligence is not intentional
     a. Nurse does not intend to cause the injury or damage that results from the negligent action; injury results from carelessness or inadvertent action or inaction
     b. Law of negligence deals with foreseeability; nurse must know when there is a risk of injury or damage and anticipate such a result might occur and act so as to prevent it; negligence is the failure to be aware of impending or inherent danger, thereby being unable to control it
     c. Standard of what should be the care may be established by nurse expert witnesses should the issue of negligence go to a court of law
  3. Standards are widely interpreted
     a. Accepted standards are more likely to be national, that is, accepted across a wide geographic area and by national professional groups
     b. The local standard, that which permits different standards of care in the varying localities, is rarely used in court decisions
     c. The local standard has fallen out of favor because of better communication among practice settings, information exchange via technology, the wider availability of technology, and the national standards of education that practitioners bring to all practice settings; all these factors permit the same standard of care to be expected no matter what the practice setting

C. Proving negligence
  1. The four elements of negligence (A, 1 to 4 above) must all be proven by a plaintiff in order to establish negligence; there are also other conditions that must be met by a plaintiff
     a. A plaintiff/patient who wishes to pursue a negligence action against a health care provider must do so within a statutorily mandated period of time called the *statute of limitations;* such laws are in place in order to promote the timely filing of lawsuits so that evidence does not become stale and that witnesses are still available; statutes of limitations on medical negligence are state-level law and usually run 1 or 2 years from the date of the injury or from the date the injured plaintiff knew *or should have known* of the injury; such laws require patients to maintain some awareness of their health and to take timely action if they believe a health care provider has caused damage by negligent conduct
     b. If a health care provider, such as a nurse, becomes aware that there has been some occurrence that may precipitate a lawsuit, it is appropriate to generate an incident report (see Chapter 44)

2. Duty
   a. Duty is said to arise when one party undertakes to provide care to another; in a health care setting, duty generally arises when a patient is admitted to the institution or accepted as a patient by a health care agency
   b. Generally, the law does not recognize the existence of a duty of one party to another commonly called a *duty to rescue;* this is *not* true if the injured party is a dependent, such as a spouse, parent, or child, if the first party caused the injury or put the second party in danger of the injury, if the first party owns, operates, or controls the premises where the injury occurred or the danger exists, or if there is some contractual agreement between the parties for providing care
   c. Duty is established for nurses at definable times, such as (1) when a patient assignment is accepted; (2) if, when a nurse is assigned to a patient unit, even if not assigned to care for a particular patient, the nurse notes a potential or actual problem with any patient; (3) a nurse notes a potentially dangerous situation anywhere in the employment situation; (4) a nurse observes a visitor with a problem
   d. Scope of duty must also be established; such duty is generally described as adhering to an established standard of care
   e. Standard of care may be established in court by an expert witness; expert witnesses are recognized by courts if they are members of the profession in question, have adequate experience in the clinical setting for which the standard is to be determined, and possess the appropriate credentials to provide credibility with the finder of fact, the jury; generally, a nurse cannot be an expert witness with regard to medical practice, nor a physician for nursing practice, although there are some exceptions in case law
   f. A nurse defending against negligence does best if it can be proven that there was no duty; it may be more difficult to show that the nurse's actions were not the proximate cause of an injury rather than proving the nurse was not part of the situation at all
   g. In a civil lawsuit, it is the plaintiff who must prove his/her case, but a defendant health care provider must defend his/her own actions
3. Breach of duty
   a. After a duty has been established, it must be shown that a breach of that duty has occurred by the failure to adhere to a standard of care either by acts of omission or commission or by an act that was supposed to be done but was done incorrectly
   b. A breach can also occur when a nurse delegates tasks improperly, fails to document assessments and actions, or provides substandard patient care
   c. The existence of a breach of duty can be established by an expert witness
4. Causation
   a. The connection between the breach of duty and the injury that permits a finding of negligence
   b. Proving causation means that it must be shown that *but for* the actions or inaction of the defendant, the injury would not have occurred
   c. The extent of the injury may be affected by intervening factors that influence what part or how much of the injury is the proximate cause of the breach of duty; therefore proving causation is a very important part of dealing with negligence; if any or all of an injury is the result of the breach of duty or the substandard care, what can be proved determines the damage award to the plaintiff
5. Injury
   a. A plaintiff who claims against a health care provider must prove the presence of an injury; such injuries may be physical, mental/emotional, interference with rights or property, damage to reputation, or invasion of a legally protected interest
   b. In many cases, courts have not permitted negligence actions based on mental/emotional injuries alone, that is in the absence of an accompanying physical injury; mental/emotional injury that is secondary to a physical injury is usually actionable

c. Courts and juries will award money damages to winning plaintiffs based on a variety of factors; such factors include extent of the injury, how much of the person's life activities will be affected in the future because of the injury, how much the medical expenses have been and will continue to be, how much pain and suffering have occurred since the injury and how much will be endured in the future

d. If a plaintiff/patient contributed in any way to his/her injury (a condition called *comparative fault*), his/her damages may be reduced by the amount of fault that can be attributed to the actions of the plaintiff; courts treat comparative fault in different ways—in some courts, the plaintiff must contribute to his/her own injury at least 50% of the attributable fault or his/her damages are not reduced; in other courts, any contribution by a plaintiff will reduce his damages by the percentage of plaintiff's own fault as determined by a jury

III. INTENTIONAL AND QUASI-INTENTIONAL TORTS

A. These civil torts are different from the negligence torts discussed previously; in negligence there is no purposeful action by the nurse to cause the harm; in intentional torts, there is purposeful action and intent to do an act or cause the effect of the act; for a tort to be intentional, however, it is not necessary for intent to be hostile or arise from a desire to harm another; there must be an understanding that the harmful outcome is highly likely or that the act was done with reckless disregard for the interests of others; the difference between intentional and quasi-intentional torts addresses the level of intentionality; sometimes quasi-intentional torts do not have the specificity of purpose that intentional torts have

B. Intentional torts include

1. Assault: putting another in apprehension of harmful or offensive touching; actual touching is not necessary nor an element of assault; usually words alone cannot be considered assault; there must be a present ability to do the threatened act; person must be aware of the assault; protects a person's interest in freedom from fear of unwanted contact

---

EXAMPLE A long-term care resident continually attempts to get out of her bed or her chair and has occasionally fallen; frustrated, the nurse brings a vest restraint into the room, shoves it into the resident's face and says, "if you try to get out again, you will find yourself tied in THIS." The nurse is guilty of assault.

---

2. Battery: unwanted and offensive touching of another person or things attached to him/her such as clothing or handbag; actual contact must occur for battery, but physical harm is not an essential element; if physical harm occurs, the person doing the touching is liable for the injury; it is important to understand that the person touched need not be aware of it, so that an unconscious patient could have a cause of action in battery; the results of the battery do not necessarily need to be intended or foreseen, the intent is to do the *act;* although a patient may consent to a touching, if it turns out to be unreasonably offensive, the nurse may still be liable for battery; there is a cause of action in battery if a medical or surgical procedure is done without informed consent

---

EXAMPLE A patient is observed to have a distended bladder because of urinary retention and the nurse tells him a catheterization is necessary; when the nurse arrives with the catheter equipment, the patient refuses the procedure; the nurse determines that the procedure is absolutely necessary, calls two staff members to restrain the patient, and inserts the catheter over the loud objections of the patient, thereby draining 1200 ml of urine; the nurse and the assisting staff members may be liable for battery

---

3. False imprisonment: an intentional restriction of a person's freedom of movement against the will of that person; inability or impossibility of escape is a necessary element of false imprisonment; present or future verbal threats or moral pressure are not actionable

---

EXAMPLE   A nurse uses a restraint to prevent an elderly woman resident from sliding out of her geriatric chair because of an inability to maintain posture; the restraint only holds her in the chair but doesn't restrict movement or mobility with the chair around the unit; as long as the restraint was properly ordered and the reasons for it documented with justification of the ongoing need and the woman's response to it, the nurse is not liable for false imprisonment; however, if the resident objects to the restraint, and, as a result and for her safety, the nurse confines her to bed, the nurse may be liable for false imprisonment

---

EXAMPLE   A patient seeks to sign himself out of the hospital against medical advice; although the nurse agrees to let him go, she actually unreasonably detains him in hopes that the family members she called will arrive and convince him to stay; if the patient becomes aware of it and objects and, if he is not permitted to leave, the nurse may be liable for false imprisonment

---

4. Intentional infliction of emotional distress: the extreme and outrageous conduct of a person that causes severe emotional distress in another; the conduct must be beyond the bounds of common decency and be fairly certain to result in emotional distress in the other person; if the person causing the distress actually knows of a specific sensitivity or weakness of the other, the conduct complained of may not necessarily have to be at the extreme level as if the intended victim was a stranger
5. Conversion of property: intentional interference with the property of another; elements include that the plaintiff must have control of the property (e.g., it is not lost or missing), and the defendant intended to remove it from the plaintiff's control

---

EXAMPLE   A patient continually loses his dentures, drops them from his mouth causing breakage, unintentionally bites caregivers, and generally has trouble with them; the institution has twice paid to repair them after being dropped; frustrated, the nurse secretly takes the dentures away while the patient is sleeping; when he asks for them, staff tells him they do not know where they are; the patient continues to complain about needing them and asking staff to find them for him; the nurse may be liable for conversion of property

---

C. Quasi-intentional torts include
   1. Defamation: this quasi-intentional tort occurs when a person interferes with the good name and reputation of another; there must be "publication" of the comments about the person, that is they must be made public either in writing (libel) or spoken (slander); the comments must be so injurious as to harm the reputation or good name of the plaintiff and that those who hear of the comments tend to have a lower opinion of the plaintiff or resist associating with him; liability for defamation can be against the person who initially made the defamatory communication and those who repeat it; public figures who voluntarily enter public life may generally not sue in defamation because the First Amendment to the Constitution permits freedom of political speech and public figures have access to the media to refute such statements; private persons have greater protection and may take action against defamatory language whether it is intentionally or negligently done

EXAMPLE   A patient who is a chef in a prominent local restaurant is admitted to the hospital for pneumonia; he is a very tall, extremely thin person; in the cafeteria and at a nursing committee meeting, his primary nurse comments about his admission and states that he looks as if he has AIDS, not merely pneumonia, and a discussion ensues; later some of the nurses who attended the meeting pass on this information within earshot of patrons and restaurant employees while dining at another neighborhood restaurant; if the chef's reputation is damaged or if his business is negatively affected, the primary nurse and all the nurses who repeated the information may be liable for defamation; damages are generally based on the person's losses, and business losses can be considerable

EXAMPLE   Nurse A is asked about a potential hire, Nurse B, by a colleague from human resources; the potential hire happens to be a woman who was dating Nurse A's boyfriend before A met him; Nurse B continues to call him and the calls have become harassing; Nurse A suggests that hiring B would be a mistake because she is dishonest and incompetent; Nurse A may be liable for defamation because she maligned the professional reputation of Nurse B and may have cost her a job

    2. Breach of confidentiality: provides for the protection of a person's private information; in health care settings, the requirement of confidentiality protects patient/client/resident information and theoretically promotes the sharing of intimate and personal facts with health care providers without fear of violating the confidentiality of that information
    3. Invasion of privacy: distinguished from breach of confidentiality, invasion of privacy occurs when a person's right to be free from intrusion on personal space and private affairs is impaired; this tort includes
        a. The use of a person's likeness or name without permission for commercial advantage
        b. Prying into personal affairs or seclusion in an unreasonable or objectionable way; no interference with privacy may be claimed if one is in a public place
        c. Publicly disclosing private facts that the public has no legitimate interest in knowing
        d. Placing a person in a false light, that is attributing to that person characteristics that are not true or are misleading

EXAMPLE   During a health fair at a local hospital, attendees are photographed as they move through the health information booths; a man from the community is photographed while speaking to a representative of the erectile dysfunction clinic and the photograph is published in the local community newspaper along with several other photographs of fair visitors; later the man claims that his privacy was violated and that the picture placed him in a false light (e.g., his friends teased him about having sexual problems); the hospital is likely not to be found liable for either intrusion into private affairs or placing in a false light because the fair was a public place; however, considering the sensitivity of the issues for most people, it was probably poor judgment to publish that particular photograph and it is possible that a critical jury might award some damages to the man

IV. Defenses to Torts

    A. If nurses are sued in civil court for intentional tortious action, they may have some defenses other than to claim the act was not done; such defenses do not claim non-action but assert that, although the action was taken, there was a good reason for it; these are affirmative defenses, which claim to a court that, although an act that caused some injury to an individual's interest was actually done, there was justification for it

B. Defenses include
   1. Privilege: the nurse or other defendant has a right to do the complained-of act or, because of the particular circumstances of the nurse-patient relationship, certain conduct is justified

EXAMPLE Nurse shares confidential information with other health care providers who need to know the information, even though the patient asked that the information not be shared; the nurse explained that such facts could not be held from other providers

   2. Self-defense: a nurse may use as much force as is reasonably necessary to defend himself/herself from attack; there must be no time to get other lawful help such as a security guard or police officer; there is no duty to retreat from the attack unless it is safe for the nurse to do so

EXAMPLE Nurse is attacked by patient trying to get access to drugs being distributed to other patients; nurse defends himself by pinning the patient against the wall with the medicine cart

   3. Defense of others: such a defense must be reasonably necessary in the situation and other help is not available; particularly important if there is some legal or social duty to the other person

EXAMPLE Home health nurse uses a baseball bat to chase out of the house and then hit a family member who was attacking the patient and the nurse with a knife; the nurse then locks the door and calls police

   4. Consent: a willingly given consent from a patient where there is no confusion as to what is being consented to may be used as a defense by a nurse to an action in intentional or quasi-intentional tort

EXAMPLE Home health nurse locks elderly man in his room after he asks for her to protect him from an intruder while she attempts to chase an attacking family member out of the house

   5. Necessity: a lawful need to interfere with the person or property of another

EXAMPLE An elderly man with dementia shows the home health nurse several loaded guns that he keeps in his bedside table at home; it is clear that he is not competent to handle them; the nurse retrieves them and locks them up until responsible family members can be notified

REFERENCES

Black HC: *Black's law dictionary,* ed 6, St Paul, MN, 1991, West Publishing Company.
Brent NJ: *Nurses and the law,* Philadelphia, 1997, WB Saunders.
Rini AG: Confidentiality; Restraint use. In Luggen AS, Travis SS, Meiner S: *NGNA core curriculum for gerontological advanced practice nurses,* Thousand Oaks, CA, 1998, Sage.
Rosenblatt RE, Law SA, Rosenbaum S: *Law and the American health care system,* Westbury, NY, 1997, The Foundation Press.

CHAPTER 44

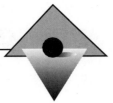

RISK MANAGEMENT

Alice G. Rini

LEARNING OBJECTIVES

Upon completion of this chapter, the reader will be able to:

- Define the term *risk management*
- Discuss the handling of variance, occurrence, or incident reports
- Identify elements of a quality improvement program

I. DEFINITIONS

A. Risk management: the process by which a business or other entity reduces its exposure to financial loss; includes the development of a self-insurance program or procuring commercial insurance to protect against losses that are a foreseeable risk of doing the business; management of risk also includes the evaluation of the risk of loss by identifying potential risks, analyzing the chances of the potential risk becoming actual, and acting to reduce the occurrence of risk or loss; in health care institutions and agencies risk of financial loss exists in

1. Inadequate patient care
2. Visitor accidents
3. Systems breakdown and equipment failure or loss
4. Employee injuries and personnel problems
5. Corporate liability for the malpractice actions of employees and others
6. Issues related to any function undertaken by the organization

B. Unplanned or unexpected loss: incidents that are known to occur but are not predictable in terms of time or scope; exposure to new risks has emerged with the advent of new technology and could exceed the ability of staff to appreciate the extent of the potential problems because of the lack of extensive knowledge about the functioning and inherent dangers in using the technology with patients

C. Risk control: the activities of persons involved in risk management, which include the development of policies to which employees must adhere to support the risk management function, educational programs that assist employees in becoming aware of and sensitive to risk management issues, analysis of institutional processes and procedures to ensure that they do not precipitate risk

1. Risks may be avoided by eliminating financially marginal services that have high potential for lawsuits; where there are good profit centers, strong process controls are useful that permit the service to function but limit the risk
2. The financial consequences of risk can be shifted to others by contracting the transfer of that risk to the party providing the service; contracting with health care provider groups to provide a particular service and also assume the risk of any liability; however, institutions that use this method of risk reduction cannot always escape all liability

3. Risk prevention is the important function of avoiding the occurrence of problems or limiting the losses associated with such events after they have occurred; educational programs, process and procedure analysis, identification of risky practices or conditions and correcting them are strategies that prevent risk; after adverse events have occurred there are actions that can be taken to prevent greater loss; immediate contact with injured parties by risk management personnel, offering financial mitigation such as waiver of institutional billing or providing additional no-cost care may be useful, although these are considered controversial by some risk managers because they seem to admit liability; approach is all important in such situations and is directed toward enhancing good will on the part of the institution and forestalling lawsuits by an injured patient or a patient who may only believe his/her care was substandard

II. Occurrence/Variance/Incident Reports

A. Occurrence/variance/incident reports are important tools of the risk manager, who is often also institutional legal counsel; such reports are required when there are occurrences that are not consistent with routine patient care
   1. If a health care provider, such as a nurse, becomes aware that there has been some occurrence that may precipitate a lawsuit, it is important to notify the health care institution or agency, which may be able to take some action to protect itself or the personnel working there; sometimes this notification takes the form of an incident or occurrence report
   2. Reports may or may not be discoverable by plaintiffs; *discovery* means that an injured party may find out that such a report was made
   3. Occurrence/variance/incident reports are institutional work product, prepared in contemplation of legal protection or to monitor quality; generally, in law, such a business work product has remained private to the institution and cannot be discovered or seen by a party suing the institution
   4. Over the last decade or so, some courts have permitted the reports to be made available to the plaintiff on a theory of fairness; the belief is that a plaintiff who is injured by the negligence of a person within an agency or institution should have enough information to pursue his/her action
   5. Health care institutions prefer to keep this work product report private and not disclose it to suing plaintiffs; often the preparer of the report has been asked to make a judgment as to the cause of the incident or problem (information that may help the plaintiff) but this judgment may not indicate the actual cause (remember, it must be proved that a breach of duty is the direct or proximate cause of the plaintiff's injury not merely a factor that may have been present in the situation)

B. Preparation of the occurrence/variance/incident report
   1. Reports are generally completed by the person who witnessed or was involved in the occurrence and are prepared for the risk manager or legal counsel of the institution
   2. Institutions have policies for the preparation and distribution of reports, policies that should be rigidly adhered to; because such reports are prepared in contemplation of litigation, the fewer personnel who receive a copy, the greater the chance that the report will remain undiscoverable (see previously)
   3. The risk manager can keep appropriate administrative personnel informed of incidents; the risk manager also compiles reports and analyses of incidents so as to identify problem areas or high-risk sectors; this knowledge helps department managers to address problems and thereby prevent errors and reduce future injuries
   4. Occurrence/variance/incident reports assist in the management of claims, either by coming to terms in private negotiations with injured patients where liability seems clear or by coordinating with legal counsel on a defense against a lawsuit by a patient
   5. Commercial insurers often require such reports before paying claims; because many institutions use commercial insurance to augment self-insurance, it is important that incident

data be made available to avoid further depletion of the self-insurance fund and commercial insurance can be used as planned

III. QUALITY AND RISK MANAGEMENT

A. Institutional quality management programs are usually closely related to risk management and are sometimes housed in the same department
   1. Quality management programs in health care settings are usually concerned with the assessment and improvement of patient care
   2. Quality management focuses more closely on patient care than does risk management, which is concerned with problems in all of the institutional functions
   3. Reports prepared for risk management purposes may be shared with quality management supervisors in order to assist them in identifying serious quality deficiencies
   4. Quality management and improvement is usually managed by committees who address the various functions within the institution

B. Risk management and quality improvement functions are outcome oriented and are involved with various legal problems
   1. Risk management, although it has a preventive and monitoring function, often has its most active involvement after a problem incident
   2. Quality management is a continuous process, including quality monitoring, retrospective review, and quality committee activity; similar to the discoverability of incident reports, there is sometimes a legal question about the discoverability of quality committee reports and minutes; this is particularly true of tissue committees, credentials committees, and infection committees
   3. Review of credentials and other reviews generally take place at hiring or granting of privileges in a health care agency; removal of an incompetent practitioner who is a risk to the institution is often more difficult
   4. Plaintiffs in actions for malpractice against health care institutions, in addition to seeking incident reports, may also seek to discover any minutes of committees in which there was discussion of the problem or the personnel involved; personnel who are dismissed from their positions for problem practice or allegations of incompetence may also want the record of committee discussion to determine what was said; such dismissed persons have attempted to sue committee members for defamation based on criticism presented in the committee meeting where incidents of problem practice were addressed
   5. Whether a plaintiff should be able to obtain copies of occurrence/variance/incident reports, committee minutes, or other documents remains a legal question and differs from one jurisdiction to another; it is understood that committee discussion or an opinion about causation in a report could confirm the negligence of a professional provider or the liability of the institution under a theory of corporate liability
   6. There are often good reasons why the reports and minutes should not be made available to plaintiffs; it is believed by many commentators on the subject that confidentiality is essential to the effective functioning of committees on quality improvement and risk management and that such committees are important to the continued improvement of care; conscientious and critical evaluation of clinical practices is a valuable function that probably cannot occur in an atmosphere of apprehension where one professional's suggestion could be used to accuse another of malpractice or where any criticism could be taken as defamation

---

EXAMPLE In a hospital skilled care unit, an elderly man was found on the floor. He seemed to be uninjured but shaken and nervous. The nursing assistant who found him notified the nurse, who measured vital signs, did an assessment of pain and movement, skin damage, and cognitive ability and completed an incident/occurrence report. The report was completed according to institutional policy. The report was given to the nurse manager who reviewed it and sent it, sealed, to the hospital legal counsel according to policy. By the next day, the elderly man developed several ecchymotic areas on his legs and elbows and complained of pain. He told his family that he fell out of his chair because he had called nurses several times but received no assistance, and so he tried to go to the bathroom without help and fell. He reported that this was a common occurrence. The family complained to the nurse manager, who in turn reported the complaint and the further development of the injuries to the legal counsel. The patient was subsequently seen by a physician, treated for the bruises, and provided with mild pain medication. He was then monitored more closely by the nursing staff. The problem of falls was later discussed at a meeting of the Falls Prevention Committee as a part of the Quality Management program. In determining whether to sue for the man's injuries, which were minor in nature, the family demanded via *interrogatories* (a discovery device consisting of written questions submitted by one party to another party who has information about a case) information about the discussion in the Falls Prevention Committee, including whether the incident was discussed and what the outcome or recommendations were regarding it. Depending on statutory and/or common law in the jurisdiction, the institution may avoid providing any information about the committee's deliberations or recommendations, but it is likely that it would need to reveal that there was such a committee and the kinds of issues it addressed.

7. The defamation issue as it relates to risk management and quality improvement committees has also been subject to statutory and common law; the Health Care Quality Improvement Act of 1986 (Public Law 99-660, Title IV) provides that in peer review procedures there is a qualified, but not absolute, privilege to criticize and comment about the practice of another; only peer reviewers who act without malice and in good faith are protected in their committee functions; although such review of practice is a risk management and quality improvement function, it may be discoverable; there is case law that permits the discovery of peer review committee discussion, minutes, and recommendations

C. Managing claims and lawsuits
1. *Alternative dispute resolution* (ADR) is one way provided by some organizations and states to deal with claims other than by a court trial with a judge and jury; trials are costly and lengthy and cost both plaintiff and defendant time and money without necessarily producing a satisfactory outcome; ADR is a process by which a less formal process is used to permit each party to present his/her case to a panel of arbitrators, who hear testimony, read and review documents and exhibits, and render a decision for one of the parties; it isn't a compromise but an expedited way for a plaintiff to be heard, particularly if the case is not one where there are extensive and expensive damages
2. Some organizations have a policy that initially requires claims be heard by ADR to promote a quick resolution; ADR doesn't preclude proceeding to trial later if the outcome is not satisfactory to one of the parties; it is important to note that the arbitration procedure will give the parties a sense, if nothing else, of how their case is perceived

REFERENCES

Black HC: *Black's law dictionary,* ed 6, St Paul, MN, 1991, West Publishing Company.

Furrow BR, Johnson SH, Jost TS, et al: *Liability and quality issues in health care.* St Paul, MN, 1991, West Publishing Company.

Kraus GP: *Health care risk management,* Owings Mills, MD, 1986, National Health Publishing, Rynd Communications.

CHAPTER 45

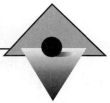

ETHICS AND VALUES

Alice G. Rini

LEARNING OBJECTIVES

Upon completion of this chapter, the reader will be able to:

- Describe the importance of ethical practice
- Discuss the development of a value system
- Analyze how the adoption of an ethical basis for practice promotes patient welfare

I. DEFINITIONS

A. Ethics: the branch of moral philosophy that deals with the standards of moral conduct and moral judgment; it deals with what is considered to be right or wrong in terms of human conduct; applied ethics deals with related decisions and actions based on ideas of right and wrong

B. Bioethics: the application of ethics and ethical theory to science and medicine

C. Values: relative worth, utility, or importance; something, such as a principle or quality, intrinsically valuable or desirable; values are also professional and personal beliefs about worth or importance; values may also guide decisions and actions

D. Value system: a personal code of conduct or organized pattern of values ·

II. ETHICS IN NURSING PRACTICE

A. There are two major ethical theories that are currently considered in answering ethical issues (if indeed they can be answered)

1. Utilitarianism: a teleological theory (from the Greek, *telos,* meaning end) that the quality of right and wrong are determined from the consequences of one's behavior; utility of action is determined by whether it tends to promote happiness or "good" and minimize suffering; greatest good for the greatest number; ends justify the means

2. Deontological theory: the quality of an act is based on the moral principle on which the act is based (from the Greek, *deon,* meaning binding duty); this theory asserts that an act is moral only if the principle governing it arises from good will; acting on the basis of a duty; an act based on good moral principle, but which causes harm, is still ethical

3. Many ethicists assert that one cannot use only one theory on which to base all practice but that elements of both are legitimate and useful

B. In medical and nursing ethics, the principles of self-determination, beneficence, and justice are major issues

1. *Self-determination* is considered the most important value in biomedical ethics and is based on the philosophical concept of autonomy

2. *Beneficence* is the obligation to do good for another, the Hippocratic obligation to do no harm

3. Justice is the concept of the dignity and worth of every individual, the right to equal treatment under the law, and the idea that all humans have rights because they are moral beings; it also means that individuals are morally and legally responsible for their own acts

---

EXAMPLE   An elderly man with inoperable prostate cancer that has metastasized to bone and liver tells the nurse he wants to die. His pain is unbearable even with medication, and he has only a short time to live in any case. His idea is to request that the doctor deprogram a pacemaker he has worn for several years for cardiac rhythm irregularities so that if he has a cardiac event, he will die quickly. He asks the nurse to support his request to the doctor and help him tell his family what he wants to do. If the nurse accepts the autonomy of the patient, he should intervene for the patient. Using the theory of deontology, the nurse would affirm that action based on the principle of autonomy, a most important principle of human relations; the concept of beneficence is also operative here in that because the patient desires his own immediate death, intervening for it could be considered doing something good. On the other hand, promoting someone's death may be considered doing harm by others. Finally, justice dictates that the patient has the right to his dignity at any point in his life. The problem is that in order to meet the patient's request, the nurse and doctor may have to take actions that violate their own values in terms of the sanctity of life in any form, or the belief that life is always preferable to non-life. There are really no clear answers to this issue, but such problems are real and need thought and wide discussion among health care professionals.

III. VALUES IN NURSING PRACTICE

A. How values are developed
  1. Observations of and experience with parents and other meaningful adults as they address and solve problems are an important way that early values are developed
  2. Role models are an essential component of values establishment
  3. Conflicting values are often experienced by young adults especially when they find that parents, teachers, clergy, and other adults hold values and attitudes that differ from the peer group
  4. The experience of nursing school, exposure to faculty, other students, and the study of philosophy and its application assist nurses in developing values about their profession and their work; nursing work itself also contributes to ongoing and evolving values development throughout one's work life
B. Values in nursing practice
  1. Self-responsibility: both ethical principles and the law require that the nurse must take responsibility for himself/herself; such responsibility includes important acts and decisions that include requirements
     a. To maintain an adequate level of competency
     b. To participate in formal and continuing education
     c. To approach patients and work with a positive attitude about both
     d. To understand one's own needs and responsibilities
     e. To accept and be accountable for one's own acts
     f. To provide quality care and assist others to do so
     g. To report substandard care to appropriate authorities
     h. To participate in and support research that expands nursing knowledge within one's own capabilities
  2. Assuming a commitment to one's patients, the profession, and one's employer
     a. Commitment to patients is managed by
        (1) Respecting patient dignity through preserving autonomy
        (2) Understanding and providing for the needs of frail older adults

        (3) Realizing that timeliness may be of utmost importance to the elderly patient who may have less time to achieve goals in life than younger adults and so understanding that delay in fulfilling that patient's needs may mean they are forever foregone

        (4) Promoting patient participation in care planning to the extent the patient is able to participate

  b. Commitment to the profession can be established by

        (1) Knowing the standards of care required in practice and adhering to them

        (2) Reporting incompetent, illegal, and unethical practice to appropriate authorities and according to one's institutional policy

        (3) Participating in professional organizations

        (4) Behaving in a manner that will maintain and improve the image and dignity of the profession

  c. Commitment to the employer is often a forgotten or ignored concept; nurses, however, have an obligation to the agency that provides their livelihood

        (1) There is a partnership between the employer and the employee and each has obligations to the other

        (2) In exchange for a salary, a safe place to work, a reasonably satisfactory environment, and other compensation, the nurse accepts assignments, is timely in terms of arrival at work, provides required care in a competent manner, and supports the employer in public situations

REFERENCES

Ahronheim JC, Moreno J, Zuckerman C: *Ethics in clinical practice,* New York, 1994, Little, Brown.

Furrow BR, Johnson SH, Jost TS, et al: *Bioethics: health care law and ethics,* St Paul, MN, 1991, West Publishing Company.

Rini AG: Values clarification. In Luggen AS, Travis SS, Meiner S, editors: *NGNA core curriculum for gerontological advanced practice nurses.* Thousand Oaks, CA, 1998, Sage.

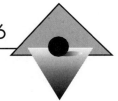

CHAPTER 46

GERONTOLOGICAL NURSING TRENDS AND ISSUES

Dianne Thames

LEARNING OBJECTIVES

Upon completion of this chapter, the reader will be able to:

- Identify specific events that have influenced the development of gerontological nursing
- Compare and contrast methods for obtaining current research findings
- Describe the roles that a gerontological nurse may assume
- Discuss the advantages and disadvantages of certification
- Explain the legal and ethical bases of nursing practice with gerontological patients
- Define the various disciplines related to the nursing care of the older adult
- Discuss the development of gerontological nursing
- List the major events in the development of gerontological nursing
- Identify the nursing leaders in the development of gerontological nursing
- Identify three educational paths available to nurses who desire to work with older adults
- Discuss two common problems associated with education of gerontological nurses
- Describe the professional organizations that affect nursing care of older adults
- Discuss the government networks that impact gerontological nursing

I. SPECIALITY ADVANCEMENT (EBERSOLE & HESS, 1998)

A. Many nurses who entered the gerontological field did so either by accident or because they were attracted to the field by federal support
B. Most had no special preparation to be gerontological nurses
C. Certification is one way to ensure minimal consistent preparation in the area of gerontological nursing
D. Approximately 11,081 nurses have been certified in gerontology, even though most nurses are engaged in some way in the care of the older adult

II. RELEVANT LITERATURE AND CURRENT RESEARCH FINDINGS AND THEIR APPLICATION (ANDERSON, 1996)

A. Journal articles
   1. Many research reports are published in refereed journals: a professional journal generally referees articles by sending them out for peer review; because there is so little space in journals for publishing articles, the peer review process assists in ensuring the reader that the highest level and most pertinent research is available for reading

2. The peer review process, however, does not guarantee that the research published is ideal work; it is the reader's and potential consumers' responsibility to evaluate the quality of the research published and determine its application to nursing practice

3. The research consumer should carefully review the article for the aspects of research; a knowledge base of research design and methodology is necessary for evaluating the printed research results; the article should be scrutinized for scientific rigor rather than merely accepted as truth because it was published (Box 46-1)

B. Research conferences

1. Research conferences are designed for the presentation of research results to a varied audience; research generally is presented by means of a poster with a written abstract or by a podium presentation; often the abstracts from all presentations are published, providing a rich resource for the research consumer to review; names and organizations are printed on the abstracts and the opportunity to network with researchers with similar interests is provided through this mechanism

2. Research conferences allow for one-on-one networking on research issues presented there; after the conference, it is possible to continue networking with researchers because of the information on the abstract

3. Box 46-2 demonstrates the basic information generally seen in an abstract at a conference

4. Review of an abstract like the one in Box 46-2 will give the research consumer the opportunity to consider new approaches to care based on established research; there is an opportunity to contact the person who did the research and potentially discuss the nuances of the research results' implementation; the abstract does not give all of the data regarding the research but should indicate to the reader if there is an interest that can be pursued

C. Current research findings

1. A wide variety of research topics is available in the current literature and through attending conferences; it is the research consumers' responsibility to make themselves available to review current research findings

2. Another opportunity for being informed on the most current data available is to be in touch with a graduate school of nursing where theses and dissertations are completed in notable numbers each year; this type of liaison would place the research consumer in the forefront of knowledge as it is initially disseminated through the written thesis or dissertation kept on file in the school library

III. ROLES OF THE GERONTOLOGICAL NURSE

A. The gerontological nurse assumes many different roles in the care of the older adult.

B. In the acute care setting, the gerontological nurse functions to prevent disease or disability that

---

BOX 46-1   Tips on Reading Research Reports

Grow accustomed to the style of research reports by reading them frequently even though not all of the technical points may be understood. Try to keep the underlying rationale for the research report in mind while reading.

Read research articles slowly; it may be useful to first skim the article to get the major points and then read the article more carefully a second time.

Do not get bogged down (or scared away) by the statistical information. Try to grasp the gist of the story without letting formulas and numbers become frustrating.

Before becoming more accustomed to the style and jargon of scientific writing, mentally translate research articles. This can be done by translating compact paragraphs into looser constructions and jargon into more familiar phrases and terms, recasting the report into active voice to get a better sense of the researcher's dynamic role in the research process, and summarizing the findings with words rather than with numbers.

From Pout DF, Hungler BP: *Essentials of nursing research: methods, appraisal, and utilization,* ed 3, Philadelphia, 1993, JB Lippincott.

BOX 46-2   **Abstract Example**

PURPOSE
To examine the use of validation therapy (VT) with demented old, old residents in a nursing home.

RATIONALE
The fastest growing population in the United States is people aged 85 years and older. In 1990, the number of people with Alzheimer's-type dementia was 2.9 million, with predictions that that number will increase to 14.3 million.

Currently, 5% of those people over 65 years of age are in nursing homes. With the increasing numbers of people over age 85 with dementia, there is a predicted increase in admissions to nursing homes.

Validation therapy is a communication technique designed to be used with old, old demented people. It requires the caregiver to validate rather than analyze the patient's feelings.

METHODOLOGY
In an effort to gather data on the use of VT with those aged 85 and older suffering from dementia in nursing homes, the following was done:

SAMPLE
A group of 8 old, old demented residents in a nursing home met with a nationally certified Validation Therapist 1 hour a week for 10 weeks.

SETTING
A local nursing home that met state criteria for licensure and was listed by the State of Utah as a citation-free facility for 5 years.

DATA GENERATION
The group activity was videotaped with three cameras to record the experience for all participants. Videotapes rather than interviews were used because of the participants' lack of short-term recall.

DATA ANALYSIS
The 30 videotapes were reviewed for global concepts and common themes. They were then coded and actual behaviors were counted per individual and in the aggregate.

FINDINGS
• Participants exhibited social behaviors within the group that they did not exhibit outside the group (i.e., greetings and handshakes, saying "please" and "thank you").
• The real world of the participants was not larger than their immediate family, even if their family members had not been physically present in their lives for months.
• Music was a common means of communication for the group.
• Residents demonstrated the ability to manage their own experiences in the group with meaningful conversations and purposeful touch. According to verbal reports from the staff, they did not do this outside of the group setting.

NURSING IMPLICATIONS
The results of this project indicate that VT promotes behavior that is more socially appropriate for this sample of people. It is a modality of communication that could be considered for use to enhance the demented elder's quality of life, rather than using restraints and isolation.

From Anderson MA, Culliton K, Brill C: *Examining the impact of validation therapy on the elderly,* unpublished abstract.

---

is the result of hospitalization, detects those diseases and/or disabilities as early as possible, and/or manages these in order to prevent further disability or complications (Burgraff & Stanley, 1995)

C. In long-term care, the nurse has a variety of roles, but the role of advocate is at the center (Burgraff & Stanley, 1995)

1. As an administrator, the nurse is responsible for management of the organization, human resources, nursing services, and professional and long-term care leadership (Lekan-Rutledge, 1997)

2. The registered nurse is responsible for assessments, care planning, supervising, and evaluating the delivery of care (Lekan-Rutledge, 1997)

BOX 46-3   Federal Law Vs. State Law

It is important to understand that federal law is the same throughout the country, but state law differs from state to state. Know the laws in your state of practice.

    D. In the community, the nurse assists the older adult to use community resources appropriately; it is essential that the nurse remain informed on the health care reimbursement system (Burgraff & Stanley, 1995)

IV. LEGISLATION AFFECTING PRACTICE (RINI, 1996)

  A. The legislature as a source of law
1. Laws are established on the federal and state levels by legislators (United States and state senators and representatives)
2. State law may not conflict with federal laws, which are superior
3. However, state law may require stricter requirements than federal laws or may address issues not considered by federal laws
4. Both federal and state laws affect nursing practice

  B. Statutes
1. Definition: rules that have been enacted by a legislative body and signed into law by the state governor or the President
2. Through statutes, regulatory agencies are established and are empowered to operate
3. State boards of nursing are regulatory agencies that govern the practice of nursing within the state; state boards regulate
    a. School of nursing curricula
    b. Licensure requirements
    c. Investigation and conduct of hearings regarding violations of regulations
4. Regulatory agencies write and publish regulations to implement statutes and carry out their legislated functions
5. Statutes at both federal and state levels affect nursing practice
    a. Social Security Act of 1965 includes Medicare and Medicaid laws (federal)
    b. Public health laws regarding hazardous substances and materials, communicable disease (federal)
    c. Child and elder abuse reporting (state)
    d. Good Samaritan laws (state) (Box 46-3)

V. HISTORY OF GERONTOLOGICAL NURSING

  A. Definitions
1. Gerontology: branch of science that studies the effects of time on human development; the study of the aged (Ebersole & Hess, 1999)
2. Gerontological nursing: uses broad scientific base to organize and formulate care of older adults; the purpose is to enhance quality of life for older adults through health promotion, support of independence and continued opportunities for development throughout life, and peaceful death (Ebersole & Hess, 1999)
3. Geriatrics: branch of medicine that deals with diseases and disabilities of older people (Miller, 1993)
4. Geriatric nursing: concerned with disease conditions of the older person; focus on illness (Ebersole & Hess, 1998)
5. Gerontic nursing: concerned with nursing care of older people; the practice of caring/curing and nurturance of older men's and women's comfort and health using basic nursing methods; involves specialized knowledge about the aged; uses established

conditions within the patient's environment that increase health-conducive behaviors and minimize and compensate for health-prejudicial losses and disabilities (Gunter, 1987)

B. Time line (Box 46-4)
1. Nursing care of older individuals has existed for many years
2. Became "official" in early 1900s
3. Slow, gradual development during the beginning of the century
4. Development increased because of technological advances, changes in demographics, and increased knowledge related to increased information in physiology, medicine, and pharmacology
5. More nurses assumed leadership roles in development of new settings and innovated cost-effective methods for delivering health care to older adults
6. Early leaders
   a. Florence Nightingale: nursing gained stature as a profession with professional goals
   b. Doris Schwartz: leader in the development of gerontological nursing practitioner program
   c. Virginia Stone: headed first masters program for clinical nurse specialist in gerontology practice (Eliopoulos, 1999)
   d. Laurie Gunter: one of the first nurses in the United States to present papers at the meeting of International Congress of Gerontology
   e. Janet Specht: first to receive the Gerontological Nurse of the Year Award sponsored by the *Journal of Gerontological Nursing*
7. Early authors
   a. Irene Burnside
   b. May Futrell
   c. Dorothy Moses
   d. Sister Marilyn Schwab
   e. Bernita Steffl
   f. Virginia Stone
   g. Lucille Taulbee
   h. Mary Opal Wolanin
   i. May Wykle

VI. Paths to Becoming a Gerontological Nurse

A. Basic education in nursing with experience in caring for older adults
B. Basic academic preparation in caring for older adults
C. Graduate academic preparation in caring for older adults
D. ANA certification: nurses demonstrate the level of expertise that they have attained
1. Identifies nurses who have demonstrated the capability of using expert clinical knowledge and skills in providing nursing care
2. Admission criteria for all levels of certification
   a. Current RN license
   b. BSN
3. Re-examination every 5 years
4. Process
   a. Application fee
   b. Establishment that nurse meets admission criteria
   c. Success on comprehensive examination
5. Levels of certification
   a. Gerontological Nurse
      (1) Admission criteria: BSN

BOX 46-4   Gerontological Nursing Time Line

1904   *American Journal of Nursing* published article on care of the aged
1920s   Many older individuals live on "poor farms"
1935   Social Security Act; federal monies made available to older individuals who were needy or who had limited financial resources
1940s   Older adults cared for in hospitals; no focused plans were made for discharging older adults home
1950   First geriatric nursing text by Newton and Anderson published
1950s   Population of older adults gradually increases; increased emphasis on wellness activities; nursing education programs moved into institutions of higher education
1960s   Nursing process defined; theoretical frameworks of nursing developed; gerontological nurses began to identify frameworks and theories that would be effective for the older individual's care; educational grants and funding for professional nurses became available, including grants for graduate nursing students to specialize in older adult care
1961   ANA recommended the formation of a special interest group for geriatric nurses
1962   70 nurses attended the first national American Nurses Association (ANA) meeting of a Conference Group on Geriatric Nursing Practice in Detroit, Michigan; the main item on the agenda was their name, indicating the "identity crisis" they were experiencing
1966   ANA Conference Group on Geriatric Nursing Practice recognized
1970   ANA developed standards of geriatric nursing practice; first publication of standards for geriatric nursing practice
1973   NANDA published first list of nursing diagnoses
1975   ANA certification in geriatric nursing practice offered; *Journal of Gerontological Nursing* became first professional nursing journal for gerontological nurses
1976   Geriatric Nursing Division changed its name to Gerontological Nursing Division; first gerontological nursing textbook published: *Nursing and the Aged* by Irene Burnside; First National Conference of Gerontological Nurse Practitioners
1979   First National Conference on Gerontological Nursing sponsored by the *Journal of Gerontological Nursing*
1980   *Geriatric Nursing Journal* first published; nursing defined in a social policy statement
1981   ANA statement on the scope of gerontological nursing practice
1984   Council of Gerontological Nursing formed (ANA); National Gerontological Nursing Association formed
1986   First conference of the National Association of Directors of Nursing Administration in Long-Term Care (NADONA)
1989   ANA certification established for Gerontological Clinical Nurse Specialist
1990s   Establishment of National Institute of Nursing Research promotes the expansion of gerontological nursing knowledge base
1991   Educators still having difficulty ensuring gerontological content in basic nursing curricula
1993   12,000 nurses certified in gerontological nursing specialties
1996   Many older adults become part of managed care systems

Modified from Ebersole & Hess, 1998; Miller, 1993; Eliopoulos, 1997; ANA, 1995.

(2) Definition: "concerned with the health needs of the older adult, planning and implementing health care to meet those needs, and evaluating the effectiveness of such care; the primary challenge is to identify and use the strengths of older adults and assist them in maximizing their independence; the older adult is actively involved as much as possible in the decision making which influences everyday living" (Burnside, 1988)

(3) Additional eligibility requirements:

    (a) 4000 hours of practice as an RN in a gerontological nursing practice (2000 of which have occurred within the past 2 years) and 30 contact hours of continuing education applicable to gerontology/gerontological nursing within the past 2 years

b. Gerontological Nurse Practitioner (GNP)
   (1) Admission criteria: varies from RN to master's degree in nursing
   (2) Definition: ". . . one who has advanced skills in assessment of the physical and psychosocial health-illness status of individuals, families, or groups in a variety of settings through health and development history-taking to physical examinations" (Burke & Walsk, 1992)
   (3) Serves in a variety of clinical settings
   (4) Additional eligibility requirements:
       (a) "Formal post-graduate GNP track or program within a school of nursing granting graduate level academic credit" OR "GNP Master's degree in nursing program" OR "completion of a gerontological, family, or adult nurse practitioner certificate program that is at least 9 months or 1 academic year of full time study or its equivalent before completing a master's degree in nursing" (Burke & Walsk, 1992)
c. Clinical Specialist in Gerontology
   (1) Admission criteria: master's degree or higher in nursing OR a master's degree or higher with a specialization in gerontological nursing
   (2) Definition: "experts in providing, directing, and influencing the care of older adults and their families and significant others in a variety of settings; specialists demonstrate an in-depth understanding of the dynamics of aging as well as the interventions necessary for health promotion and management of health status alterations; specialists provide comprehensive gerontological nursing services independently or collaboratively with a multidisciplinary team; through theory and research, specialists advance the health care of older people and the specialty of gerontological nursing; specialists are engaged in practice, education, consultation, research, and administration" (Burke & Walsk, 1992)
   (3) Additional eligibility requirements: have practiced a minimum of 12 months following completion of the master's degree and if:
       (a) "Specialist, provided a minimum of 800 hours (post master's) of direct [client] care or clinical management in gerontological nursing within the past 24 months" (Burke & Walsk, 1992)
       (b) "Consultant, researcher, educator, or administrator, provided a minimum of 400 hours (post master's) of direct client care or clinical management in gerontological nursing within the past 24 months" (Burke & Walsk, 1992)

VII. PROBLEMS WITH GERONTOLOGICAL NURSING EDUCATION

A. No uniformity in nursing curricula, which leads to the concern that there is no real guarantee that graduates will have the basic knowledge or clinical background to provide nursing care to older adults
B. Geriatric content often lost in nursing curricula because it is said to be "integrated" throughout the curriculum
C. Lack of appropriate role models

VIII. PROFESSIONAL ORGANIZATIONS IMPACTING GERONTOLOGICAL NURSING

A. National Gerontological Nursing Association (NGNA)
   1. Purpose
      a. Provides forum to identify and explore issues of interest to gerontological nurses
      b. Sponsors and conducts educational programs of importance to gerontological nurses
      c. Educates the public on health issues affecting older adults

2. Membership includes all nurses who are involved or foster the development and improvement of nursing and nursing education in relation to the care of the older adult

B. American Association of Retired Persons (AARP)
   1. Purpose
      a. To improve all aspects of living for older adults aged 55 years and older
      b. Sponsors community service programs
      c. Analyzes legislative policy and makes recommendations

C. American Society on Aging (ASA)
   1. Provides networking, education and training, advocacy
   2. Membership includes older adults, academic community, policy makers, business community

D. Association for Gerontology in Higher Education (AGHE)
   1. Supports development of academic community in the field of gerontology and aging through education, research, public service
   2. Membership includes academic institutions and organizations committed to gerontological education

E. Gray Panthers
   1. Activist group working to combat ageism
   2. Membership includes older adults and younger adults

F. National Council on Aging
   1. Information and consultation center addressing concerns of older adults
   2. Conducts research and demonstration programs
   3. Educates via conferences and workshops

G. Hartford Institute for Geriatric Nursing
   1. Purpose: setting a national agenda and shaping the quality of health care for elderly Americans by promoting the highest level of competency in the nurses who deliver care
   2. Initiatives
      a. Practice
      b. Education
      c. Research
      d. Public policy/consumer education

IX. GOVERNMENT NETWORKS

A. Administration on Aging (AOA)
   1. Function: oversees service to nation's older adults; provides programs promoting independence in older adults; coordinates federal policies on aging
   2. Location: Department of Health and Human Services (DHHS)

B. Division of Nursing, Bureau of Health Professions, DHHS
   1. Administers Title VIII: Nurse Education and the Public Health Service Act
   2. Provides resources, staff for National Advisory Council on Nurse Training
   3. Plans and supports development and utilization of U.S. nursing personnel resources, improvement of nursing services, educational programs

C. Federal Council on Aging
   1. 15-member, President-appointed, Senate-confirmed advisory committee on federal programs on aging

REFERENCES

American Nurses Association: *American Nurses Credentialing Center Certification Catalog,* Washington, DC, 1995, The Association.

Anderson MA, Culliton K, Brill C: *Examining the impact of validation therapy on the elderly,* unpublished abstract, 1994.

Burgraff V, Stanley M: Nurses' role with the elderly in acute care settings. In Stanley M, Beare PG, editors, *Gerontological nursing,* Philadelphia, 1995, FA Davis.

Burnside IM: *Nursing and the aged: a self-care approach,* ed 3, New York, 1988, McGraw-Hill.

Ebersole P, Hess P: *Toward healthy aging: human needs and nursing responses,* ed 5, St Louis, 1998, Mosby.

Eliopoulos C: *Gerontological nursing,* ed 4, Philadelphia, 1997, JB Lippincott.

Gunter LM: Nomenclature: what is in the name "gerontic nursing?" *J Gerontol Nurs* 13:7, 1987.

Lekan-Rutledge D: Gerontological nursing in long-term care facilities. In Matteson MA, McConnell ES, Linton AD, editors: *Gerontological nursing: concepts and practice,* ed 2, Philadelphia, 1997, WB Saunders.

Miller CA: *Nursing care of older adults,* ed 2, Philadelphia, 1993, JB Lippincott.

Rini A: Legislation affecting nursing practice. In Luggen AS, editor: *Core curriculum for gerontological nursing,* St Louis, 1996, Mosby.

PRACTICE EXAMINATIONS AND ANSWERS

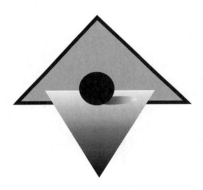

PRACTICE EXAMINATION A

UNIT ONE: PRIMARY CARE CONSIDERATIONS

1. The fastest growing age group is:
   a. Under age 65
   b. Age 85 and over
   c. Over age 90
   d. Between the ages of 65 and 80
2. The most needed home health service for older adults over age 65 is:
   a. Physical therapy
   b. Social services
   c. Homemaker/companion services
   d. Skilled nursing care
3. Aging results in a thinned epithelial layer of skin that appears dry and wrinkled. One reason for this is:
   a. Increase in subcutaneous fat
   b. Fewer and more rigid collagen fibers
   c. Increased pigmentation
   d. Thickening of the dermis
4. Normal phenomena occurring with aging include:
   a. Decreased hearing but increased sound discrimination
   b. Decreased peripheral vascular resistance
   c. Decreased ventilation/perfusion ratio with more gas exchanged
   d. Decrease in sleep stages 3 and 4
5. Musculoskeletal changes producing loss of height are the result of:
   a. Decreased muscle tone
   b. Decreased fibrous tissue
   c. Limited joint activity
   d. Narrowed intervertebral spaces
6. Decreased numbers of olfactory receptors in the mouth, decreased renewal of taste buds, and decreased sensory cells in the nasal lining have the potential to:
   a. Cause difficulty in chewing food items
   b. Enhance the appetite of the elderly patient
   c. Increase salivary gland production
   d. Place the elderly patient at risk for injury
7. An intervention that can assist the patient to decrease glare is:
   a. Use of high wattage light bulbs at all times
   b. Use of several soft indirect lights
   c. Use of nightlights
   d. Wearing sunglasses even when indoors
8. Ageism means:
   a. Any prejudice or discrimination against or in favor of an age group
   b. Negative stereotypes only against persons over 65
   c. Political bias toward older persons
   d. Prejudice or discrimination in favor of the aged
9. In teaching a 72-year-old woman about screening for breast cancer, the nurse should tell the woman that:
   a. Monthly breast self-exam is sufficient
   b. A yearly mammogram should be done
   c. The risk for breast cancer is low unless pathology has been detected earlier
   d. Mammography is unnecessary

10. Which of the following older adults would be most at risk for nutritional deficiencies?
    a. 68-year-old female with hypertension and diabetes
    b. 75-year-old female who is alcoholic
    c. 80-year-old male with Alzheimer's disease who is living in long-term care
    d. 90-year-old male with chronic congestive heart failure

11. When doing diet teaching with an older adult, it is important to stress what dietary need?
    a. Minimum of 2000 cal/day
    b. Fat intake of 15% of the diet
    c. Maintaining a low-fiber diet
    d. Limiting sodium intake to 2400 mg/day

12. Walking is recommended for a 70-year-old female with type II diabetes. This type of exercise is most beneficial for her if done:
    a. 3 times per week for 30 minutes
    b. At a slow, even pace
    c. Before meals and in the evening
    d. Whenever possible

13. Orem, in her theory about self-care, recommends that, when illness occurs, nurses need to assess the patient's status and intervene to:
    a. Decrease stress in the patient
    b. Promote a change in the patient's environment
    c. Strengthen the patient's ability to participate in self-care
    d. Teach patients how to prevent illness

14. Strategies to reduce the negative effects of relocation include:
    a. Making the move as quickly as possible
    b. Involving the older adult in planning the relocation
    c. Providing recreational activities during relocation
    d. Beginning the "new life" with bright new possessions

15. Studies involving relocation of cognitively impaired people have demonstrated:
    a. They adjust much faster than noncognitively impaired individuals
    b. If they have familiar possessions, they don't notice the change in environment
    c. They take much longer to adjust to change
    d. Not enough studies of this group have been conducted

16. During the nursing assessment of an ethnic minority older adult, the nurse needs to determine:
    a. Spiritual influences of alternative healers
    b. The patient's interpretation of symptoms of the illness
    c. The nurse's own feelings regarding the ethnicity of the patient
    d. The differences between western medicine and ethnic practices

17. A patient from an cultural/ethnic minority group who values tradition, especially the past, would most likely:
    a. Reject all new treatments recommended by a "western practice" nurse
    b. Need little instruction and teaching about a new treatment intervention
    c. Be very compliant with all instructions without questions
    d. Need considerable explanation and preparation for a new treatment intervention

18. Orem's nursing theory focuses on:
    a. Care demands
    b. Care deficits
    c. Self-care
    d. Patient dependency

19. Sr. Callista Roy's nursing theory is useful to gerontological nurses. Its focus is:
    a. Adaptation
    b. Regulator and cognator systems
    c. Stimuli: contextual, focal, residual
    d. Modes: physiological, self-concept, role function, and interdependence

20. The biological theory known as cross-link theory postulates that:
    a. Each of us has a predetermined number of cell divisions that are influenced by heredity
    b. Each of us has one or more harmful genes that activate over time, causing cell mutations
    c. We have substances, produced during normal metabolism, that are not eliminated and can cause cell damage
    d. Connective tissue and DNA interact with free radicals to damage the DNA
21. The biological theory that explains graying of hair, menopause, and thymus atrophy is:
    a. Error theory
    b. Biological clock theory
    c. Gene theory
    d. Free radical theory

Scenario: Mr. J. is 72 and in reasonably good health. He is mildly diabetic and hypertensive. His primary care provider has asked the nurse to talk with him about diet modifications. After some discussion, Mr. J. announces that he eats four twinkies a day and that even though they have fat in them he has no intention of giving them up.
Questions #24 and #25 refer to this scenario.

22. How should the nurse proceed?
    a. Assure Mr. J that the twinkies are not a problem and let it go
    b. Agree with Mr. J. that the twinkies are high in fat and strongly suggest the twinkies should be eliminated from his diet to prevent disease complications or exacerbation
    c. Suggest that Mr. J. give up one twinkie and substitute it with a low-fat snack alternative such as fresh apple or celery
    d. Help Mr. J. plan the rest of his meals around the twinkies so that his fat consumption is lowered overall
23. In the preceding question 22, answer b is representative of which learning theory?
    a. Adult education
    b. Cognitive
    c. Behavioral
    d. Humanistic
24. The philosophy of hospice is:
    a. Extending the life of the patient
    b. To provide comfort for the patient
    c. To provide high-quality comfort care for the dying patient and family
    d. To provide comprehensive care for the dying patient and family
25. Where is the setting for hospice care?
    a. Hospitals only
    b. Nursing home, provided by staff members
    c. The patient's home or other health care setting
    d. In a special hospice facility
26. All of the following are diagnoses eligible for hospice services except:
    a. HIV-related conditions
    b. Depression
    c. Cancer
    d. End-stage dementia

Unit Two: Major Health Problems

1. During a physical assessment of an 82-year-old woman, environmental modifications may be needed. Select the most appropriate environment for this examination:
    a. Busy clinic examination room with several areas separated by curtains
    b. An examination room that is next to the emergency driveway

    c.   A room with indirect soft lighting to create an environment of rest

    d.   A quiet private area with a toilet immediately off of the room

2. When determining the social support network of your 78-year-old male patient, the following information is helpful:

    a.   Does he do his own grocery shopping and cooking?

    b.   Is he a member of any private organizations or church groups?

    c.   Is his second floor apartment accessible by an elevator?

    d.   Does he enjoy going to movies or reading in the library?

3. Select the patient answer that would identify a potential deficit in daily nutrition:

    a.   I eat foods that I do not have to do anything to but warm on my stove or eat cold

    b.   My dentures have been broken for a month, and I can't afford to get them fixed just now

    c.   I always drink about a half glass of water every time I go to the kitchen, which is often

    d.   I have a light lunch everyday because I eat a late breakfast

4. Which of the following best describes the signs and symptoms of left-sided heart failure?

    a.   Dyspnea, rales, and anxiety

    b.   Rales only

    c.   Peripheral edema

    d.   Anxiety and abdominal distention

5. Which of the following best describes the signs and symptoms of right-sided heart failure?

    a.   Jugular venous distension, dyspnea, tachycardia

    b.   Dyspnea, abdominal distention, absent bowel sounds

    c.   Peripheral edema and abdominal distention

    d.   Abdominal distention, flatus, belching

6. Ms. Elizabeth Joy, 85 years old, is taken to the local clinic by her family for complaint of a dry cough. After obtaining a history from Ms. Joy and her family, it is discovered she has increased weakness, decreased appetite, is increasingly more fatigued, and has been confused the past few days. She is sleeping less and appears to be more anxious. Ms. Joy is most probably experiencing which of the following conditions:

    a.   Acute myocardial infarction

    b.   Acute congestive heart failure

    c.   Angina

    d.   Arrhythmias

7. There are four determinants of myocardial performance. Which is **not** a determinant?

    a.   Preload

    b.   Heart rate

    c.   Left ventricular ejection fraction

    d.   Afterload

    e.   Contractility

8. Which of the following conditions is not included under the blanket term *COPD*?

    a.   Asthma

    b.   Chronic bronchitis

    c.   Emphysema

    d.   Tuberculosis

9. A lifestyle change imperative for any patient with emphysema is:

    a.   Not to exercise

    b.   Lose weight

    c.   Stop smoking

    d.   Stop eating sweets

10. A patient with emphysema is short of breath and uses accessory muscles of respiration. The nurse recognizes that the patient's difficulty in breathing is caused by:

    a.   Spasm of the bronchi that traps the air

    b.   An increase in the vital capacity of the lungs

    c.   A too rapid expulsion of the air from the alveoli

    d.   Difficulty in expelling the air trapped in the alveoli

11.   Select the appropriate nursing management for a nursing home patient with dysphagia:

    a.   Serve only liquid foods that do not need to be chewed

    b.   Maintain a low Fowler's position in bed for all meals

    c.   Instruct the patient and family that tube feedings are the safest and most effective method for nutrition

    d.   Prepare food so that its consistency is not so thin that it will potentiate aspiration

12.   Ulcer disease in older adults can be caused by different reasons. Select the reason that is **not** associated with ulcer disease:

    a.   Oral ingestion of aspirin several times a day for arthritis pain

    b.   Identification of *Helicobacter pylori* in the stomach tissue

    c.   Habituation with alcoholic beverages

    d.   Use of antacids 1 hour before or 2 hours after meals

13.   A patient with a hiatal hernia asks the nurse how best to prevent esophageal reflux. The nurse's best response would be:

    a.   "Increase your intake of fat with each meal."

    b.   "Lie down after eating to help your digestion."

    c.   "Reduce your caloric intake to foster weight reduction."

    d.   "Drink several glasses of fluid during each of your meals."

14.   A normal age-related change in the female reproductive organs is:

    a.   Increased acidity of vaginal secretions

    b.   Increase in breast size

    c.   Narrowing and shortening of the vagina

    d.   Thickening of the urethral mucosa

15.   Which of the following is a *true* statement about the prostate gland?

    a.   A thin clear fluid is produced on ejaculation

    b.   Hyperplasia of the prostate gland proceeds slowly

    c.   The gland is located above the bladder and around the urethra

    d.   Testosterone decreases the incidence of hyperplasia

16.   Which of the following teaching instructions would be most appropriate following a TURP?

    a.   Teach the patient Kegel exercises

    b.   Instruct the patient that he may resume normal activity

    c.   Instruct the patient that his urine should be clear and yellow after 12 hours

    d.   Instruct the patient to limit his fluid intake for the first 24 hours

17.   Which of the following is a risk factor in the development of prostate cancer:

    a.   Minimal sexual activity

    b.   Diet high in cholesterol

    c.   Decreased levels of DHT (5ax-dihydrotestosterone)

    d.   Genetics, especially in first-line relatives

18.   Which of the following assessment data would be highly suspicious of prostate cancer?

    a.   PSA 2 mg/ml

    b.   Priapism especially at night

    c.   Digital rectal exam revealing a hard nonmovable nodule

    d.   Increase in libido

19.   Mrs. Mark, age 88, has just had abdominal surgery. She begins to hemorrhage. The nurse should observe the patient for signs of progressive hypovolemia, which include:

    a.   Oliguria

    b.   Bradypnea

    c.   Pulse deficit

    d.   Hyperkalemia

20. During the administration of a unit of packed red cells, an older patient complains of lumbar pain that is new. The nurse should:
    a. Increase the flow of normal saline to dilute the blood infusion
    b. Obtain a full set of vital signs and report any abnormal values
    c. Perform an indepth musculoskeletal assessment
    d. Stop the transfusion immediately and increase the saline drip

21. Type I osteoporosis is:
    a. Osseous disease
    b. Premenopausal bone loss
    c. Postmenopausal bone loss
    d. Caused by osteoarthritis

22. Many older women are now taking alendronate (Fosamax) for osteoporosis. What teaching would you give to a woman who receives this prescription?
    a. Take before meals on an empty stomach
    b. Take at bedtime with an 8-ounce glass of water; avoid exercise after medication is taken
    c. Take at dinner time with the meal
    d. Take on arising in the morning 30 minutes before breakfast, with a glass of water

23. Thermoregulation is essential to survival in climate variances either below or above 74° to 78° F. Age-related changes can often place the older adult at risk for hypo- or hyperthermia. Select the mechanism that is **not** associated with normal age changes of thermoregulation:
    a. Diminished shivering
    b. Diminished sensory perception of temperatures
    c. Diminished thirst perception
    d. Diminished dryness in skin tissue

24. When obtaining a health history from a patient recently diagnosed with non–insulin-dependent diabetes mellitus (NIDDM), the nurse should expect the patient to mention symptoms associated with the classic signs of DM such as:
    a. Polydipsia, polyuria, irritability
    b. Polyphagia, confusion, polyuria
    c. Polydipsia, polyphagia, polyuria
    d. Polydipsia, nocturia, weight loss

25. Mr. Baker, age 82, is diagnosed as having NIDDM. The priority teaching goal is to have the patient:
    a. Perform foot care
    b. Administer insulin
    c. Test urine for sugar and acetone
    d. Identify hypoglycemia/hyperglycemia

26. All of the following statements concerning HIV/AIDS among women are correct **except:**
    a. Decreased vaginal lubrication may contribute to vulnerability to the HIV virus
    b. Older women are very likely to be diagnosed late in the disease progression
    c. Older women's long-term partners are less likely to have "come out" than their younger counterparts
    d. Gradual loss of memory is likely to indicate HIV/AIDS in an older woman

27. Education about HIV/AIDS for older persons:
    a. Should be targeted where older persons congregate
    b. Will not increase their awareness of risky behaviors
    c. Is not necessary because messages and programs for younger persons will decrease the prevalence in the older population
    d. Should not address sensitive issues such as sexuality and condom use

28. A/an _____ stimulates the production of a specific immune response.
    a. T cell
    b. B cell

    c.   Antibody

    d.   Antigen

29. HIV/AIDS is a disease primarily of which system?
    a.   Cardiovascular
    b.   Respiratory
    c.   Immune
    d.   Reproductive

30. In planning activities for an older adult diagnosed with vascular dementia and living in a nursing home, the nurse should:
    a.   Plan varied activities that will keep the resident occupied
    b.   Provide familiar activities that the resident can successfully complete
    c.   Offer challenging activities to maintain the resident's contact with reality
    d.   Make sure that the resident actively participates in the unit's daily activities

31. An older adult with a diagnosis of dementia of the Alzheimer's type likes to talk about olden days and at times has a tendency to confabulate. The nurse should recognize that confabulation serves to:
    a.   Prevent regression
    b.   Prevent embarrassment
    c.   Attract the attention of others
    d.   Reminisce about achievements

32. Mrs. Homer has suddenly had a change in personality that includes yelling incoherently at her roommate and not being able to find the dining room for lunch. The nurse recognizes that this rapid onset of irritability and confusion is most probably a sign of:
    a.   Delirium
    b.   Alzheimer's disease
    c.   Multi-infarct dementia
    d.   Depressive reaction

33. What are the modifiable risk factors for stroke that nurses need to teach patients?
    a.   Smoking, hypertension, TIAs, dysarthria
    b.   Diabetes, cardiovascular disease, TIAs, dysarthria
    c.   High cholesterol, diabetes, hypertension, dysarthria
    d.   Hypertension, smoking, high cholesterol

34. Symptoms of stroke include:
    a.   Headache, hemiparesis, shortness of breath, orthopnea
    b.   Hemiparesis, monoparesis, dysarthria, dysphasia
    c.   Headache, orthopnea, double vision, weakness
    d.   Orthopnea, dysarthria, shortness of breath, dysphasia

35. Your patient has a history of insomnia and has asked for advice. As the nurse, you suggest interventions that include all but one of the following. Select the *incorrect* instruction:
    a.   Keep a strict record of sleeping patterns for 1 week and return to discuss the record
    b.   Before bedtime, take a brisk walk, enjoy a hot bath, and listen to soft music
    c.   Discourage sleeping during the day hours or immediately after the evening meal
    d.   Avoid caffeine but drink an alcoholic cocktail to help relax before bedtime

36. Which of the following is a critical factor in response to a crisis in the older adult?
    a.   Translocation
    b.   Self-destructive behavior
    c.   Perception of the event
    d.   Ineffective coping

37. Which of the following assessment tools would be appropriate when assessing the older adult for cognitive abilities?
    a.   MiniMental State Assessment Tool
    b.   Geriatric Depression Scale
    c.   Hamilton Anxiety Scale
    d.   IADL Assessment Tool

38. Which of the following characteristics is typical of a wanderer?
    a. Quick to enter into unfamiliar territory
    b. Can be aimless or nonpurposeful
    c. Not aware of changes in memory and recall
    d. Becomes very social in the milieu
39. Pathological signs of grieving include:
    a. Crying
    b. Failure to acknowledge and accept losses
    c. Grieving lasting at least 3 months
    d. Diminished social activities and church attendance
40. Which of the following would be a drug of choice for an older adult who is experiencing anxiety?
    a. Buspar (Buspirone)
    b. Xanax (Alprazolam)
    c. Anafraril (Chloipramine)
    d. Zoloft (Sertraline)
41. Xerosis is
    a. Dry skin
    b. A burrowing mite
    c. A topical medication for dry skin
    d. A type of eczema
42. Your patient has been diagnosed with scabies. She complains bitterly of pruritus. Interventions you might suggest to soothe her skin include:
    a. Oatmeal compresses and Epsom salts baths
    b. Giving Vistaril, which is very useful for pruritus
    c. Skin wraps with elastic dressings
    d. Vaseline followed by elastic wrap dressings
43. Seborrheic keratoses are:
    a. Benign lesions
    b. Precancerous lesions
    c. Cancerous lesions
    d. Pus-filled crusty lesions
44. Your patient describes a wart-like gray nodule with raised borders that used to be flesh colored. You suspect:
    a. Basal cell carcinoma
    b. Melanoma
    c. Squamous cell carcinoma
    d. Seborrheic keratoses
45. Cerumen in the ear is a cause of
    a. Sensorineural loss
    b. Conduction loss
    c. Mixed loss
    d. Ototoxic effect
46. Drugs can cause ototoxicity and sensorineural hearing loss. Nurses should be aware of the following drugs that may cause this problem:
    a. Gentamycin and pungent salves
    b. Salicylates and gentamycin
    c. Furosemide and oral tolbutamide
    d. Furosemide and diphenhydramine
47. Management of the patient with hearing loss includes using communication patterns such as:
    a. Speaking louder than normal with a slightly higher tone of voice
    b. Speaking softer than usual, enunciating clearly with a lower tone of voice
    c. Speaking to the "good ear" with a higher tone of voice
    d. Speaking face to face with lowered tone of voice

48. Vision correction is a need of:
    a. 25% of older adults
    b. 50% of older adults
    c. 75% of older adults
    d. 90% of older adults

49. Definition of the term *arcus senilis* is:
    a. Diminished pupil size resulting from sclerosis of the pupil sphincter
    b. Normal age change in eyes with calcium and cholesterol deposits in the edge of the iris
    c. Increased light scatter causing glare
    d. Failure of the lacrimal pump

50. An important intervention after your patient has had cataract surgery is to teach the patient:
    a. To avoid intraocular pressure increases for the next 2 to 3 weeks
    b. To avoid all cholesterol-containing foods
    c. To avoid night driving
    d. About the need to keep diabetes in good control for the next 2 to 3 weeks

51. Glaucoma is a major cause of blindness. It can be treated if diagnosed early. Diagnosis is made by:
    a. Measuring the angle of the eye
    b. Measuring peripheral vision of the visual fields
    c. Testing intraocular pressure
    d. Conducting an examination for corneal edema

52. Failure to discontinue medications that are ineffective or no longer necessary places an elderly patient at risk of:
    a. Polypharmacy
    b. Pharmacokinesis
    c. Alterations in the drug's half-life
    d. Liver insufficiency

53. Movement of a drug from the site of administration into the body is:
    a. Distribution
    b. Bioavailability
    c. Absorption
    d. Clearance

54. Dehydration affects the amount of fluid required to distribute a drug evenly throughout the body. This aspect of pharmacokinetics is called:
    a. Clearance
    b. Volume of distribution
    c. Excretion/elimination
    d. Perfusion

55. An elderly patient taking digoxin is at risk for an adverse drug reaction (ADR) because:
    a. He/she is likely to experience interindividual variability in drug effects
    b. This is a drug with a narrow toxic-therapeutic range
    c. The patient is likely to be old
    d. The patient is likely to be taking numerous other medications

56. Pain is:
    a. Related to an injury
    b. Related to a perception of injury
    c. A sensory and emotional experience related to tissue damage
    d. Whatever the patient says it is

57. Pain is present in about what percentage of older adults in the community?
    a. 5% to 10%
    b. 10% to 20%
    c. 25% to 50%
    d. 75% to 100%

58. Pain is present in about what percentage of residents of long-term care facilities?
    a. 20% to 30%
    b. 50%
    c. 60% to 70%
    d. 85%
59. Chronic pain common to elderly people may be differentiated from acute pain by:
    a. The lack of change of vital signs with acute pain
    b. The lack of change of vital signs with chronic pain
    c. Increased pulse with acute pain
    d. Increased pulse and blood pressure with acute pain
60. A new patient is being assessed for pain. You should ask about:
    a. Location, intensity, quality, duration, variation, consequences, and aggravating factors
    b. Sleeping pattern, location, tension, depression, level of irritability, effect on marital relations
    c. Intensity, duration, variation, loss of sense of humor
    d. Quality of the pain, variation, location, effects on social life

UNIT THREE: ORGANIZATIONAL AND HEALTH POLICY ISSUES

1. The funding of senior centers falls under the Administration on Aging (AOA) programs. Select the Title program that funds these centers:
    a. Title 18
    b. Title IV
    c. Title 19
    d. Title 20
2. Home-delivered meals for older adults unable to obtain adequate nutrition is available through a variety of community sources. Select the statement that is accurate about home-delivered meals:
    a. Provides a home-health aid to cook meals for home-bound older adults
    b. Delivers meals to needy, home-bound older adults
    c. Delivers meals to the homes of older adults who desire them
    d. Delivers groceries to home-bound older adults who are able to cook their own meals
3. The interdisciplinary team approach to assisting patients with health care issues is preferable to an individual discipline approach because:
    a. Individual disciplines promote integrated problem-solving
    b. The individual discipline will focus on expert planning
    c. Teams with an interdisciplinary focus promote integrated problem-solving
    d. The interdisciplinary team will promote fragmented care delivery
4. Housing problems of older adults is provided for by:
    a. Ombudsman program of 1987
    b. OBRA Title X (Omnibus Budget Reconciliation Act)
    c. Older Americans Act of 1973
    d. Health Care Financing Administration (HCFA)
5. Mrs. Jones was admitted to Happy Acres Nursing Home last month. She is accustomed to eating six small meals a day at home. At Happy Acres, she is offered three main meals. Snacks do not seem to be available. She is complaining but without results. This may be an issue for:
    a. An ombudsman
    b. A social worker
    c. A nutritionist
    d. Nursing
6. Diagnosis-related groups (DRGs) is which type of payment reimbursement system?
    a. Retrospective
    b. Fee for service
    c. Prospective
    d. Per diem

7. Medicare Part B will reimburse for which service?
    a. Meals on Wheels
    b. Outpatient therapy
    c. Medications for older adults
    d. Personal care attendant
8. Prospective payment system (PPS) is a type of Medicare Part A reimbursement for which health care provider?
    a. Home health
    b. Physicians
    c. Skilled nursing facility
    d. Personal care facility
9. Medicare Select is what type of insurance plan?
    a. Health maintenance policy
    b. Medigap policy with restrictions
    c. Preferred service policy
    d. Medigap policy with highest premium prices
10. The Resident Assessment Instrument (RAI) is mandated for all nursing home residents **except:**
    a. Those in intermediate care beds
    b. Those in skilled care beds
    c. Those in personal care beds
    d. Those who have Medicare as the payor

UNIT FOUR: PROFESSIONAL ISSUES

1. Select the statement that best describes the purpose of an audit:
    a. To determine if quality criteria of patient care are met
    b. To determine promotions and merit pay raises
    c. To satisfy third-party insurance companies for reimbursement
    d. To be used as a vote of confidence for the administration
2. An audit team is established to determine the number of patients being readmitted with post–operative infections following orthopedic surgery. This is an example of which type of audit?
    a. Structure
    b. Process
    c. Outcome
    d. Departmental
3. Patient records are audited to determine how discharge teaching of foot care (with diabetic patients) is being done. This is an example of which type of audit?
    a. Structure
    b. Process
    c. Outcome
    d. Supervisory
4. Select the best description of a retrospective audit:
    a. It is performed while the patient is receiving services
    b. It is done with several patient interviews by the audit team
    c. It is aimed at future interventions after changes in nursing care
    d. It is performed after the patient receives the service
5. A nurse manager is asked by the director to develop a policy on absenteeism. The manager will:
    a. Assign it to the assistant head nurse who is closer to the staff nurse and grasps the problems of absenteeism better
    b. Develop a tool for standardization and evaluation
    c. Seek input from administration
    d. Seek input from those who are most frequently absent

6. The operating budget in an acute care setting:
   a. Is the budget for the operating room
   b. Is the budget for the operating room and PAR (post-anesthesia/recovery)
   c. Is the budget for the operating room, PAR, and surgical units
   d. Is the budget for the day-to-day activities of a unit or organization

7. Fixed costs are different from variable costs in budget preparation. Fixed costs include:
   a. Costs related to patient volume such as linens, supplies, and some salaries
   b. Equipment depreciation and interest on loans
   c. All full-time equivalents (FTEs)
   d. Major purchases such as cardiac monitors

8. Three major styles of leadership are:
   a. Autocratic, democratic, theocratic
   b. Autonomous, democratic, laissez-faire
   c. Transactional, intractable, theocratic
   d. Autocratic, democratic, laissez-faire

9. The first-line manager:
   a. Is the director of nursing over clinical nursing
   b. Is the vice president or chief nursing executive
   c. Is the head nurse
   d. Is any management title that is the highest in the organization

10. Manager tasks are:
    a. Planning, organizing, directing, delegating, and controlling
    b. Visionary, motivator, trustee, decision-maker
    c. Figurehead, spokesman, negotiator, decision-maker, delegator
    d. Leader, organizer, trustee, controller, delegator

11. The nurse manager identifies a problem on the unit that is compromising quality of care. Using the problem-solving or decision-making process, the manager analyzes the situation, determines possible solutions and alternatives, selects one, and implements it. The outcome is evaluated. What step in the process is missing?
    a. Focusing on the objectives
    b. Gathering data relating to the problem
    c. Organizing a workgroup
    d. Developing a strategic plan

12. Choose the answer that best describes the reason why nursing research is important:
    a. Improves nursing practice
    b. Competes with the medical knowledge base
    c. Changes health policy
    d. Both a and c

13. The purposes of nursing research are to:
    a. Describe, predict, and compare to medical studies
    b. Explain the processes of the nursing plan of care
    c. Identify, describe, explore, explain, predict, and control
    d. Control the patterns of investigation into practice issues

14. Which of the following steps is **not** within the conceptual phase of the research process:
    a. Identify the problem
    b. Review the literature
    c. Define the theoretical framework
    d. Interpret the results

15. Experimental and quasi-experimental designs have at least one thing in common:
    a. Manipulation of the independent variable
    b. One or more controls, including a control group
    c. Random assignment to groups
    d. Experimental results

16. Which of the following steps are within the empirical phase of the research process?
    a. Collect data, transcribe qualitative data, and code quantitative data
    b. Omit qualitative data
    c. Define the theoretical framework and select a research plan
    d. Communicate the findings
17. Which of the following steps are **not** within the analytic phase of the research process?
    a. Analyze the data
    b. Review the literature
    c. Interpret the results
    d. Examine the implications
18. Patients' rights in health care settings:
    a. Are ethics-based and have no force in law
    b. Include the right to refuse any treatment
    c. Are specified by the Constitution
    d. Are available only to those who have become incompetent
19. The right of privacy is:
    a. A constitutional interpretation
    b. Guaranteed by ANA standards
    c. Difficult to sustain in health care facilities
    d. Not a nursing responsibility
20. The notion of confidentiality:
    a. Protects an individual from unwanted visitors
    b. Promotes trust in professional relationships
    c. Provides punishment for nurses who disclose private information
    d. Arises from certain constitutional provisions
21. A nurse has a duty to prevent falls, which includes:
    a. Duty to assess the patient
    b. Duty to restrain persons with fall potential
    c. Duty to constantly observe all behavior
    d. Duty to give minimal assistance in ADLs
22. Responsibilities of the nurse include:
    a. Clean and repair equipment used on a daily basis
    b. Modify special equipment to meet the needs of each patient
    c. Select and use equipment in a responsible manner
    d. Enter into a maintenance agreement with private companies
23. The Uniform Anatomical Gift Act of 1987:
    a. Permits the taking of major organs without specific consent
    b. Provides a model for state acts regarding organ donation and distribution
    c. Has eliminated the shortage of organs
    d. Has had little effect on the decision to donate organs of loved ones who die
24. Organ donations may be made by:
    a. Anyone with a living will
    b. The family members of a person with a terminal illness
    c. Anyone over the age of 18 years
    d. A statement in a testamentary will
25. A donor of an organ:
    a. May not change his/her mind after consenting to a donation
    b. Can designate to whom the organ will go
    c. Can choose the physician/surgeon who will harvest the organ
    d. Is treated carefully in order to preserve the health of potentially donatable organs
26. Health care institutions must:
    a. Harvest all organs from patients who die in case they are usable by others
    b. Notify family members of the option to avoid donation of organs

c.   Inform the local organ procurement agency of all impending deaths

d.   Encourage organ donation by all terminally ill persons

27.   Organs donated by hepatitis-positive donors:

a.   Are immediately destroyed

b.   May be transplanted to AIDS patients

c.   Could be available to other hepatitis-positive patients who need organs

d.   Are used for research only

28.   The American Nurses Association Code of Ethics is:

a.   A law

b.   A nursing law

c.   Evidence of a practice standard

d.   All of the above

29.   The Code of Ethics:

a.   Demands certain behaviors in practice

b.   Provides guidance in dealing with ethical issues

c.   Describes required patient behaviors

d.   None of the above

30.   Code statements are based on:

a.   Medical ethics

b.   Legal tenets

c.   Beliefs about persons

d.   Hard-to-follow regulations

31.   Code statements deal with:

a.   Nursing responsibilities

b.   Patient behaviors

c.   Ethical dilemmas

d.   End-of-life issues

32.   Nurses are accountable for:

a.   Excellent patient care

b.   Communicating on a daily basis with other care providers

c.   Making hourly entries in the official patient record

d.   Providing safe care in a timely manner

33.   Nursing accountability means that:

a.   It is generally unwise to delegate nursing tasks

b.   Nurses are responsible for all of their own actions

c.   Nurses can transfer liability to physicians when physician orders are not appropriate for the patient

d.   Nurses will probably live in constant fear of lawsuits

34.   Safe and appropriate patient care includes:

a.   Timely assessments of patient status

b.   Weekly assessment of mental status

c.   Measurement of intake and output

d.   Contacting family members for authorization of all care

35.   Delegation:

a.   Includes assigning patient care to other staff members

b.   Means transferring the responsibility for certain tasks to unlicensed personnel

c.   Requires that the nurse teach the delegatee how to provide care assigned

d.   Cannot be done with nursing assistants

36.   When delegating nursing tasks:

a.   All authority for the task and its outcome are delegated

b.   It is always to other duly licensed personnel

c.   The nurse must evaluate whether the task can be safely delegated based on patient health status

d.   The nurse should directly observe the completion of the task

37. Bioethics is:
    a. The ethical study of life science
    b. The application of ethical theory to medical situations
    c. Not particularly useful to nursing
    d. Related to nursing values
38. Values may:
    a. Be related to bioethics
    b. Conflict with care
    c. Guide decisions and actions
    d. Not be appropriate to consider in care situations
39. Utilitarianism espouses:
    a. The greatest good for the greatest number
    b. The greatest good for important leaders
    c. Equal good for all law–abiding people
    d. Utilizing appropriate values
40. Deontological ethics espouses
    a. Firm moral principles
    b. Situational ethics
    c. Greatest good for the greatest number
    d. Moral acts in health care
41. In biomedical ethics, one of the most important principles is:
    a. Patient safety
    b. Adequate care for the elderly
    c. Patient self-determination
    d. Justice for all
42. Most nurses who enter the field of geriatric nursing do so for which of the following reasons?
    a. They have a sincere love of working with older adults
    b. An opportunity presented itself
    c. It was the only position they could secure
    d. Pay and benefits were better than other job offers
43. All of the following are true about research conferences **except:**
    a. Networking is usually a waste of time
    b. Research is presented for a varied audience
    c. Either poster or podium presentations may occur
    d. Publication of abstracts provides a rich source for research review
44. Which of the following best describes the role of the gerontological nurse in the acute care setting?
    a. Manager of human resources
    b. Advocate for use of community resources
    c. Early detector of diseases caused by hospitalization
    d. Organizational manager
45. State Boards of Nursing are regulatory agencies that are responsible for all of the following **except:**
    a. School of nursing curricula
    b. Licensure requirements
    c. Conducting hearings regarding violations of regulations
    d. Passing laws affecting the practice of nursing

Answers with Rationales: Practice Examination A

Unit One: Primary Care Considerations

1. b. According to the U.S. Census Bureau's mid-decade report, the fastest growing age group is the 85 and over group.

2. d. Skilled nursing care is required for 81% of older adults needing home health care services, while physical therapy is needed by 17%, social services by 9%, and homemaker/companion services by 23%.

3. b. The skin shows aging because of an absence of subcutaneous fat, decreased and less elastic collagen fibers, and thinning of the epithelial layer (Ebersole & Hess, 1998).

4. d. Normal phenomena of aging include loss of hearing and sound discrimination, increased peripheral vascular resistance because of less elasticity in arteries and veins, decreased ventilation/perfusion ratio with less gas exchange because of decreased chest wall compliance, change in AP diameter, and limited thoracic movement (Lueckenotte, 1996).

5. d. Intervertebral disk spaces narrow and the spinal column becomes compressed with aging. Slowed metabolic processes, which are normal with aging, affect bone as well as muscle tissue (Lueckenotte, 1996).

6. d. With fewer taste buds and decreased sensory cells, the elderly have less sensation in their oral cavity, reduced ability to sense hot and cold, and decreased sensitivity to smell, placing them at a safety risk (Luggen, et al, 1998).

7. b. Indirect or filtered light cuts glare, which is a problem because of decreased ability of the pupil to constrict. There is also lens and vitreous clouding, which causes light to scatter through the lens (Ebersole & Hess, 1998; Eliopoulos, 1997).

8. a. *Ageism* is a term that describes discrimination solely attributable to old age (Ebersole & Hess, 1998).

9. b. Suggested screening for preventive health maintenance is a yearly mammogram for women after age 50.

10. b. Alcoholism is a risk factor for malnutrition (Nutrition Screening Initiative, 1992).

11. d. Sodium intake should not exceed 2400 mg/day (Tyson, 1999).

12. a. Regular exercise at least three times per week is recommended (Tyson, 1999).

13. c. Orem's theory focuses on the patient's return to self-care (Orem, 1995).

14. b. "Residents' responses indicated that if they had actively participated in the decision to be admitted, the adjustment to the long-term care facility was easier." (Iwasiw, Goldenberg, MacMaster, et al, 1996)

15. d. "Relocation is a stressor, but there is not enough evidence to determine if the stress of intra-institutional relocation for people with dementia is harmful, beneficial, or neither." (Kovach, 1998)

16. b. Perception of the illness may have cultural/ethnic influences on the way in which the patient interprets the symptoms and meaning of the illness. The nurse needs to have examined personal feelings regarding care for people of differing cultural/ethnic backgrounds before direct patient contact.

17. d. Older adults who are oriented to the past as a cultural legacy are reluctant to try new treatments but will if the explanation is thorough and done with sensitivity.

18. c. Orem's theory is entitled *self-care deficit theory*. There are many terms that are used in the theory such as *self-care deficit, self-care demands*. Other nursing systems involve wholly compensatory, partly compensatory, and supportive-educative care. Because independence of older adult patients is promoted, Orem's focus on self-care is useful in gerontological nursing.

19. a. All answers are part of Roy's adaptation theory, but the focus is on adaptation in the different modes, systems, and stimuli.

20. d. Only d is correct; all others are definitions of other theories; cellular DNA and connective tissue interact with free radicals damaging DNA; normal defense mechanisms are weakened over time and eventually irreparable damage occurs.

21. b. Biological clock theory proposes that we inherit a program of predetermined cell divisions that "play out," as seen in graying hair, thymus atrophy, menopause, etc.

22. d. By helping Mr. J. use his diet knowledge to meet his needs, the nurse is allowing Mr. J. to make his own decisions and to relate new information to old information. Once he understands meal planning, Mr. J. might decide to eliminate or reduce the twinkies.

23. c. Behavioral theory is based on reward and punishment. The reward for giving up twinkies is potential wellness; the punishment for not giving them up is exacerbation of the disease process.

24. c. High-quality comfort or palliative care is the main goal of hospice services.

25. c. Hospice services can be provided wherever needed by the patient and family if the criteria for services are met.

26. b. Depression may become life threatening (suicide) if not treated, but it does not qualify for hospice services because it is not considered to be a terminal condition with less than 6 months of expected survival.

UNIT TWO: MAJOR HEALTH PROBLEMS

1. d. Conducting an interview with an 82-year-old should include sensitivity for a potential of a hearing deficit and the need for personal responses to remain private.

2. b. Memberships in church or social organizations can provide a foundation for receiving social support when family members are unavailable for any reason.

3. b. The loss of chewing, whether because of poor dental condition or lack of dentures, has a negative effect on the nutritional state of the elderly patient.

4. a. The most common signs and symptoms of left-sided heart failure are those related to pulmonary congestion, dyspnea, rales, anxiety, cough, cyanosis, frothy white sputum, and mental status changes secondary to hypoxemia.

5. c. The most common signs and symptoms of right-sided heart failure are peripheral edema, jugular venous distension, enlarged liver and spleen, and distention of the abdomen. Right-sided failure is the inability of the right side of the heart to effectively pump blood from the body into the lungs, resulting in a back-up of blood into the venous circulatory system.

6. b. Because of an increased sedentary lifestyle, many older adults will not experience exertional dyspnea with acute congestive heart failure. Orthopnea and nocturnal dyspnea also may not occur in older adults. Usually the presenting symptom will be a dry cough. When symptoms are present, there is usually a complaint of generalized weakness, anorexia, and fatigue. Increased insomnia, nightmares, and anxiety are not uncommon.

7. c. Changes in *preload* can lead to peripheral edema, pulmonary vascular congestion, pulmonary edema, and/or decreased alveolar oxygenation complications. Decreased *afterload* is linked to decreased arterial oxygenation and decreased oxygen saturation while increased afterload can cause reduced peripheral tissue perfusion, resulting from arterial vasoconstriction. Reduced *contractility* is linked to increased cardiac workload, fluid volume excess, increased sodium retention, and activity intolerance. Increased *heart rate* leads to reduced myocardial oxygen demand complications. Left ventricular ejection fraction is not a determinant.

8. d. *Chronic obstructive pulmonary disease (COPD)* is a blanket term for three separate yet overlapping conditions: asthma, chronic bronchitis, and emphysema. Tuberculosis is not considered a chronic obstructive pulmonary disease because it is a disease caused by infection with the mycobacterium *Tuberculosis hominis*.

9. c. Smoking contributes to the risk of developing emphysema and other chronic lung and cardiac conditions. Smoking damages the elastic nature of lung tissue, leading to emphysema.

10. d. Enlargement of the air spaces results in hyperinflation of the lungs and increased total lung capacity. However, once the air is in the alveolar sacs, it is trapped and there is great difficulty in exhaling the air volume.

11. d. Food consistency should not be so thin that it will potentiate aspiration; liquid food is inappropriate unless other conditions require it; bed level needs to be elevated to near sitting position during meals; tube feedings are reserved for specific deficits in cognition, consciousness, or aspiration.

12. d. All other answers are associated with peptic ulcer disease except for the use of antacids before or after meals.

13. c. Weight reduction decreases intra-abdominal pressure, thereby decreasing the tendency to reflux into the esophagus; fats decrease emptying of the stomach; lying down increases pressure and is a cause of reflux; fluids should be limited during meals.

14. c. Normal age-related changes in the older female include a decrease in vaginal acidity, decreased breast size, narrowing and shortening of the vagina, and a thinning of the vaginal wall (Ebersole & Hess, 1998).

15. b. The prostate gland is located below and under the bladder. A thin milky fluid is produced on ejaculation, and hyperplasia of the gland is a slow process. Testosterone increases the risk of BPH (Ebersole & Hess, 1998).

16. a. Postoperative teaching after TURP includes the following: teach the patient that he should not lift heavy articles for at least 7 to 10 days after surgery as bleeding can occur; instruct the patient that his urine may be slightly pink-tinged with some burning initially; advise the patient that there are no fluid restrictions; and teach the patient Kegel exercises to increase perineal muscle strength and decrease the incidence of incontinence (Ebersole & Hess, 1998).

17. d. Multiple sexual partners and a diet high in fat and low in beta-carotene increase the risk of prostate cancer. Genetics are a factor, especially in first-line relatives (Zaccagnini, 1999).

18. c. A PSA >4 ng/ml may signify prostate cancer. New onset of impotence, decrease in libido, and a hard nonmovable nodule on digital rectal exam may also signify prostate cancer (Miller, 1997).

19. a. The decreased blood volume leads to a decreased glomerular filtration and reduction in urinary output; respiratory rate would increase; apical and radial pulse should remain the same; hypokalemia occurs because sodium is retained while potassium is excreted.

20. d. The lumbar pain is a sign of an acute hemolytic transfusion reaction; the pain is caused by hemolysis, agglutination, and capillary plugging in the kidneys; all other choices would permit additional blood to be infused, leading to potential irreversible damage and/or death.

21. c. Type I is a diagnostic category for osteoporosis that occurs in women who are postmenopausal or have had an oophorectomy.

22. d. Clinically, the patient will tolerate Fosamax better if it is given on an empty stomach, without taking medications or food for 30 minutes following the dose and without lying down for at least 30 minutes after the dose.

23. d. Skin dryness is common among older adults but does not place them at risk of a thermoregulatory crisis; all other answers are true for risk factors of hypothermia or hyperthermia.

24. c. Excessive thirst, excessive hunger, and frequent urination are caused by the body's inability to correctly metabolize glucose; irritability and confusion are associated with hypoglycemia; frequent urination occurs throughout the 24-hour day.

25. d. Knowledge of the signs and treatment for hypoglycemia or hyperglycemia is critical for patient's health and well-being and essential for survival; foot care is important but not critical; insulin is not a factor in NIDDM; blood glucose monitoring with a finger-stick is preferred.

26. d. Memory loss is not a symptom that is exclusively associated with HIV/AIDS in the older person.

27. a. Educational programs related to HIV/AIDS and the older adult should be distributed to senior centers, AARP, social groups, and other organizations that are primarily aimed at older and/or retired persons.

28. d. Antigen.

29. c.   HIV/AIDS is a disorder of the immune system.
30. b.   Routines and familiarity with activities or the environment provide for a sense of security; change is poorly tolerated; challenging activities can be frustrating; attention span limits activities.
31. b.   Confabulation is used as a defense mechanism against embarrassment caused by lapse of memory; the patient fills in the blanks in memory by making up details.
32. a.   Delirium is an acute transient confusional state having a rapid onset and brief duration. It is often associated with an infection; delirium reverses on initiation of treatment for the underlying cause.
33. d.   Modifiable risk factors are hypertension, cholesterol elevation, and smoking.
34. b.   Everything listed is a possible symptom of stroke except orthopnea and shortness of breath.
35. d.   Alcohol is a stimulant that will prevent sound sleep; all other choices are recommended to be included in patient teaching plans.
36. c.   The critical factor is personal perception of an event. The impact on self-esteem and sense of capability will be greater than the magnitude of the event (Ebersole & Hess, 1998).
37. a.   The MiniMental State (MMS) Assessment Tool measures orientation and cognitive function. It is designed to identify four levels of functioning. If a clinical screening on cognition is to be performed, MMS will likely be the most valid and reliable (Ebersole & Hess, 1998).
38. b.   Wanderers move from place to place aimlessly. They tend to walk away without purpose (Luggen, 1996).
39. b.   Pathological grieving involves inability to express feelings about losses, failure to acknowledge and accept losses; there are alterations in social adjustments, inability to re-establish relationships (Isaacs, 1996).
40. a.   Drugs most commonly used in the older adult for anxiety are buspirone and ativan (Luggen, 1996).
41. a.   Dry skin.
42. a.   Oatmeal and Epsom salts are very soothing for itchy skin that results from a variety of causes.
43. a.   Benign lesions; actinic keratoses are pre-cancerous lesions that must be surgically removed.
44. c.   Squamous cell carcinoma presents as flesh-colored nodule, progresses to red, then a hard, wart-like gray ulcerating or indurating lesion with raised borders. It metastasizes and requires surgical excision. A general rule for melanoma is a lesion that changes shape, size, and color.
45. b.   Cerumen, or ear wax, accumulates in the external ear and blocks sound transmission to the inner ear, a conduction loss.
46. b.   Some of the drugs known to cause ototoxicity are gentamycin, furosemide, salicylates, streptomycin, ibuprofen.
47. d.   High tones are not heard well; use low tones. Speak so lip reading can be "part of hearing"; speak to the good ear or the ear that hears best.
48. d.   More than 90% of those >65 years of age need vision correction.
49. b.   Only b is correct definition of arcus senilis; all other answers are incorrect definitions.
50. a.   Avoid increased IOP for 2 to 3 weeks after cataract surgery; for example, straining during bowel movements, bending down, lifting heavy objects.
51. c.   Eye professionals should check IOP in all people >40 years of age; glaucoma is the #1 cause of blindness among African Americans (second leading cause in the United States).
52. a.   Polypharmacy is the excessive or unnecessary use of medications (Pepper, 1999).
53. c.   Drug absorption is the first element of pharmacokinetics (Podrazik & Schwartz, 1999).
54. b.   Although a hypothetical volume, the concept of volume of distribution is necessary to understand how a drug is distributed evenly throughout the body (Podrazik & Schwartz, 1999).
55. b.   The loss of lean body mass (digoxin is largely muscle bound) and loss of renal clearance with advanced age create the need for careful monitoring of serum levels in a drug with a narrow toxic-therapeutic range (Podrazik & Schwartz, 1999).

56. d. Nurses have long known that pain cannot always be linked to actual injury or tissue damage. Pain is whatever, whenever, wherever the patient says it is.

57. c. A number of studies have been conducted on the prevalence of pain in community-based older adults. Results are that 25% to 50% have pain.

58. d. Most residents in long-term care facilities have a number of chronic health problems that cause pain. Research data reveals that up to 85% of residents have pain. It also appears that many of these residents do not receive pain medication for their pain.

59. b. Acute pain produces changes in vital signs: increase in pulse, blood pressure, respirations. It also produces symptoms not present in chronic pain such as diaphoresis, tension, facial grimacing, crying, guarding, restlessness, and immobility of the painful part.

60. a. All are correct, but a. is more complete and thorough an assessment for a new patient.

UNIT THREE: ORGANIZATIONAL AND HEALTH POLICY ISSUES

1. d. Title 20 funding from the AOA supports senior centers and their programs.

2. b. Home-delivered meals are available for those older adults unable to obtain adequate food from other sources and who are needy and home-bound.

3. c. The interdisciplinary team can provide multiple insights into total goal setting; this team approach is not fragmented. Although individual planning and problem-solving are important, the team approach is most effective, especially with older adults who have complex health problems.

4. c. The Older Americans Act (1973) provides programs for nutrition, transportation, mental health services, housing, ombudsmen, training, etc.

5. a. Resident rights, including the availability of snacks, are protected by ombudsmen in nursing facilities. Ombudsmen are provided for by the Older Americans Act (1973).

6. c. DRGs is a system that has predetermined a cost for services; it does not consider exceptions for standard conditions. It provides a set amount of dollars for a specified condition.

7. b. Part B of Medicare is limited to medically necessary doctor's services, outpatient hospital care, and some services provided as medical support services (radiology).

8. a. In 1996, PPS was mandated to include payment to home health agencies for services (with restrictions).

9. b. Medicare Select is a Medigap policy that provides services within a specific physician/health facility network at a lower cost than a standard Medigap policy.

10. c. RAI includes the minimum data set (MDS), and is not necessary for residents in personal care beds.

UNIT FOUR: PROFESSIONAL ISSUES

1. a. Audits provide a guide to determine if the designated quality criteria of patient care are being met.

2. c. Outcome audits determine the results of nursing interventions and changes in patients' health status.

3. b. Process audits measure how care is provided and are task oriented.

4. d. The retrospective audit is done following a patient's discharge. It is less time-consuming and costly, and accuracy depends on documentation in the medical record.

5. c. Policy is a comprehensive statement used to guide decision-making. It is usually developed at the highest level of management with input from managers and staff.

6. d. Operating budget includes revenues and expenses that occur daily on units, departments, and organizations.

7. b. Fixed costs include management and some staff salaries; for example, minimal staff requirements in an intensive care unit. Fixed costs include equipment depreciation, interest on loans, and any items that do not change when the patient census changes.

8. d. The *autocratic* leader does not consider group input; he/she makes all decisions. The *democratic* leader considers group input and includes the group in decision-making. The *laissez-faire* leader allows autonomy in the group.

9. c. The first-line manager is the head nurse or the manager who is one level higher than the staff employees who are supervised by the manager. The first-line manager's primary responsibility is the service/product, which is patient care.

10. a. There are five tasks of any manager: planning, organizing, directing or leading, delegating or empowering, and controlling or evaluating.

11. b. After clear identification of a problem to be solved or decision to be made, the manager must gather data relating to the problem or issue. The third step is analysis of the situation or problem and studying the influences. Step four is determining potential solutions and alternatives, then choosing one to implement. And, finally, the outcome is evaluated.

12. d. Nursing research is important for improvement and accountability of nursing practice, credibility of the nursing profession, and changes in health policy.

13. c. The purposes of nursing research are to identify, describe, explore, explain, predict, and control.

14. d. The conceptual phase involves reading, thinking, discussing, and conceptualizing.

15. a. Quasi-experimental designs involve manipulation of the independent variable but no control group or randomization.

16. a. The empirical phase involves the collection of data and the preparation of these data for analysis.

17. b. The analytic phase involves analysis and interpretation to make the data meaningful.

18. c. Patients' rights belong to every citizen of the state or country (United States) and are capable of being enforced by law.

19. a. The right of privacy is considered a constitutional protection as interpreted by the Supreme Court.

20. b. The statutory foundation assigned to confidentiality provides a legal status to relationships between and among professionals.

21. a. Assessment is a primary duty of a nurse in determining risk for falls.

22. c. When equipment is selected for a specific use with a patient, the nurse must be familiar with and able to operate the equipment effectively.

23. b. Uniform Anatomical Gift Act (1987) was enacted to alleviate the shortage of donated organs and to provide a model for states.

24. c. Anatomical gifts of all or any part of the human body may be made by any person over the age of 18.

25. b. A donor of an anatomical gift may designate a recipient.

26. c. Mandatory notification of all deaths by hospitals and health care agencies became law in 1998.

27. c. Organs donated by hepatitis-positive donors may go to similar patients in the belief that a relatively healthy organ is better than a failing organ in an ill patient.

28. c. The ANA can set practice standards as the professional association representing the nursing profession.

29. b. Guidelines for dealing with ethical issues can be found in the ANA Code of Ethics.

30. c. The ANA code for professional behavior is based on beliefs about people and the way in which they expect to be given nursing care.

31. a. The Code of Ethics deals with nursing responsibilities to be fulfilled that follow accepted professional standards and ethics.

32. d. Accountability includes providing safe care that is delivered in a timely way. Perfection may not be possible, but communication can be continuous.

33. b. Accountability of nursing actions requires that nurses accept responsibility for all of their actions.

34. a. Nurses have a duty to perform timely assessments of the patient's status and follow through on untoward findings.

35. a. Delegation is a method for organizing patient care in a safe manner by assigning care-giving personnel specific duties.

36. c. Patient care delegation must be done with an understanding of the patient's needs and the staff members' qualifications.

37. b. Bioethics is the application of ethical actions in medical situations.

38. c. Values are the result of making decisions based on an understanding of right and wrong.

39. a. Utilitarianism is a system of ethical decision-making that is based on the "greatest good" principle.

40. a. Deontological ethics is a system of ethical decision-making based on the discovery and confirmation of a set or morals or rules that govern ethical dilemmas.

41. d. Biomedical ethics involves justice for all without favoritism.

42. b. While some nurses are attracted to the field because of their love for working with older adults, most are in the field by accident or because of the federal funds support.

43. a. Networking is one of the long-lasting benefits of attending a research conference.

44. c. Options a and d are primarily roles in long-term care; b is the role of the community nurse. Only c is carried out in acute care.

45. d. Options a, b, and c are functions of the State Boards of Nursing. Boards of Nursing cannot pass laws.

PRACTICE EXAMINATION B

UNIT ONE: PRIMARY CARE CONSIDERATIONS

1. Admission to a nursing home is prompted by which of the following conditions in older adults:
   a. Inability to shop and cook for themselves
   b. Following discontinuance of driving a car
   c. When bowel and bladder incontinence are present
   d. Following the immediate family members moving out of the area
2. An age-related change that affects kidney function is:
   a. Decreased bladder capacity
   b. Decreased number of functioning nephrons
   c. Increased glomerular filtration rate
   d. Increased reabsorption of tubules
3. Normal aging changes within the cardiovascular system include:
   a. Decreased peripheral vascular resistance and increased pumping action
   b. Fewer numbers of pacemaker cells and decreased elasticity of vessels
   c. Increased blood flow and increased cardiac output
   d. Increased contractility and hypertrophy
4. The elderly patient is unable to resist disease processes as readily as the younger patient because of:
   a. Enhanced WBC production
   b. Increased inflammatory response
   c. Increased response to immunization
   d. Reduced T-cell activity
5. Which of the following factors can have a negative affect on relationships among the elderly population?
   a. Close sustaining relationships
   b. Community resource allocations
   c. Organizations and neighborhoods
   d. Shrinking social networks
6. Which individual action will help to prevent or eliminate ageism?
   a. Be informed about facts on aging
   b. Encourage older persons to retire when they reach age 65
   c. Ignore your own attitudes about growing old
   d. Avoid discussing age-related issues with the elderly
7. Prejudice is:
   a. A process of stereotyping against or in favor of an age group
   b. Beliefs or attitudes based on a stereotype about older persons
   c. Inappropriate negative treatment of older persons as a result of a negative belief
   d. A negative emotion toward older people
8. A patient is newly diagnosed with diabetes. The identified nursing diagnosis is "health maintenance, altered: related to knowledge deficit of treatment regimen." The best goal for this nursing diagnosis is:
   a. Patient will accurately administer insulin by 3/1/02
   b. Patient will understand how to give medication by time of discharge
   c. Patient will receive instruction about insulin 15 minutes each day
   d. Patient will learn about signs/symptoms of hypoglycemia and hyperglycemia
9. Knowing that older adults have a high degree of osteoporosis, the nurse should urge older adults to make which of the following adjustments in diet?
   a. Limit coffee intake to 2 cups/day
   b. Take calcium supplements after age 70

    c.   Limit time outdoors

    d.   Sit with legs elevated during the day

10. The influenza vaccine should be recommended for which of the following adults?

    a.   A 75-year-old woman newly admitted to a nursing home

    b.   A 50-year-old male with glaucoma

    c.   A 60-year-old newly diagnosed patient with emphysema who has had the vaccine within the last 3 months

    d.   Those adults who have had the pneumovac vaccine

11. In discussing complementary healing methods with older adults, it would be important to include which of the following?

    a.   None of the complementary healing methods should cause any harm and might be worth a try

    b.   It is important that medications you are taking be discussed with your doctor, whether they are prescription or over-the-counter medications

    c.   It has been shown that the placebo effect may be responsible for the outcomes of most complementary therapies

    d.   At this time, none of the complementary therapies are covered by health insurance

12. When doing an inservice at your nursing home, the nurse emphasizes which of the following as *true* regarding tuberculosis?

    a.   Screening for TB is needed because of concern for the safety of health care workers and patients

    b.   The immune function of older adults makes them less susceptible to TB than younger adults

    c.   Biannual testing for TB is recommended

    d.   Reactivation of an earlier exposure/infection does not generally occur

13. Territoriality can be defined as:

    a.   Definite visible borders surrounding an individual's possessions and home

    b.   Limiting a person's autonomy and self-identity

    c.   Protection of the invisible space surrounding a person and seen as an extension of that person

    d.   Space surrounding an individual that the person feels comfortable having others invade

14. Autonomy:

    a.   Is of the highest value to older adults

    b.   Cannot be provided for without sacrificing safety

    c.   Is guaranteed by law

    d.   Is characterized by disinterest in others' needs

15. Cumming and Henry in 1961 developed a theory that social equilibrium is achieved by reciprocal withdrawal between society and older adults to their mutual satisfaction. This theory is entitled:

    a.   Continuity

    b.   Activity

    c.   Subculture

    d.   Disengagement

16. Rose's subculture theory is based on the belief that:

    a.   Older adults come from a cohort that does not change and is distinct as a subculture in their later life

    b.   The subculture is a response to a loss of status

    c.   Older adults prefer their own company and choose to belong to a subculture of peers

    d.   Forming a subculture is a positive response to aging

17. In Erikson's developmental theory of aging:

    a.   The person accepts the past and maintains integrity or cannot and despairs

    b.   The person has an innate hierarchy of needs that must be accepted to maintain integrity

    c.   The person has certain tasks, such as adapting to change, changing roles, death

    d.   To maintain integrity, the person must be creative, have values, be spiritual

18.   The family life cycle includes six stages, one of which is:

    a.   The family unit as a complex social system

    b.   The provision of basics, belonging, and self-actualization

    c.   The adjustment to the specific tasks of aging, such as adjusting to loss

    d.   Later life, or accepting shifting generational roles and death

19.   In assessing the learning needs of a patient, what might be a good first question?

    a.   What do you know about high blood pressure?

    b.   Do you understand the nature of hypertension?

    c.   What did your primary care provider tell you about high blood pressure?

    d.   Does hypertension run in your family?

20.   When an educator asks a patient to take a written test after a teaching session, what is the educator doing?

    a.   Validating the learning that has occurred

    b.   Determining what the learner has learned and how well the teacher has taught

    c.   Demonstrating the value of the teaching that took place

    d.   Showing the learner his/her progress

21.   In a normal learning situation, who ultimately determines what and how much the learner learns? The:

    a.   Educator

    b.   Patient

    c.   Primary care provider

    d.   Patient's family

Scenario: M. W. is an 80-year-old woman with a past medical history of hypertension, congestive heart failure, and dementia. She has been a resident at Golden Days Nursing Home for 3 years. The staff nurses report than when M. W. was first admitted to the nursing home she was very active and constantly walked the halls and participated in the daily programs such as bingo and crafts. In the last 6 months, however, her functional and cardiovascular status have declined and she is unable to ambulate independently. She has poor nutritional intake, which has resulted in her losing 15 pounds during the last 3 months. M. W.'s daughter is her legal guardian and has stated that her mother told her that she did not want any extraordinary measures taken to extend her life—"When it is my time, please let me go peacefully." Her daughter asked if her mother could be cared for by the hospice teams that she has seen some of the other nursing home residents and their families receive services from.

22.   What are the admitting diagnoses that would qualify M.W. for hospice services?

    a.   Failure to thrive

    b.   End-stage cardiovascular disease

    c.   End-stage dementia

    d.   All of the above

23.   Select the order in which phases of grief usually occur when an older adult encounters a significant loss:

    a.   Denial, anger, bargaining, depression, and acceptance

    b.   Shock, denial, anger, separation, and acceptance

    c.   Denial, bargaining, separation, and resolution

    d.   Shock, anger, depression, acceptance, and resolution

24.   Pathological signs of grieving include:

    a.   Feeling of sadness on the first anniversary of the significant loss

    b.   Suicide ideation, weight loss

    c.   Increased social activity with volunteerism

    d.   Increased number of losses

UNIT TWO: MAJOR HEALTH PROBLEMS

1. Which of the following are important considerations when choosing a functional assessment tool/instrument?
    a. Reliability and validity
    b. Time required to administer
    c. Safety concerns in administering the tool
    d. All of the above

2. When performing a cultural assessment with a non-English-speaking immigrant, newly arrived in the United States, the best type of assessment tool is:
    a. The one generally used for all patients to reduce the embarrassment of being an immigrant
    b. Referring all non-English-speaking patients to an interpreter in their native language
    c. Using a structured assessment tool that is specific for "non-English as a first language" patients
    d. Having a family member who speaks some English help with the assessment

3. Which statement best describes a physical assessment:
    a. Is a process to gather objective data about the patient
    b. Involves being completed in one brief session
    c. Requires minimal observation of the patient
    d. Involves one method to gather needed information

4. Current research suggests that significant differences exist between men and women in the manifestation and clinical features of coronary artery disease. Which of the following statements is *false?*
    a. The most common initial symptom of coronary artery disease in women is angina
    b. Women tend to have fewer Q waves and ST segment changes with chest pain
    c. Men experience chest pain longer than women before diagnosis
    d. Initial signs and symptoms of coronary artery disease are more atypical (including epigastric pain and shortness of breath)

5. There are many risk factors for cardiovascular disease. Four of these risk factors are considered the "deadly quartet." Which of the following is *not* one of these four?
    a. Hypertension
    b. Cigarette smoking
    c. Diabetes
    d. Obesity

6. Which of the following statements regarding hypertension is *true?*
    a. Isolated systolic hypertension is the result of normal aging so therapy is rarely indicated
    b. Hypertension in the older adult is associated with reduced peripheral vascular resistance and normal renin
    c. According to the Sixth Report of the Joint National Committee on Detection, Evaluation, and Treatment of High Blood Pressure, a 80-year-old woman with an average blood pressure of 158/92 is considered hypertensive
    d. Nonpharmacological treatment of hypertension is achievable if salt is restricted to 1 g a day

7. Mr. Christopher Lee, an 83-year-old nursing home resident, is found on the floor at 4:00 AM, presumed to have had a syncopal episode. He is confused and short of breath and begins vomiting. You recall the day nurse reported he had been complaining of increased weakness. Mr. Lee is experiencing:
    a. An acute myocardial infarction
    b. Acute congestive heart failure
    c. Angina
    d. Third-degree heart block

8. Mrs. Joy is complaining of severe pain in her lower extremity. You suspect she probably has peripheral arterial disease with a possible occlusion. Before you telephone the physician, what are the other symptoms you would assess for?
    a. Pallor when limb is dependent, red when elevated; warm and shiny skin
    b. Brawny (reddish-brown), cyanotic if dependent; cold with stasis ulcers

    c.   Brawny in color, cyanotic if dependent; cold, shiny skin; stasis ulcers

    d.   Pallor when limb is elevated, red when dependent; cold, shiny skin; pulselessness

9.   While listening to Mr. J's lungs, you hear adventitious sounds. He has told you that he has been losing weight lately, has night sweats, with a dull chest ache that never seems to go away. He states that he often has red-streaked sputum. Your first nursing action is to:

    a.   Excuse yourself and seek an isolation mask before continuing the assessment

    b.   Call for a STAT chest x-ray to rule out bacterial pneumonia

    c.   Report Mr. J. to the infection control officer before any further contact

    d.   Take a specimen of the sputum and continue the assessment as you were doing

10.   Mrs. Lang is being treated in the home for pulmonary tuberculosis. To help control the spread of the disease to her children and grandchildren, the nurse should instruct the patient and family to:

    a.   Have all family members sit at least 8 feet away from Mrs. Lang

    b.   Keep all personal articles away from the family members

    c.   Open windows in each room slightly to allow a good airflow throughout the house

    d.   Avoid putting used dishes in the dishwasher with the rest of the family's dishes

11.   When performing the initial history and physical assessment of a patient with a tentative diagnosis of peptic ulcer, the nurse would expect the patient to describe the pain as:

    a.   Gnawing epigastric pain or boring pain in the back

    b.   Sudden, sharp abdominal pain, increasing in intensity

    c.   Heartburn and substernal discomfort when lying down

    d.   Located in the right shoulder and preceded by nausea

12.   The primary care provider orders enteric precautions for a patient with hepatitis A. In addition to standard precautions, the isolation procedures that must be followed are:

    a.   A private room is required and the door must be kept closed

    b.   Persons entering the room must wear a gown, a mask, and gloves

    c.   Gowns and gloves must be worn only when handling the patient's soiled linen, dishes, or utensils

    d.   A gown and gloves must be worn when handling articles possibly contaminated by urine or feces

13.   When teaching a patient about the signs of colorectal cancer, the nurse stresses that the most common complaint of persons with colorectal cancer is:

    a.   Abdominal pain

    b.   Rectal bleeding

    c.   Change in bowel habits

    d.   Change in caliber of stools

14.   Which of the following is a *true* statement about older adults and sexual intercourse?

    a.   The response to sexual stimulation is slower, less intense, and shorter in duration

    b.   Refractory time shortens for the male

    c.   Hormonal changes in the female result in inability of the uterus to respond during intercourse

    d.   The older adult male is able to have another erection within 3 to 4 hours after the first orgasm

15.   Which of the following would be the most appropriate goal for a patient with urinary incontinence?

    a.   Patient will use Attends as needed

    b.   Patient will lessen the risk factors that potentiate the occurrence of incontinence

    c.   Patient will receive instruction in bladder training

    d.   Patient will receive instruction in Kegel exercises for urge and stress incontinence

16.   Bacterial count in a midstream specimen that indicates a UTI is:

    a.   100 colonies per 100 ml/urine

    b.   1000 colonies per 100 ml/urine

    c.   10,000 colonies per 100 ml/urine

    d.   100,000 colonies per 100 ml/urine

17. Which of the following would be a correctly stated nursing diagnosis for end-stage renal disease (ESRD)?
    a. Decubitus ulcers related to pruritis
    b. Electrolyte balance due to decreased kidney function
    c. Coping, ineffective individual: depression with suicidal ideation related to extreme stress from chronic life-threatening disease
    d. Altered family coping because of chronic illness; feelings of hopelessness about patient's destiny of death

18. Schilling test is ordered for an older patient suspected of having pernicious anemia. The nurse recognizes that the primary purpose of the Schilling test is to determine the patient's ability to:
    a. Produce vitamin B_{12}
    b. Absorb vitamin B_{12}
    c. Store vitamin B_{12}
    d. Digest vitamin B_{12}

19. Osteoarthritis is a disease that primarily affects:
    a. The spinal vertebrae
    b. Knees, hips, and fingers
    c. Toes, spine, and cervical vertebrae
    d. Fingers and toes

20. When assessing a patient with Graves' disease, the nurse should expect to find:
    a. Constipation, dry skin, and weight gain
    b. Lethargy, weight gain, and forgetfulness
    c. Weight loss, exophthalmos, and restlessness
    d. Weight loss, protruding eyeballs, and lethargy

21. A practice that will help an older adult lower dietary sodium intake is:
    a. Avoiding the use of carbonated beverages
    b. Using an artificial sweetener in coffee
    c. Increasing the use of dairy products
    d. Using catsup for cooking and flavoring foods

22. Mrs. Able is diagnosed with an electrolyte imbalance. When monitoring for hyponatremia, the nurse should assess for:
    a. Dry skin
    b. Confusion
    c. Tachycardia
    d. Pale coloring

23. Older persons may not be diagnosed until late in the course of AIDS infection because:
    a. Older persons do not seek medical attention as often as younger people
    b. Symptoms of AIDS may be confused with other conditions commonly seen in older persons because providers do not routinely screen this age group for HIV
    c. AIDS is very rare in older persons
    d. Older persons do not develop symptoms of AIDS until very late in the disease

24. An opportunistic infection is one that:
    a. Occurs only in persons 50 years of age or above
    b. Will result in serious illness and death within a very short period of time, usually less than 30 days
    c. Never causes serious illness, even in the immunocompromised
    d. Is an infection commonly occurring in patients with decreased immune function but rarely seen in persons with a normal immune system

25. Risk factors for HIV/AIDS infection in older persons include all of the following **except:**
    a. Failure to be screened for the bacteria causing AIDS
    b. Blood transfusion before 1985

    c.   Homosexual and/or bisexual behaviors

    d.   Declining use of condoms in older persons

26.   Changes in the immune functioning of older persons include:

    a.   Diminished response to vaccines

    b.   Decreased resistance to bacterial, fungal, and viral infections

    c.   Delayed or diminished hypersensitivity reaction

    d.   All of the above

27.   Each of the following is true related to infections in the elderly **except:**

    a.   Older persons are less likely to exhibit classic signs and symptoms of infection

    b.   Mortality rates are higher for older persons with serious infections than for other age groups

    c.   Elderly persons are less likely to report illness, take medication, and follow health care provider recommendations when they become infected

    d.   Elderly persons are more likely to become infected than younger persons

28.   Serious complications of stroke are common, and nurses have a strong role in prevention of these complications. They are:

    a.   Incontinence, pulmonary emboli, dysphagia

    b.   Dysarthria, incontinence, vein thrombosis

    c.   Urinary incontinence, depression, pressure sores

    d.   Labile affect, dysphagia, incontinence

29.   Incidence of Parkinson's disease is:

    a.   Greatest in 50- to 60-year-old adults

    b.   Greatest in 61- to 70-year-old adults

    c.   Greatest in 71- to 84-year-old adults

    d.   Greatest in 85- to 94-year-old adults

30.   Parkinson's disease is caused by:

    a.   Increased dopamine, resulting in tremor and muscle rigidity

    b.   Decreased dopamine, resulting in motor deficits and motor rigidity

    c.   Diminished serotonin receptors, resulting in tremor and rigidity

    d.   Increased serotonin production that overwhelms receptors, blocking transmission and causing motor deficits and muscle rigidity

31.   Mrs. James is an 80-year-old woman who has had Parkinson's disease for 15 years. She has masked facies, bradykinesia (slowed movements), resting tremor of the fingers on her left hand, muscle rigidity, and depression. She takes levodopa and benadryl at night for sleep. Nursing management of Mrs. James should include:

    a.   Assessing her diet for protein, which inhibits levodopa absorption; determining that she takes levodopa on an empty stomach; looking for drug toxicity because of the benadryl; supporting physical therapy in her treatment regimen

    b.   Assessing her diet for acid products, which slow levodopa absorption; ensuring that she takes levodopa after meals or with milk; looking for levodopa enhancement with the benadryl

    c.   Assessing her diet for protein content because high protein enhances levodopa absorption; ensuring that she takes levodopa on an empty stomach with 6 to 8 oz water; looking for toxicity of levodopa with benadryl, an anticholinergic

    d.   Assessing her diet for fat content because fat decreases absorption of levodopa; ensuring that she takes levodopa after meals to prevent nausea; supporting the physical therapy in her treatment regimen

32.   Mr. Jasper reports that his sleep is frequently interrupted with a gasping feeling of not getting enough air. His wife says that he snores with increasing loudness until he stops breathing for about 15 seconds. As his nurse, you understand that the cause could be:

    a.   A side effect of antihypertensives taken at bedtime

    b.   Commonly caused by abdominal sleeping

    c.   Associated with obesity

    d.   Taking too many naps during the day

33.   Which of the following nursing interventions would be most appropriate for a patient who has screaming episodes?
   a.   Leave the patient alone till the screaming subsides
   b.   Assist patient to a quiet room
   c.   Develop a plan of care that anticipates and fulfills patient needs
   d.   Implement reality orientation, assuring patient of safety

34.   In which of the following situations would electroconvulsive therapy be most appropriate?
   a.   First-line treatment once the diagnosis of depression has been confirmed
   b.   Contraindicated in patients over 65 years of age
   c.   Used for patients with dysthymia
   d.   Used when a patient has debilitating depression and other modalities have failed

35.   The nurse should inform the older adult who abuses alcohol, ativan, and Zoloft that this combination can lead to:
   a.   Loss of respect from significant others
   b.   Death from drug interactions
   c.   Reduced self-esteem
   d.   Abuse of other street drugs

36.   Which of the following statements is *true* about suicide rates?
   a.   Suicide rates decrease after the age of 65
   b.   The suicide rate is six times higher in African-American males than in the general population
   c.   Older adults express their thoughts of suicide more readily than other age groups
   d.   Eighty percent of older adults who threaten suicide follow through on the threat

37.   Which behavior would you consider of primary concern in an older adult diagnosed with major depression?
   a.   Expressing guilty feelings
   b.   Consuming alcohol
   c.   Asking the family to take favorite possessions
   d.   Negative statements and hyperactivity

38.   Pressure ulcers are caused by:
   a.   *Staphylococcus aureus*
   b.   Persistent hyperemia of skin tissues
   c.   Poor nutrition, lack of subcutaneous fat
   d.   Ischemia and anoxia of skin tissue

39.   Of primary importance in the care of your elderly patient's pressure ulcers is:
   a.   Improving nutrition, including protein, carbohydrates, and vitamins
   b.   Debridement
   c.   Sheepskin pads
   d.   Identifying areas of potential breakdown

40.   Assessment of the debilitated patient's skin should be:
   a.   Visual
   b.   Tactile
   c.   To establish a baseline for future documentation
   d.   Visual and tactile

41.   Herpes zoster is caused by:
   a.   Reactivation of varicella zoster
   b.   Reactivation of herpes simplex zoster virus
   c.   Reactivation of *Staphylococcus aureus*
   d.   A dorsal root ganglion virus

42.   The nurse can identify shingles or herpes zoster early because it may be accompanied by:
   a.   An onset of fever with vesicular lesions along a dermatome
   b.   A positive Tzanck test of fluid in vesicles

    c.   Pain, itching, and burning along a dermatome
    d.   Post-herpetic neuralgia, which can last for years
43.   Macular degeneration is a major cause of blindness in the United States. In this disorder, there is:
    a.   Loss of central vision
    b.   Loss of peripheral visual fields
    c.   Corneal edema with blurring of vision
    d.   Bright lights across visual fields, obscuring vision
44.   Diabetic retinopathy is a major cause of blindness. Nursing management of patients with diabetes includes:
    a.   Teaching how to maintain good diabetes control
    b.   Assessing for "floaters" in the eye
    c.   Teaching the need for eye examinations every 2 years
    d.   Testing the visual fields
45.   Dysgeusia means:
    a.   Dry mouth
    b.   Taste
    c.   Loss of taste or change in taste
    d.   Unpleasant smell affecting taste
46.   Some causes of diminished taste are:
    a.   Smoking, systemic infections
    b.   Leukoplakia, head injury
    c.   Head injury, cranial nerve I disorder
    d.   Vitamin deficiencies, nasal polyps
47.   A disturbing taste or taste hallucination may be indicative of:
    a.   Local cancer
    b.   Psychosis
    c.   Severe depression
    d.   Nasal polyps
48.   Many diseases affect taste and smell; these include:
    a.   Allergies, Alzheimer's disease, and asthma
    b.   Allergies, zinc deficiency, and magnesium deficiency
    c.   Allergies, liver disease, and magnesium deficiency
    d.   Allergies, chronic renal failure, and magnesium deficiency
49.   Medications should be reviewed at least:
    a.   Every 3 months
    b.   Every 6 months
    c.   Every 9 months
    d.   Every year
50.   The aphorism "start low, go slow" is based on the understanding that:
    a.   Older adults need time to understand how to take medication properly
    b.   Pharmacokinetics and/or pharmacodynamics are not easily predicted for aged patients
    c.   Most older adults weigh less than younger patients
    d.   Allergies to medications may be unknown
51.   Failure of the primary care provider and the patient to agree on a therapeutic endpoint often results in:
    a.   Polypharmacy
    b.   Adverse drug effects
    c.   Allergic responses
    d.   Organ failure
52.   Pill dispensers, calendars, alarm systems, and check-off systems associated with medication administration are considered:
    a.   Surrogate nurses
    b.   Surrogate family members

    c.   Memory prosthetics

    d.   Self-care crutches

53. All of the following are necessary principles of pharmacoeconomics **except:**

    a.   Considering the unit cost of the drug

    b.   Estimating the cost associated with managing the side effects of a drug

    c.   Considering patient/family caregiver inconvenience

    d.   Considering special skills or assistance needed to administer the drug

54. Some pain medications should be avoided in older adults. These are:

    a.   Chloral hydrate, benzodiazepines, pentazocine (Talwin)

    b.   Meperidine (Demerol), chloral hydrate, propoxyphene (Darvon)

    c.   Meperidine (Demerol), methadone, chloral hydrate

    d.   Meperidine (Demerol), methadone, pentazocine (Talwin)

55. Nurses have the reputation (in the literature) of withholding pain medications and giving low doses of pain medications. They fear addicting patients. In fact:

    a.   Only 10% ever become addicted

    b.   Only 5% become addicted

    c.   Only 1% become addicted

    d.   Only 1/2 of 1% become addicted

56. A drug to use for Mrs. J's degenerative arthritis accompanied by mild-to-moderate pain—a 3.5 on the pain scale of 0 to 10—is:

    a.   Acetaminophen for its antiinflammatory effect

    b.   Aspirin for its antiinflammatory effect

    c.   Acetaminophen for its analgesic effect

    d.   Indomethacin (Indocin) for treatment of arthritis accompanied by mild-to-moderate pain

57. When Mrs. G. is given oxycodone for her severe arthritis pain, you will want to:

    a.   Watch for narcotic abuse

    b.   Watch for a sedative effect

    c.   Start a bowel regimen

    d.   Give it orally because of expense

58. Nonpharmacological methods of pain management include:

    a.   Radio, TV, puzzles

    b.   Chemotherapy

    c.   Radiotherapy and chemotherapy

    d.   Education and medications

UNIT THREE: ORGANIZATIONAL AND HEALTH POLICY ISSUES

1. If the patient/family perceive that a referral is not needed, then the patient will have problems with:

    a.   Accessibility

    b.   Affordability

    c.   Reciprocity

    d.   Receptivity

2. In case management, services are based on assessment and need determination. Identify those areas that are consistent with this determination:

    a.   Assessment of the acuity of the older adult's need for services uses physical, cognitive, functional, social, and economic parameters

    b.   Assessment of older adult's need for services requires economic screening before physical and functional screening

    c.   Cognitive and functional assessments should be done before physical assessment to determine service needs

    d.   Physical, functional, and cognitive assessments are the only parameters done by the nurse case manager

3. Nursing interventions that promote geriatric rehabilitation require:
   a. Advanced courses in rehabilitation techniques
   b. A physician's order for physical and/or occupational therapy
   c. Attention to basic nursing care interventions to support self-care and prevent secondary complications
   d. The use of seat belts to ensure safety and prevent injuries that may slow the rehabilitation process
4. The MDS (Minimum Data Set) was mandated by OBRA (Omnibus Budget Reconciliation Act) in 1987. It is:
   a. An interdisciplinary assessment tool
   b. The physician's assessment form used in the long-term care setting
   c. Used to identify resident problem areas
   d. To be completed within 60 days of admission
5. Certified nursing assistants (CNAs):
   a. Are licensed by the state
   b. Are graduates of professional nursing schools
   c. Are registered by the state
   d. Are certified by the HCFA (Health Care Financing Administration)
6. The Omnibus Budget Reconciliation Act mandated all the following **except:**
   a. Nurse aide training requirements
   b. Capitated payment model for many health care providers
   c. Resident assessment instrument
   d. Fee-for-service payment plan
7. The main reason for the changes in health care financing is primarily:
   a. Projected lack of funding for the Medicare program
   b. Desire to tie clinical assessments to financial reimbursement.
   c. Consumer pressure to improve conditions in nursing homes
   d. Fraudulent billing practices of health care providers
8. The switch from fee-for-service reimbursement to a capitated reimbursement happened first in which health care service?
   a. Nursing homes
   b. Home health agencies
   c. Physician practice
   d. Hospitals
9. Resident assessment protocols (RAPs) are clinical guidelines for evaluating areas of concern and are generated through which of the following:
   a. OASIS
   b. MDS
   c. RAI
   d. PPS

UNIT FOUR: PROFESSIONAL ISSUES

1. Which organizations have developed guidelines and standards for quality assurance in nursing practice?
   a. America Nurses Association (ANA) and National League for Nursing (NLN)
   b. NLN and Joint Commission for Accreditation of Hospitals and Organizations (JCAHO)
   c. ANA and JCAHO
   d. JCAHO and American Medical Association (AMA)
2. The standards and scope of gerontological nursing practice are set by:
   a. The National League for Nursing (NLN)
   b. The American Nurses Association (ANA)
   c. National Gerontological Nursing Association (NGNA)
   d. Each agency that hires gerontological nurses

3. Select the best description regarding research in gerontological nursing practice:
    a. The gerontological nurse uses research findings in practice
    b. The gerontological nurse routinely establishes hypotheses-testing projects
    c. The gerontological nurse does not need to practice research findings
    d. The gerontological nurse evaluates the validity of research projects

4. The standards of clinical gerontological nursing care are:
    a. Assessment, nursing diagnosis, planning, interventions, and evaluation
    b. Assessment, planning, outcome identification, interventions, and evaluation
    c. Assessment, planning, nursing diagnosis, interventions, implementations, and evaluation
    d. Assessment, diagnosis, identifying outcomes, planning, implementing, and evaluation

5. When Nurse Jones delegates patient care responsibilities to the nursing assistant, Miss Turner, she should:
    a. Describe the goals of the assignment and the rationale for the assignment
    b. Set limits especially in terms of time
    c. Have the right to give orders and to expect obedience
    d. Do an assessment of Miss Turner's competence

6. Nonverbal communication:
    a. Is 90% of communication and includes gestures and clothing
    b. Is 25% of communication and includes touching behavior and culture
    c. Is 50% of communication and includes body types and personal artifacts
    d. Is 75% of communication and includes facial expression and spatial arrangement of the environment

7. Grapevines:
    a. Are slow and change often during the flow from one person to another
    b. Are present in all organizations and contain mainly correct information
    c. Are an informal flow of information, which is slower than direct communication
    d. Are considered horizontal communication flows

8. Nurse Manager Morton is developing a new performance appraisal tool for his unit. He will use the following:
    a. The standard for performance
    b. The job description
    c. The job analysis
    d. The job evaluation

9. QA is different from QI in that QA is:
    a. Focused on clinical problem-solving and QI on continuous improvement of performance
    b. Focused on continuous improvement of performance and QI on clinical outcomes
    c. Focused on each department and QI on each person
    d. Hospital-wide and QI is individual-focused

10. Adult education principles used by staff education departments include:
    a. The teacher is the expert and the learner is motivated to learn
    b. The teacher provides learning experiences and the learner gains from the experience.
    c. The learner is self-directed and is internally motivated
    d. The learner has experiences that are varied and the teacher provides a task that is a new learning experience

11. Classic change theory processes, according to Kurt Lewin, include:
    a. Unfreezing, moving, and refreezing
    b. Changing the status quo, changing, retraining
    c. Unfreezing, changing, evaluating change
    d. Educating about change, changing, evaluating change

12. Which of the following steps are **not** within the dissemination phase of the research process?
    a. Recommend how the findings can be used in practice
    b. Review the literature

    c.   Use the findings

    d.   Communicate the findings

13. From the following items, choose the question that pertains to critiquing the introduction of a research article:

    a.   Did the researcher present the descriptive statistics for the participants in the study?

    b.   Is the design appropriate for answering the research question/hypothesis?

    c.   Did the researcher present explanations for the results?

    d.   Do the research questions match the problem statement and the purpose?

14. From the following items, choose the question that pertains to critiquing the methods of a research article:

    a.   Did the researcher present the descriptive statistics for the participants in the study?

    b.   Is the design appropriate for answering the research question/hypothesis?

    c.   Did the researcher present explanations for the results?

    d.   Do the research questions match the problem statement and the purpose?

15. From the following items, choose the question that pertains to critiquing the results of a research article:

    a.   Did the researcher present the descriptive statistics for the participants in the study?

    b.   Is the design appropriate for answering the research question/hypothesis?

    c.   Did the researcher present explanations for the results?

    d.   Do the research questions match the problem statement and the purpose?

16. From the following items, choose the question that pertains to critiquing the discussion of a research article:

    a.   Did the researcher present the descriptive statistics for the participants in the study?

    b.   Is the design appropriate for answering the research question/hypothesis?

    c.   Did the researcher present explanations for the results?

    d.   Do the research questions match the problem statement and the purpose?

17. Select the answer that describes an aspect of the research utilization process:

    a.   Select a sample population

    b.   Decide if the findings are appropriate for use in practice

    c.   Conduct a pilot study

    d.   Select a research design

18. Confidential information may be disclosed:

    a.   To a patient's family

    b.   If a patient is incompetent to decide about disclosure

    c.   To obtain a professional license

    d.   If the patient has an infectious disease

19. Select the response that is **incorrect** concerning the patient's medical record:

    a.   Is only available to facility personnel caring for the patient

    b.   May be released to the patient on request

    c.   In terms of the information therein, belongs to the patient

    d.   Belongs to the attending physician

20. In supporting the right of self-determination, the standard of substituted judgment may be used. This means:

    a.   Any decision must support the current welfare of the patient

    b.   The preferences of the patient are respected

    c.   The patient ombudsman must be involved

    d.   The family's wishes are considered equally with the patient's preferences

21. When an intentional tort is charged, it means:

    a.   A criminal action was performed in a medical facility

    b.   Negligence was the result of an unintentional act

    c.   An act was performed that required immediate arrest of the perpetrator

    d.   A willful act that violated the rights of others

22. The term *medical battery* refers to:
    a. Physical injuries sustained from fighting among medical workers
    b. Actions performed by a surgeon during an operation that result in abnormal bruising
    c. The informed consent issue
    d. No term exists such as "medical battery"
23. Research reveals that:
    a. Families usually respect the wishes of a family member who chooses to donate an organ
    b. Religious persons tend not to donate organs
    c. A spouse must always confirm the desire of the dying spouse to donate an organ
    d. Many people do not donate organs because they are not asked to do so
24. Local organ procurement agencies are required to achieve a certain number in terms of organs donated. This could:
    a. Encourage stronger efforts to obtain organs from questionable sources
    b. Precipitate the acceptance of lesser quality organs in order to meet expectations
    c. Help families who are unsure about donation to do so
    d. Reduce the cost of organ transplantation
25. In allocating organs:
    a. Persons with liver disease are excluded from consideration
    b. Persons whose needs are most urgent have priority when organs become available
    c. Physicians decide whether an organ should be transplanted locally or sent to another regional hospital
    d. Patients can refuse to allow an organ to leave the local community
26. Organs can be:
    a. Sold privately under certain circumstances
    b. Donated to other family members who are in need of the organ
    c. Advertised in local media before being offered to other communities
    d. Transplanted up to 1 year after harvesting
27. The Organ Procurement and Transplant Network (OPTN):
    a. Provides information to health care providers and the public about transplant programs
    b. Evaluates patients for transplantation
    c. Is composed of physicians and other health care personnel who do transplants
    d. Is a governmental organization dedicated to organ transplants
28. Interpretive statements for the Code:
    a. Direct nurses how to use the Code
    b. Are written by ethical experts
    c. Expand on the Code tenets and provide guidance
    d. Provide legal references for the statements
29. The Code and Standards of Care:
    a. Are difficult to use in practice
    b. May be cited in care plans
    c. Are sometimes found in statutes and regulations
    d. None of the above
30. Documentation:
    a. Should be completed at the end of the nurse's shift
    b. May be used to justify reimbursement from insurers
    c. Provides an opportunity for the nurse to list assumptions about the patient's behavior
    d. Cannot be used against the writer in a lawsuit
31. In case of a legal action against a health care institution, the patient record:
    a. Is not discoverable because it is a business record
    b. Will be reviewed for regular, timely assessments and actions
    c. Is generally ignored because it is self-serving to the institution
    d. May not be used to prove or disprove care quality

32. The standards of care for nursing practice are determined by which of the following: (1) standards promulgated by the American Nurses Association, (2) regulations of boards of nursing at the state level, (3) federal government guidelines for practice, (4) specialty nursing organizations:
    a. 1 and 2
    b. 2 and 3
    c. 1, 2, and 4
    d. All of the above

33. Standards of care that are developed by health care institutions:
    a. Are standards to which nurse employees must adhere
    b. Are not evidence of a legal standard of care
    c. Are only important if they are required by licensing and accrediting agencies
    d. May not be introduced in court

34. Nursing competence:
    a. Is based on education completed
    b. Cannot be determined from a typical employee evaluation
    c. Is a quality based on many factors, including skill, knowledge, and intent
    d. None of the above

35. The concept of moral justice means that:
    a. Everyone is entitled to equal amounts of health care
    b. There is a right to equal treatment under the law
    c. People have a right to justice only if they act in moral ways
    d. People need help to act in moral ways

36. Ethical principles hold that:
    a. Nurses are responsible for the acts of their subordinates
    b. Patients cannot be held to the same moral standards as health care providers
    c. A nurse must adhere to the ethics dictated by the professional organization
    d. Nurses must take responsibility for their own acts and decisions

37. An ethical responsibility of nurses is to:
    a. Correct the inappropriate values of others
    b. Study ethical theory
    c. Report substandard care to appropriate authorities
    d. Maintain an adequate standard of care in one's work situation

38. An important ethical consideration in working with elderly persons is to:
    a. Recognize that timeliness may be of great importance because a patient is near the end of life
    b. Be sure that one's patients understand they can ask for assistance in dying
    c. Obtain consent for care from family members because most elderly persons are unable to make such decisions
    d. None of the above

39. In the employer-employee partnership, the nurse has an ethical obligation to:
    a. Lobby for the employer's interests to the state legislature
    b. Provide safe, competent care to one's patients
    c. Reduce costs in the provision of care
    d. Speak only about the good qualities of the employer

40. The author of the first gerontological nursing textbook was:
    a. Irene Burnside
    b. Priscilla Ebersole
    c. Dorothy Moses
    d. Mary Opal Wolanin

41. Which group of nurses have advanced assessment skills?
    a. Gerontological Nurse Specialists
    b. Gerontological Nurse Practitioners

    c.   Certified Gerontological Nurses

    d.   Masters in Gerontological Nursing

42. Which of the following is a criterion for certification in gerontological nursing?

    a.   At least an MSN

    b.   Documented background in nursing research

    c.   Two years of clinical work with older adults

    d.   Membership in National Gerontological Nursing Association

43. What is the professional organization whose membership includes licensed practical nurses and registered nurses?

    a.   Association for Gerontology in High Education

    b.   American Association for Retired Persons

    c.   Gray Panthers

    d.   National Gerontological Nursing Association

44. What is the government program that supports research on aging and diseases associated with aging?

    a.   Bureau of Health Professions

    b.   U.S. Division of Nursing

    c.   Administration of Aging

    d.   National Institute on Aging

ANSWERS WITH RATIONALES: PRACTICE EXAMINATION B

UNIT ONE: PRIMARY CARE CONSIDERATIONS

1. c. Nursing home admission for individuals with bowel and bladder incontinence make up 44% of admissions.

2. b. The kidney shrinks in size and weight and loses working nephrons and glomeruli, decreasing filtration, concentration, and dilution (Luggen, et al, 1998).

3. b. The cardiac system shows thickened valves, loss of vessel elasticity because of collagen stiffness and cross-linkage, decreased blood flow and decreased cardiac output, decreased contractility, increased peripheral vascular resistance, and loss of pacemaker cells. Hypertrophy indicates a pathological process (Luggen, et al, 1998).

4. d. T-cell function is decreased. Dysregulation of the immune system occurs because of increased autoantibodies and reduced response to foreign antigens (Ebersole & Hess, 1998).

5. d. Loss resulting from death among peers increases a person's aloneness and social isolation. Social contact is associated with positive life satisfaction and mental health (Luggen, et al, 1998).

6. a. Being informed about the multiple facets of aging can replace stereotypes of aging with facts (Ebersole & Hess, 1998).

7. b. Prejudice is to prejudge another person based on images that are not accurate (Burke & Walsh, 1997).

8. a. Goals must be specific, measurable, and include a target date (Carpenito, 1997).

9. a. Caffeine promotes the excretion of calcium (Ebersole & Hess, 1998).

10. a. Because of communal living arrangements, it is important for residents of long-term care facilities to receive the influenza vaccine (Miller, 1997).

11. b. Because some herbal remedies can interfere with conventional medications, patients need to inform health professionals of all the pharmaceuticals they are taking (Yen, 1999).

12. a. Because of a resurgence in TB, all residents of long-term care should have a 2-step PPD on admission; health care workers should also be tested on a routine basis (Ebersole & Hess, 1998).

13. c. Territoriality is a state where an individual demonstrates possessiveness, control, and authority over a physical space. The space is an extension of the individual and includes home, place of work, etc. Territoriality is a way of providing privacy, autonomy, security, and self-identity (Edwards, 1998).

14. a. Being able to conduct daily living in the manner it was done during mid-life is a goal that most older adults hope to maintain. When autonomy is lost, physical and mental decline can be identified.

15. d. Disengagement theory was developed by Cumming and Henry.

16. b. Rose, 1965, believed that older adults have their own norms, habits, and beliefs, which make a subculture. They interact better among themselves than other age groups. This subculture is a response to loss of status.

17. a. Erikson believes that aging is a normal stage in life in which the elder accepts his/her past life and maintains integrity or cannot accept it and experiences despair.

18. d. The only correct answer; others come from systems theory or Havighurst's developmental theory.

19. a. This question gives the patient a nonthreatening opportunity to demonstrate knowledge and lets the educator know the patient's level of knowledge.

20. b. Evaluation of a session with a written posttest provides important information about the interaction for both learner and educator.

21. b. The patient is the ultimate learner and decides what and how much to learn.

22. d. All of the diagnoses given are potentially fatal conditions and would qualify for hospice services.

23. a. While not all phases may be experienced, the most common sequence of grieving is denial, anger, bargaining, depression, and acceptance.

24. b. Weight loss can be a signal of depression. Deepening depression can lead to suicide ideation and possibly a suicide attempt. Pathological grieving persists continuously for more than 6 months, while sadness is to be expected on anniversary or special days related to the deceased.

UNIT TWO: MAJOR HEALTH PROBLEMS

1. d. Reliability, validity, time involvement, and safety are all factors in a functional assessment tool.

2. c. Interpreters and family members may add or not relate information for one reason or another. While they are preferable to not having an acceptable communication with a non-English speaking patient, the use of a structured instrument is the best solution to this dilemma.

3. a. Objective data is obtained from a physical assessment/examination, following obtaining subjective information from the health history and interview process.

4. c. The significance of chest pain in women is often unappreciated. Women historically have had a greater prevalence of non-coronary artery disease cause of chest pain, including mitral valve prolapse, coronary artery spasm, and rheumatic heart disease. Treatment algorithms for chest pain are based on findings in men. Older women also delay seeking treatment from the time of onset of symptoms. Women also have a higher incidence of silent myocardial infarctions.

5. b. Although cigarette smoking is certainly a risk factor, the four risk factors considered the "deadly quartet" include hypertension, hypercholesterolemia, diabetes, and obesity. Individuals with one of the four risk factors are at increased risk for having any of the other three.

6. c. According to the Sixth Report of the Joint National Committee on the Detection, Evaluation, and Treatment of High Blood Pressure, stage I (mild) hypertension is a systolic blood pressure of 140 to 159 and a diastolic blood pressure of 90 to 99. Diastolic blood pressure increases the age and continues to rise until approximately the sixth decade and then remains constant. Systolic blood pressure increases with age and continues to rise after the sixth decade.

7. a. The presenting signs and symptoms of an acute myocardial infarction in the elderly are atypical. An older adult experiencing an acute MI will present with a change of mental status, dyspnea, syncope, weakness, or vomiting rather than chest pain.

8. d. The signs and symptoms of peripheral arterial disease are the limb is usually pale, pulseless, cold, and has very little hair with shiny skin.

9. a. All of the symptoms are indicative of pulmonary tuberculosis, which is spread through airborne droplets. Wearing a mask is essential if the assessment will bring the nurse within touching distance of the patient.

10. c. Fresh airflow into the house changes the air and lowers the concentration of microorganisms. Only articles contaminated with infected sputum should be contained. Dishwashers have extreme heat that can kill the mycobacterium.

11. a. Classic symptoms of peptic ulcer include gnawing, boring, or dull pain located in the mid-epigastrium or back; pain is caused by irritability and erosion of the mucosal lining; b more likely indicates a perforated ulcer; c is more likely a hiatal hernia; d is more likely cholecystitis.

12. d. Hepatitis A is transmitted via fecal-oral route; enteric precautions must be used when there are articles that have potential fecal and or urine contamination.

13. c. Constipation, diarrhea, and/or constipation alternating with diarrhea are the most common symptoms of colorectal cancer; pain is reported in less than 25% of patients; rectal bleeding is the second most common sign; the caliber of stools is a much later sign.

14. a. In the older adult the refractory time in the male lengthens, hormonal changes in the female cause the uterus to contract resulting in painful intercourse, and the older adult male may not be able to have another erection for 24 hours (Miller, 1997).

15. b.   The first action by the nurse needs to be assisting the patient to the highest quality of life. This is best achieved if the risk factors for developing incontinence are decreased (Lueckenotte, 1994).

16. d.   The bacterial count for a midstream specimen, which indicates a UTI, is 100,000 colonies per 100 ml/urine (Luggen, et al, 1998).

17. c.   All other statements are not written according to NANDA.

18. b.   Pernicious anemia is caused by the inability to absorb vitamin B_{12}, resulting from a lack of intrinsic factor in gastric juices. The Schilling test requires that radioactive vitamin B_{12} be administered with detection of absorption and monitoring of excretion.

19. b.   Osteoarthritis can affect many body joints, including all those mentioned in the question. However, it primarily and most commonly affects the knees, hips, and fingers.

20. c.   These are the classic signs associated with hyperthyroidism; weight loss and restlessness occur because of an increased basal metabolic rate; exophthalmos occurs because of parabulbar edema. Choices a and b are associated with hypothyroidism; lethargy is not a sign of Graves' disease.

21. a.   Carbonated drinks are generally high in sodium and should be avoided.

22. b.   Cellular swelling and cerebral edema are associated with hyponatremia; as the extracellular sodium level decreases, the cellular fluid becomes relatively more concentrated and pulls water into cerebral cells. All other choices are not associated with hyponatremia.

23. b.   Providers do not routinely screen this age group for HIV or associate AIDS-type symptoms with HIV; instead other conditions, more commonly seen in older persons, are suspected.

24. d.   Patients with decreased immune system function are at high risk for opportunistic diseases that rely on the body's inability to fight infectious processes.

25. a.   HIV/AIDS is not a bacterial process; it is caused by a virus.

26. d.   The older person may have age changes in immune function that include a diminished response to vaccines along with a corresponding decreased resistance to bacterial, fungal, and viral infections and a delayed or diminished hypersensitivity reaction.

27. c.   Although elderly persons seek care for illness, take medication, and follow health care provider recommendations, screening for HIV/AIDS is not routinely done.

28. c.   Common complications include urinary incontinence, pressure sores, depression, dysphagia (difficulty swallowing), and deep vein thrombosis.

29. d.   Parkinson's disease incidence is highest in the oldest age group (85- to 94-year-old adults).

30. b.   This is the only correct answer; decreased dopamine (a neurotransmitter) can result in motor deficits, tremor, muscle rigidity, bradykinesia, gait and balance disturbances, depression, anxiety, and dementia.

31. a.   A high protein diet blocks levodopa effect, and alkaline products, such as milk, slow the absorption of levodopa. The drug should be taken on an empty stomach for best effect. Drug toxicity occurs when levodopa is given with anticholinergics; symptoms such as confusion, nightmares, hallucinations, reversed sleep-wake patterns may occur. Physical therapy is very important for PD patients; it helps prevent immobility and maintains muscle ability and tone.

32. c.   Sleep apnea is associated with respiratory depressant medications, snoring, obesity, dementia, depression, hypothyroidism, alcohol and tobacco use.

33. c.   Screaming is a form of communication and often is done in relation to unmet needs. It is important to determine when screaming occurs in relation to whether a patient is tired, hungry, or needs to be toileted (Carson & Arnold, 1996).

34. d.   Electroconvulsive therapy may be used in patients with life-threatening depression if antidepressants have not been effective (Lueckenotte, 1996).

35. b.   Multiple drug use by older adults is common because of chronic illnesses and medication sharing. OTC drugs are also a common abuse. Teaching the older adult about the effects of alcohol with other drugs is of utmost importance. In general, psychoactive drugs, as with most other drugs administered to the elderly, are metabolized much more slowly than at any other stage of life. This results in greater intensity of the drugs' effect and longer duration, which could lead to death (Isaacs, 1996).

36. d. Older adults have more losses than any other age group. Severe loss is thought to be the major cause of suicide in the elderly. The wish to control the circumstances, timing, and method of one's death is a strong factor in the decision to commit suicide. Suicide pacts between spouses are not uncommon. Older adults also have decreased socialization and a network of support and community services. Older adults have feelings of hopelessness and loss of control, which are strong factors in the decision to commit suicide (Haber, Krainovich, Miller, et al, 1997).

37. c. Giving away favorite belongings is a key factor in determining depression and possible suicidal ideation in an older adult (Carson & Arnold, 1996).

38. d. Ischemia and anoxia from persistent pressure of skin tissue result in pressure ulcers. Contributing factors are poor nutrition, loss of subcutaneous fat, immobilization, heat, and moisture.

39. a. Improving nutrition is primary; debridement may be done if the ulcer is severe; sheepskin pads are very useful and are primarily used for prevention as is the identification of areas of potential breakdown.

40. d. Visual and tactile evaluation of skin should be done. The assessment findings are then documented to evaluate prevention interventions.

41. a. Herpes zoster or shingles is caused by reactivation of the chickenpox virus, varicella zoster.

42. c. In determining herpes zoster, before vesicular lesion eruption, there may be symptoms of pain, itching, and burning along the dermatome that will later exhibit the characteristic vesicular lesions. With early suspicion, consultation can be arranged and treatment can begin, which may prevent later complications.

43. a. In macular degeneration, there is degeneration of the macula in the center of the retina, which has the best vision. Central vision is lost although peripheral vision is retained.

44. a. Nursing management of diabetes includes keeping the diabetes in good control and emphasizing the need for professional eye exams every year.

45. c. Loss of taste begins about age 60 with a decrease in the number of taste buds; taste buds are diminished by 30% at age 70.

46. d. Other causes of diminished taste include smoking, poor oral hygiene, medications, sinusitis, head injury, oral infections.

47. a. Cancer of the pharynx or esophagus and CNS disorders can cause taste or smell hallucinations.

48. a. 23% of those with allergies lose the sense of smell. Other illnesses affecting taste and smell are Alzheimer's disease, asthma, cancers, epilepsy, diabetes, liver disease, Parkinson's disease, chronic renal failure, viral infections, vitamin deficiencies, and zinc deficiency.

49. b. The drug regimen of every patient must be reviewed at least every 6 months to monitor for effectiveness, determine the achievement of the therapeutic goals, and prevent the hazards of polypharmacy (Miller, 1998; Pepper, 1999).

50. b. Many of the pharmacokinetics and pharmacodynamics of drugs commonly prescribed for older adults are not well understood for older populations whose members experience a variety of age-related and idiosyncratic responses to treatment (Podrazik & Schwartz, 1999).

51. a. The benefits of a drug must be measured against the therapeutic endpoint established by the patient and his/her provider (Pepper, 1999).

52. c. A *memory prosthetic* is the term used to describe an artificial device to enhance memory (Pepper, 1999).

53. c. Measures of economic burden typically do not include the cost of inconvenience, time, or burden to the patient and his/her informal supports (American Medical Directors Association, 1998).

54. d. Demerol, methadone, pentazocine, and propoxyphene should be avoided in older adults because of the number and severity of their side effects.

55. c. Only 1% of patients ever become addicted to pain medications. In older adults, this is often a purely physiological dependence that is managed without difficulty.

56. c. Degenerative arthritis usually does not have an inflammatory component. Acetaminophen for mild-to-moderate pain will be useful as an analgesic. Acetaminophen is not an antiinflammatory drug.

57. c. Always, always start a bowel regimen when giving opioids. Constipation can be a major problem of pain management with opioids.

58. a. Radio, TV, and puzzles are among the many distractions that are very useful nonpharmacological adjuncts in pain management.

UNIT THREE: ORGANIZATIONAL AND HEALTH POLICY ISSUES

1. d. Receptivity of a referral source is predicated on acceptance; accessibility is an environmental concern; affordability is not a concern for a situation where a service is not wanted as much as it is for a service desired when funding sources are unknown; reciprocity is incorrect.

2. a. Assessment of the acuity of the older adult's need for services using physical, cognitive, functional, social, and economic parameters is the standard in case management; none of the other answers meet the parameters.

3. c. Nursing interventions in rehabilitation focus attention on basic nursing care that will support self-care and prevent secondary complications; nursing interventions in a rehabilitation setting are the same as in an acute care setting; the rehabilitation setting is for physical and/or occupational therapy so admission to the setting is paramount to a physician's order; seat belts are not the issue with nursing interventions.

4. a. The MDS is a standardized interdisciplinary assessment tool used in all nursing homes. It is completed within 14 days after admission with input from all disciplines.

5. c. The Omnibus Budget Reconciliation Act (OBRA) of 1987 requires certification of aides and standardized training. The states maintain records of CNAs. They are unlicensed personnel.

6. d. The Omnibus Budget Reconciliation Act changed Medicare from a "fee-for-services" to a capitated payment model.

7. a. Health Care Financing Administration (HCFA) reorganized the financial aspects of Medicare in order to safeguard the overall funds available to older Americans and others entitled to benefits.

8. c. Capitation began with physician practice.

9. b. RAPs are problem-oriented frameworks for additional assessment. The MDS does not provide a comprehensive assessment; it identifies potential problems that are further developed by the RAPs.

UNIT FOUR: PROFESSIONAL ISSUES

1. c. ANA and JCAHO have developed guidelines for quality assurance in nursing practice. NLN has guidelines for educational programs, and the AMA is an organization for physicians only.

2. b. The organization that establishes the standards and scope of clinical gerontological nursing care and professional gerontological nursing performance is the ANA.

3. a. Standard VII of the Standards of Professional Gerontological Nursing Performance states that the gerontological nurse uses research findings in practice.

4. d. Standards I through VI include assessment, diagnosis, outcome identification, planning, implementation, and evaluation.

5. a. Choice a is most correct and the best way without establishing barriers to delegation.

6. a. Communication is 93% nonverbal, unspoken, unwritten. It includes gestures and clothing, touching behaviors, culture, body types, personal artifacts, facial expression, spatial arrangement, eye behaviors, voice characteristics, and more.

7. b. Grapevines are always present in organizations on an informal basis. They cannot be eliminated and are more rapid than other communication methods. About 75% of grapevine information is correct.

8. a. The standard for performance is derived from job description, job analysis, and job

evaluation. It is a qualitative and quantitative analysis of job activity. It may be a standard established by the institution or by a professional organization or association such as the ANA.

9. a. QA is clinical problem-solving oriented, involving clinical departments and focused on the individual. QI has the focus of continuous improvement of performance and is hospital-wide. Its focus is on process and systems rather than individuals.

10. c. Adult education principles include the following: learning is a continual process in life; learners are self-directed and internally motivated; learner experiences are varied and valued; learning experiences are task- or problem-centered.

11. a. Three steps in the change process include unfreezing or changing the status quo, moving or changing, and refreezing or stabilizing and maintaining the change.

12. b. The dissemination phase of the research process involves communicating and using the findings.

13. d. The introduction of a research article includes the research problem/question and purpose, review of the literature and theoretical framework, and hypotheses.

14. b. Methods used in a research article include the research and sampling design, methods for data collection, description of the intervention, and description of the instruments.

15. a. Results of a research article involve examining the statistical analyses of a quantitative study and the categories/themes of a qualitative study.

16. c. Discussion of a research article involves review of the findings, explanations for the results, implications, and recommendations.

17. b. A decision should be made regarding the use of each study in the synthesis of the research findings. The decision should involve overall scientific merit, type of participants used in the study and similarity to the population to which the findings will be applied, and relevance to the research problem/question.

18. d. Certain health-related information is required to be disclosed for the public's protection. Infectious diseases and violent injuries are among the reportable events.

19. d. The medical record of a patient does not belong to a physician but is held as information related to treatment. The patient can obtain copies of the record when the proper protocol is followed.

20. a. The best interest standard requires that all decisions be made that promote the patient's current welfare without consideration of previously stated preferences.

21. d. An intentional tort is a wrongdoing that violates another person's rights through a willful action.

22. d. Informed consent requires that the person receiving medical care (or responsible guardian) be told about the actions planned, side effects, other treatment, and projected outcome of a medical intervention.

23. a. A decision by a family member to donate an organ on death is usually honored by other family members.

24. b. Health Care Financing Administration makes organ procurement organizations responsible for obtaining numbers of organs. Some critics feel this may result in less quality organs.

25. b. Priority of need is set as one of the highest reasons for an organ becoming available to a specific recipient.

26. b. Organs can be made available by family members to other family members when life is not in jeopardy for the donor and the donation is discussed with the planned recipient.

27. a. The Organ Procurement and Transplant Network operates by a contract with the Department of Health and Human Services, which requires that information is made available to health care providers and the public concerning transplantations.

28. c. Interpretive statements for the Code expand on it and provide guidance for nurses.

29. c. Although the Code and Standards of Care are not law, they are often adopted into statutes and regulations.

30. b. Among other things, documentation provides a means to justify reimbursement from insurers.
31. b. Medical records are reviewed for legal purposes. This may include review for safe and timely assessments.
32. d. All choices in this question are correct (1 to 4).
33. a. The actual practice of employees is measured against institutional standards. If the standards are not met, then a breach has occurred.
34. c. Competency of practicing nurses requires requisite knowledge, ability, skill, and interest to perform certain activities.
35. b. Moral justice means that everyone is entitled to equal treatment under the law.
36. d. Nurses are responsible for their own acts and decision-making.
37. c. Reporting substandard care is an ethical responsibility of nurses.
38. d. None of the other answers are appropriate.
39. b. Nurses are ethically obligated to provide safe, competent care to their patients.
40. a. In 1976, Irene Burnside authored *Nursing and the Aged*.
41. b. By definition, the NP specializes in use of advanced assessment skills.
42. c. Two years of clinical practice with older adults is required to be eligible for the certification exam.
43. d. According to the by-laws of National Gerontological Nursing Association, LPNs and RNs are eligible for membership.
44. d. National Institute on Aging is a government program that supports research on aging and diseases associated with aging.

INDEX

Unplanned loss, defined, 261
Unstable angina, 58
Upward communication, 202
Urethra, age-related changes, 96
Urethritis, 93, 96–97
Urge incontinence, 91
Uric acid crystal accumulation in gout, 109
Urinary incontinence, 91–93
Urinary system
    age-related changes, 84
    diabetes mellitus' effect on, 114
    diseases of
        benign prostatic hyperplasia, 84–87
        end-stage renal disease, 95–96
        incontinence, 91–93
        prostate cancer, 87–88
        urethritis, 96–97
        urinary tract infection, 93–95
Urinary tract infection, 93–95
    during menopause, 122
    in Parkinson's disease, 139
Urine creatinine, 47
Urine culture and sensitivity, 93
Uterus, age-related changes, 6, 84
UTI; *see* Urinary tract infection
Utilitarianism, 265

V

Vaccination
    hepatitis A, 78
    hepatitis B, 78
    Medicare reimbursement, 188
    for preventive health maintenance, 20
Vagina
    age-related changes, 96
    dryness in menopause, 122
Vaginitis, 96–97
    atrophic, in menopause, 122
Value added services, 190
Value system, 265
Values, ethics and, 265–267
Valve, cardiac, 5
Variable cost, 198
Variables in research, 210, 211, 212
Variance analysis in research, 213
Vascular disease, peripheral, 61–62
Vascular system, normal aging changes, 5
Venous disease, 62

Ventilation/perfusion ratio, 5
Verapamil, 162
Vertebral compression fracture, 106
Villers Foundation, Inc., 13
Vision
    loss of, 159–162
        community resources, 28
    normal aging changes, 4–5
Visiting nurse, 178
Visual laser ablation, 86
Visualization, 21
Vital capacity, 5
Vital signs
    in chronic obstructive pulmonary disease, 66
    in pneumonia, 68
Vitamin A, 162
Vitamin D
    intake for health promotion and
        disease/disability prevention, 18
    ocular toxicity of, 162
VLAP; *see* Visual laser ablation
Volume of distribution, 167
Vulva, normal aging changes, 6

W

Walker as assistive device, 136
Wandering, 144–145
Water exercise, 18
Weakness in stroke, 134
Wellness, 14
Wheelchair, 136
White blood cell count, 101
Withdrawing treatment, 229
Withholding treatment, 229
Women; *see* Female population
Wrist, rheumatoid arthritis of, 108

X

Xanax; *see* Alprazolam
Xerosis, 154

Y

Year, fiscal, 198
Yoga, 22

Z

Zoladex; *see* Testosterone-ablating drug
Zung's Self-Rating Scale, 148